PSYCHOSOCIAL ISSUES IN DAY CARE

PSYCHOSOCIAL ISSUES IN DAY CARE

Edited by
Shahla S. Chehrazi, M.D.

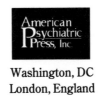

Washington, DC
London, England

Note: The authors have worked to ensure that all information in this book concerning drug dosages, schedules, and routes of administration is accurate as of the time of publication and consistent with standards set by the U.S. Food and Drug Administration and the general medical community. As medical research and practice advance, however, therapeutic standards may change. For this reason and because human and mechanical errors sometimes occur, we recommend that readers follow the advice of a physician who is directly involved in their care or the care of a member of their family.

Copyright © 1990 American Psychiatric Press, Inc.
ALL RIGHTS RESERVED
Manufactured in the United States of America
First Edition

90 91 92 93 4 3 2 1

American Psychiatric Press, Inc., 1400 K Street, N.W., Washington, D.C. 20005

The paper used in this publication meets the minimum requirements of the American National Standard for Information Sciences—Permanence of Paper for Printed Library Materials, ANSI Z39.48—1984.   ∞

Library of Congress Cataloging-in-Publication Data

Psychosocial issues in day care / edited by Shahla S. Chehrazi.—1st ed.
      p. cm.
   Includes bibliographical references.
   ISBN 0-88048-310-5 (alk. paper)
   1. Day care centers—United States—Psychological aspects. 2. Day care centers—Health aspects—United States. 3. Child abuse—United States—Prevention. I. Chehrazi, Shahla S., 1945–   .
   [DNLM: 1. Child Abuse. 2. Child Care. 3. Child Day Care Centers. 4. Child Development. 5. Child, Preschool. WS 105 P9775]
      HV854.P79 1990
      362.7′12′019—dc20
      DNLM/DLC
      for Library of Congress   90-561
                                                              CIP

British Library Cataloguing in Publication Data

A CIP record is available from the British Library.

Contents

PART I:
DEVELOPMENTAL CONSIDERATIONS AND DAY CARE

PART II:
THE RELATIONSHIP BETWEEN PARENTS
AND CHILD CARE PROVIDERS

PART III:
PEDIATRIC ISSUES IN DAY CARE

PART IV:
CHILD ABUSE AND DAY CARE

PART V:
NATIONAL POLICY AND DAY CARE

About the Contributors

SUSAN S. ARONSON, M.D., F.A.A.P., is a practicing pediatrician in the Philadelphia area and is Clinical Professor of Pediatrics at Hahnemann University. She became involved in early childhood programs as a pediatric consultant to the Howard University Head Start Program and the District of Columbia Parent and Child Center in 1970. Since then she has served as consultant to many individual child care programs, to systems of child care programs, to numerous state child care licensing agencies, and to the federal government. She currently serves as a member of the Steering Committee for the federally funded joint American Academy of Pediatrics–American Public Health Association project to establish national reference standards for health, safety, sanitation, and nutrition for child care programs. Dr. Aronson is the mother of Lori, a medical student, and Bruce, a college student.

CATHERINE AYOUB, M.N., Ed.M., is Clinical Fellow in Psychology at Boston Children's Hospital and Judge Baker Children's Center. She holds a master's degree in psychiatric nursing and is a doctoral candidate in counseling and consulting psychology at the Harvard Graduate School of Education. Ms. Ayoub has written numerous publications in the field of child maltreatment and serves on the editorial board of *Child Abuse and Neglect, the International Journal.*

JAY BELSKY, Ph.D., received his doctorate from Cornell University in 1978 in the field of human development and family studies. In 1984, he was awarded the Boyd McCandless Distinguished Early Career Award from the Division of Developmental Psychology of the American Psychological Association. In 1985, he received a Research Scientist Development Award from the National Institute of Mental Health (NIMH). He is currently professor of human development in the College of Health and Human Development at Pennsylvania State University. In addition to day care, Dr. Belsky's scholarly interests include child maltreatment, the parent-child relationship, the transition to parenthood, and, more broadly, the ecology of human development.

SHAHLA S. CHEHRAZI, M.D., is a psychoanalyst and child psychiatrist who works with children and their families. She is assistant clinical professor of psychiatry at the University of California, San Francisco, Medical School, and a member of the faculty at the San Francisco Psychoanalytic

Institute. She has been interested in and has written about children's development, especially female development. Her interest in day care is a natural outcome of her clinical work and her research on early development, as well as her own parenting experience. Dr. Chehrazi lives in Kentfield, California, with her husband and two sons.

STEVEN A. FRANKEL, M.D., associate clinical professor of psychiatry at the University of California Medical School, San Francisco, is a member of the San Francisco Psychoanalytic Institute and is board certified in both child and general psychiatry. Dr. Frankel is in private practice in Kentfield, California.

JOHANNA FREEDMAN, M.Phil., is a graduate student in child, clinical, and community psychology at Yale University, and a student fellow of the Bush Center in Child Development and Social Policy.

MARTIN GLASSER, M.D., F.A.P.A., is a child psychiatrist and the former director of the University of California, San Francisco, Child Study Unit. He has consulted to courts, departments of social services, and attorneys regarding youth for the past 15 years. He currently holds a joint appointment in pediatrics and psychiatry as associate clinical professor at the University of California, San Francisco, Medical School. Dr. Glasser has extensive experience in the evaluation of children who have been victims of physical or sexual abuse. He is in private practice in San Diego.

PENELOPE GRACE, D.S.W., has worked with maltreated children and their families since 1975. After earning her doctorate, she held a postdoctoral fellowship in family violence at Harvard Medical School and Boston Children's Hospital. She currently holds an appointment as an Instructor in Pediatrics at Harvard Medical School. Dr. Grace has a private practice in Wellesley, Massachusetts, and consults to day care centers and agencies on issues involving children and violence.

CAROLLEE HOWES, Ph.D., is associate professor in the Graduate School of Education, University of California at Los Angeles (UCLA). She received her doctorate in psychology from Boston University in 1979 and completed 2 years of postdoctoral training in social psychiatry at Harvard University. She has published two books and numerous articles on children's peer relations and play, and on children's experiences in child care.

BARBARA KALMANSON, Ph.D., has been on the staff at the Infant-Parent Program, Department of Psychiatry, University of California, San Francisco, at San Francisco General Hospital for 9 years. Recently, she has been supervising a mental health team that provides consultation to day care providers and parents. Dr. Kalmanson is a past fellow of the National

Center for Clinical Infant Programs. She is in private practice in San Francisco.

ROBERT J. KELLY, Ph.D., received his doctoral degree in clinical psychology from the State University of New York at Buffalo. After completing his internship at the University of Southern California Medical Center in 1984, he became an NIMH postdoctoral research fellow in the Department of Psychology at UCLA, where he also became co-principal investigator of a large-scale study of sexual abuse in preschools, funded by the National Center on Child Abuse and Neglect. In addition to his position at UCLA as assistant research psychologist, Dr. Kelly maintains a private practice and, since 1986, has co-led a group at the UCLA Psychology Clinic for male survivors of sexual abuse.

ALICIA F. LIEBERMAN, Ph.D., is associate professor at the University of California, San Francisco, and senior psychologist of the Infant-Parent Program at San Francisco General Hospital. Dr. Lieberman received her doctoral degree from Johns Hopkins University with a focus in attachment theory. Her postdoctoral training was in infant mental health. She is currently engaged in teaching, clinical work, and research exploring the clinical application of attachment theory.

CONGRESSMAN GEORGE MILLER (D-California) serves as chairman of the Select Committee on Children, Youth, and Families, United States House of Representatives, a position he has held since the committee's creation in 1983. The committee is charged with providing an ongoing assessment of the conditions of American children and families, and making recommendations to Congress and the public about how to improve public and private policies. Congressman Miller also chairs the Water and Power Subcommittee of the Committee on the Interior and is a senior member of the Committee on Education and Labor. He has represented the 7th Congressional District in California since 1974.

PATRICIA A. NACHMAN, Ph.D., is director of the Margaret S. Mahler Observational Research Nursery and adjunct assistant professor in graduate psychology at the New School for Social Research in New York. She is clinical instructor in psychiatry at New York University Medical Center and is research associate at the Margaret S. Mahler Psychiatric Research Foundation.

CAROLYN M. NEWBERGER, Ed.D., graduated from Sarah Lawrence College and the Harvard Graduate School of Education. She is a specialist in children's cognitive development. Since completing her clinical training at the Judge Baker Children's Center, she has been working on applying developmental theory to clinical problems. Dr. Newberger directs a federally funded study of the impact of child sexual abuse on children's development and holds an academic appointment at the Harvard Medical School.

EVELYN K. OREMLAND, Ph.D., is director of the Child Life Program and assistant professor in the Department of Education at Mills College in Oakland, California. Her professional activities have included holding offices at the national level in the Association for the Care of Children's Health and the Child Life Council. Dr. Oremland's research and publications have focused on issues of children's health care, specifically on chronic illness during childhood. She co-edited two books with her husband, Jerome D. Oremland, M.D.: *The Effects of Hospitalization on Children* and *The Sexual and Gender Development of Young Children: The Role of the Educator*.

DEBORAH PHILLIPS, Ph.D., is assistant professor of psychology at the University of Virginia. Her areas of specialty are community psychology, public policy, and developmental psychology. Most recently, her research has focused on the effects of child care on children's social and emotional development; factors that influence the quality of child care, particularly the role of child care staff; and parents' influence on children's developing perceptions of their academic abilities. She has also written extensively on public policies in the area of child care and has testified numerous times before the U.S. Congress on child care issues. Immediately before joining the faculty at the University of Virginia, Dr. Phillips was a midcareer fellow at Yale University's Bush Center in Child Development and Social Policy. She was also the first director of the Child Care Information Service of the National Association for the Education of Young Children.

CAROL S. STEVENSON has been a staff attorney at the Child Care Law Center since 1981. She is an honors graduate of the University of Kansas and Hastings College of the Law. In her work at the Child Care Law Center, she has written and spoken extensively about zoning laws affecting child care facilities, regulation of child care, and child abuse prevention. She serves on the national advisory boards for the Child Care Initiative Project, the National Family Day Care Association, and the Child Care Action Campaign, and is a member of the Board of Directors of the Child Care Employee Project. She lives and works in San Francisco and is the mother of two children.

MARCY WHITEBOOK, M.A., is the founding member and executive director of the Child Care Employee Project, a resource and advocacy organization dedicated to improving the quality of child care by increasing child care staff salaries and benefits. She is also project director and principal investigator for the National Child Care Staffing Study, a comprehensive examination of center-based child care in the United States in the 1980s. Ms. Whitebook worked for many years as a child care teacher and received her master's degree in early childhood education from the University of California at Berkeley in 1976. She is the mother of a 7-year-old son, who has been in center-based child care since he was 7 months old.

EDWARD F. ZIGLER, Ph.D., is Sterling Professor of Psychology at Yale University, where he also serves as director of the Bush Center in Child Development and Social Policy. In addition, he is head of the psychology section of the Yale University Child Study Center and Yale University School of Medicine. Professor Zigler is the author or editor of more than 20 books and has published more than 400 scholarly articles. Dr. Zigler has received numerous honors, including awards from the American Psychological Association, the American Academy of Pediatrics, the National Head Start Parents Organization, and the American Academy of Child and Adolescent Psychiatry.

Foreword

This volume provides a much-needed comprehensive review of day care/child care. With 53% of American women now in the work force and the number expected to increase during the next decade, day care has become a reality and a necessity. Such care, however, is unregulated and unlicensed in too many states. Child care providers are often inadequately trained and poorly paid. Working parents face emotionally and financially difficult demands, and sometimes have little choice in the type of care their child receives. There is no comprehensive national child care policy, nor are there uniform standards to ensure the quality of care.

Social realities make untenable the position that mothers be returned to the home to care for their children. The situation today is reminiscent of the early 1920s, when an effort was made to ratify a constitutional amendment restricting child labor. The amendment failed because it was labeled a "Bolshevist plot" advocating "destruction of the family." Although that particular measure was not passed, the slow, tedious process of legislation restricting child labor did begin. We are currently in similar straits regarding day care. Although the social reality of day care is evident, national policy lags behind. It is an historical fact, however, that when powerful social necessity dictates policy, seemingly insuperable disadvantages can be overcome. There are numerous examples to illustrate this process: for example, the kibbutz experience in Israel, nurseries and schools in China, the entry of women into the marketplace and factories during World War II, and the Head Start programs. Urgent social need can produce positive outcomes.

A comprehensive day care policy is desperately needed. Planning should begin immediately to provide the best of programs rather than merely to piece together stop-gap measures to meet minimal standards. We should adopt standards that ensure a safe and healthy nurturing environment, with age-appropriate programs tailored to meet the developmental needs of preschool children. Quality must be the watchword if we are to achieve success. We do not tolerate shoddy workmanship in the production of aircraft, nor permit ourselves to fly with poorly trained pilots. So, too, should we insist on enforceable standards for the care of our children. There will always be questions: At what age should day care start? What is the best educational approach? What training is necessary for personnel? What parent education should complement care? But these should not deter us from our appointed task.

Day care is an opportunity for great good for children and families if undertaken with knowledge, enthusiasm, and sufficient resources. All aspects of the problem are considered in this volume. The authors provide a comprehensive and much-needed overview of the psychological, developmental, and social implications of substitute child care, along with a blueprint for positive action. It is a truism that our children are the hope of the future. They deserve the best. We should settle for no less.

Irving Philips, M.D.

Preface: On Day Care

Day care centers formally came into being in this country during World War II, when women needed to be freed from household duties to work in defense plants and other industries related to the war effort. Following the war, most of these centers either closed or functioned, with more limited goals, as nursery schools. It was not until 1964, when President Johnson declared a war on poverty and Project Head Start was born, that the impetus was renewed for women to consider the benefits of activity outside the home for their preschool children. In most advanced industrial countries of the world, day care has been and continues to be a national commitment rather than a controversial and privately developed and financed system.

The impact of day care on children has been continually debated in the popular press as well as in the research literature. Arguments range from predictions of dire consequences for children to forecasts of nothing but benefits. Much of the literature has focused on studies from selected day care facilities that were generally considered inadequate rather than from representative or random samples. Moreover, the studies of developmental parameters, including verbal responsiveness, attachment behavior, social interaction, and play, occurred in a relatively short-term framework with neither consideration of family and home nor alternatives to day care. Longitudinal data have not been available. Much of the literature that has focused on the impact of maternal work on children has not attended to the availability of other adults in the household, what other resources were available, and the relationships between mothers and children. The effect of maternal employment has been confounded with data on maternal separation and deprivation and has not addressed the complexity of sociocultural factors. In an early review paper, Murray (1975) concluded that developmental progress in infants appeared to be related to the strength of the mother-infant attachment and the level of stimulation in the home, regardless of the setting of rearing. Separations, the author noted, were not harmful as long as they were accompanied by predictable substitute care. Predictability and reliability, then, became a focus in day care centers and were considered of paramount importance.

Fraiberg (1977), drawing on the work of Spitz, Bowlby, and others, stressed the importance of the child's first attachments to the mother for later cognitive development and for the ability to form relationships and maintain control later in life. Her generalization implied that maternal work in itself led to attachment failure and that this degree of separation could be linked with failure to thrive and psychopathology later in life. Her argument polarized the loving mother on the one hand and the impersonal, inadequate day care facility on the other. Kenniston (1977), in reviewing Fraiberg's book, noted that the link between maternal employment and the failure of bonding and development was not supported. Indeed, the link to psychopathology is even more tenuous.

In 1982, Brazelton and Keefer (p. 108) wrote as follows:

> The use of the positive developmental model (based on an understanding of the important reciprocal interaction) may help stimulate programs to redirect their efforts toward supporting the mother-infant relationship rather than just the infant's cognitive or motor skills. This framework may also enable day care workers to capitalize on their potential for being a cohesive rather than a divisive influence on young families. The competition that inevitably develops between adults who care for young children (and that is understandable because it reflects the extent of their commitment to the children) may be more effectively dealt with in both of these situations.

In the mid-1960s, when I was part of a group of young working mothers trying to start the first day care center in Boston, the attitudes we encountered contrasted dramatically with today's. We constantly met with derision, negativism, and outright hostility. At every turn, our motives were questioned and impugned. Were we really concerned about the welfare of our children? Why was working so important to us? Did we know the negative consequences, especially the emotional ones, of day care?

It was only because we counted among our group a number of women who were experts in this area and who were confident that we could do what we had planned in a careful, thoughtful, and innovative way that we were able to meet each obstacle and bring our dream to fruition: attending as our first priority to the well-being of our children.

We have come a long way in the two decades since that experience. To see day care as a national political agenda topic now is enormously rewarding. Our determined group has long since dispersed across the country, and we and our children have generally done very well. As we travel the country, we often encounter each other. We reminisce and share memories. We are gratified and enthusiastic. The bulk of our efforts in the context of the early feminist movement of the 1960s enabled us to fulfill our own aspirations, and our children benefited from the care and attention they received. The mothers have had opportunities they might not otherwise have had, and they have largely been successful. The fathers' careers were less overtly affected. The children run the gamut of promises and problems and achievement and disappointment that we see in their peers.

We all—mothers, fathers, teachers, children—cleaned floors, painted, put in fence posts, and cooked together. We built a dream.

Today we have entered a new era. We no longer ask why we should have day care or what harm will it do, but how we can do it best. Obstacles, however, continue to exist. Most often they are economic and legal. But the challenge continues; we must provide optimal quality day care if we are to ensure the future for our children.

Carol Nadelson, M.D.

REFERENCES

Brazelton B, Keefer C: The early mother-child relationship, in The Woman Patient, Vol 2. Edited by Nadelson C, Notman M. New York, Plenum, 1982, pp 95–109

Fraiberg S: Every Child's Birthright: In Defense of Mothering. New York, Basic Books, 1977

Kenniston K: Book review of Every Child's Birthright: In Defense of Mothering. New York Times, Dec 11, 1977, Sec 7

Murray A: Maternal employment reconsidered: effects on infants. Am J Orthopsychiatry 45:773–790, 1975

Editor's Preface

Although I had practiced child psychiatry for many years and had been professionally concerned about children's early development, child care, and parenting in our society, it was only after having my own children that I confronted the reality of child care. Only then, in struggling to create a balance between my career and my family, did I fully experience the challenge facing working parents. I talked to my female friends and female colleagues and found that they were struggling with the same issues. I gradually became more aware of how decisions concerning children's upbringing and, in particular, those concerning child care have a powerful impact on our lives.

My personal experience affected my practice as well. I became more keenly aware of many of my patients' dilemmas. My increasing interest in this area led to my organizing a symposium on the subject of child care with the goal of bringing the best current information to professionals as well as to parents, much needed because the field of child care is so complex that even experts are reluctant to make clear recommendations. The information that is offered can be confusing and ambiguous to parents and professionals alike. Throughout my at times painful struggle about having my own children in child care, there were no clear guidelines on when, how much, or what type of child care to choose.

The symposium was a complete success and was received with great interest and enthusiasm, confirming my belief that we, as mothers and professionals, needed to take a more active role in the social dilemma of child care. The symposium provided me with new information and resources. Dr. Edward Zigler, the keynote speaker, was particularly impressive. In a world reluctant to make definitive scientific statements, his clarity was refreshing. He noted that "while high-quality day care does not appear to be detrimental to children's development, and even in some particular cases appears to be beneficial, there is little question or doubt that low-quality day care is detrimental to children's development." Also of great value were the clear guidelines presented by several contributors for evaluating the quality of care.

The excitement and interest in response to the symposium motivated me to publicize it in synopsis. Once I was involved, however, the project became more ambitious. Because I was fortunate to be able to work part-time, I felt I could juggle creating a book, working, and parenting. I decided to put together a book offering the most recent knowledge and findings on day care from as inclusive a perspective as possible. And I was determined not to get trapped in the polarizing arguments over day care. It seemed clear that the question had gone beyond whether child care per se is good or bad, to how we can create the best child care possible. To offer a real contribution toward this end, I contacted workers from a variety of fields, including psychoanalysis, child psychiatry, developmental psychology, early childhood education, pediatrics, and politics. The outstanding contributors to this volume offer a wide range of perspectives, which together present a comprehensive view of the issues surrounding child care in the United States today.

My hope was to publish a scientific and comprehensive guide to child care that could help parents who feel overwhelmed and helpless when trying to cope with working and parenting, as well as to empower professionals who work with children and families. This, I believe, has been accomplished with the support and contributions of many who have helped me during the past 2 years.

In the early stages of this project, my friends and colleagues Stanley Steinberg, M.D., and Joseph Afterman, M.D., offered support and encouragement. I thank Cici Peters for her valuable editorial assistance and April Kaskey for her administrative skills and enthusiasm.

In the later stages of this project, the feedback and criticism from Carol Nadelson, M.D., and the editorial staff of the American Psychiatric Press helped me through many revisions of the book. I owe much to Daniel Silver for his careful and insightful reading of the chapters and his invaluable editorial work.

Finally, my gratitude goes to Stephen Raffle, my husband, for his patience and support and to our two sons, Alexander, 6, and Phillip, 4, from whom I learned about child care.

Shahla S. Chehrazi, M.D.

Introduction

This volume is a comprehensive overview of current child care issues facing parents and professionals. The 16 chapters of the volume are organized into five parts: developmental considerations and day care, the relationship between parents and child care providers, pediatric issues in day care, child abuse and day care, and national policy and day care. Although these divisions are useful for heuristic purposes, we should not lose sight of the ultimately interconnected nature of the many issues facing us in providing high-quality care for children.

PART I: DEVELOPMENTAL CONSIDERATIONS AND DAY CARE

Chapter 1, by Edward Zigler and Johanna Freedman, is an authoritative overview of the growing day care crisis in the United States. The authors analyze its evolution and propose innovative solutions to the problem. In the midst of the current ambiguity and disagreement surrounding the psychological-developmental effects of day care on children, the authors provide a clear view: Although high-quality day care does not appear to have an adverse effect on children's development, "low-quality child care can have a detrimental effect on the development of children." Quality care, they argue, not only must be consistent and reliable but should also meet children's varying needs at different developmental stages, which are defined as infancy (birth to 2 years), preschool (2–5 years), and school age. Zigler and Freedman warn that day care must not be allowed to degenerate into a two-tiered system in which economically privileged children are adequately supplied with "environmental nutrients," while the many children whose parents cannot afford high-quality care are developmentally disadvantaged. The authors conclude by offering recommendations for a national parental-leave policy and a comprehensive national child care plan.

Day care research in the 1960s focused on whether substitute care was detrimental to children's development. This work was heavily influenced by studies of institutionalized children. Day care research in the 1970s framed its concerns somewhat differently: Does the child's relationship to the caregiver interfere with the development of secure attachment to the parent? In the 1980s, researchers began to recognize the complexity of the variables involved in assessing the effects of day care. Recent studies have examined the multiple factors that contribute to the quality of care and acknowledge that day care must be studied in the context of children's family situations. Current research, however, still suffers from a lack of substantial longitudinal studies.

In Chapters 2 and 3, differing views are presented on the effects of day care in the first year of life on infant-parent attachment. In Chapter 2, Carollee Howes suggests that the influence of infant care on children's development is complex and multidimensional, but that the age of entry into child care is less important than the stability and quality of the care and the nature of the child's family situation. On the other hand, in Chapter 3, Jay Belsky presents data suggesting a higher incidence of insecure attachment in infants with extensive first-year day care experience and proposes several possible explanations for these findings.

In exploring this controversy, it is helpful to keep in mind the tentative nature of our present state of knowledge, the absence of conclusive data, and the need for further validation and documentation of existing studies. Despite any differences, both researchers agree on the synergistic risk effects of poor-quality day care, low socioeconomic status, and family stress, and are concerned about the accumulation of such risk factors beginning in infancy.

The authors of Chapters 4 and 5 bring a clinical perspective to bear on the discussion of potential developmental risks of early day care. In Chapter 4, Alicia Lieberman presents a discussion of the implications for early day care issues of the two dominant models of infant development—the anxiety-based and competency-based models. She then presents an integrative view in which both models are seen to contribute to a richer understanding of the developmental issues in day care. Her clinical focus leads to the conclusion that careful attention must be paid to the individual child and to whether the stresses of day care are exceeding that child's coping capacities.

In Chapter 5, Steven Frankel reviews both attachment research and psychoanalytic developmental theory to discuss the nature of early parent-infant and caregiver-infant relationships and the deep and potentially long-term effects of various early care situations. Frankel, like Lieberman, stresses that early day care must be viewed within a developmental framework that takes family situations into account. In addition, both authors caution against oversimplifying the complex issues and unresolved questions involved in existing research and point out that further empirical work with long-term follow-up is essential before a conclusive picture can emerge.

PART II: THE RELATIONSHIP BETWEEN PARENTS AND CHILD CARE PROVIDERS

The four chapters of Part II explore the critical relationship between parents and child care providers, with an emphasis on separation issues. In Chapter 6, Shahla Chehrazi explores parents' subjective experiences of juggling working and parenting and emphasizes the importance of the parents' relationship with the provider in enhancing the quality of the child care experience. The author addresses the role of the father in day care and stresses the need for studies that include fathers. A valuable set of guidelines is included to enable parents to assess and evaluate the quality of substitute care, to develop a working relationship with the care provider, and to help the child master separation.

In Chapter 7, Deborah Phillips and Marcy Whitebook review demographic characteristics of providers, job satisfaction among child care workers, and the crucial relationship between child care quality and caregiver job satisfaction. Because most American families cannot afford to pay the high costs of child care, providers are expected to subsidize fees and accept salaries far below the value of the service they perform. Thus, the disparity between the actual importance of child care and its low economic and social position points toward a crisis in the availability, quality, and cost of care providers. The chapter concludes with the suggestion that public funds be used to provide salary and training supplements for caregivers.

In Chapter 8, Patricia Nachman describes an observational study conducted at the Margaret S. Mahler Research Nursery. The findings indicated differences in groups of children cared for by mothers and alternative caregivers in the areas of socialization, symbolization, and identification. The author focuses on children's adaptive capacities in coping with daily separations, centering on their ability to identify with peers and to maintain internal emotional connectedness to the absent parent. The particular contribution of this work is its attention to the child's inner mental world of representation, defense, and adaptation. As with any study with small numbers of subjects, there is a need for follow-up and replication. But the intensive observations reported here are a powerful method for gaining insight into the effects of substitute caregiving.

Barbara Kalmanson focuses specifically on children's reactions to separation in Chapter 9, presenting concrete ways in which parents and caregivers can assess children's subjective experience of daily separations. "Normal" as well as problematic responses to separation are carefully explored. The author integrates theoretical and empirical work into a set of guidelines for evaluating the nature, magnitude, and pattern of separation distress, emphasizing ways in which parents and caregivers can ease the child's pain at separation and promote his or her mastery of the experience.

PART III: PEDIATRIC ISSUES IN DAY CARE

Although health and safety are among the central issues in day care, pediatricians and health care professionals are hampered by insufficient data on the incidence of infectious disease and illness in day care settings. A number of studies note an association between day care attendance and increased frequency of illness. Others report no difference in the overall burden of illness but suggest that although younger children in day care suffer more frequently than their counterparts cared for at home, the illness rate diminishes with age, so that by age 2, it is actually lower than for children cared for at home.

In Chapter 10, Susan Aronson presents the view that in the absence of any conclusive studies, the significance of these reported changes in illness rates is unknown. Nevertheless, an integrative and interdisciplinary approach to improving health conditions in day care settings is important. The author offers clear and concise guidelines on how to assess a day care setting for safety and health, and suggests ways in which child care professionals, health care professionals, and parents can work together to improve health conditions in day care centers.

In Chapter 11, Evelyn Oremland notes the limited facilities and options available to sick children and their parents and suggests various possible alternatives. In addition, the chapter examines regression and psychological vulnerability during illness and offers measures to promote children's capacity for coping with illness. The author notes that the presence of caregivers with whom children have well-established relationships, supportive and understanding care, and an opportunity to engage in therapeutic play are all critical in attending to sick or injured children's emotional as well as physical needs.

PART IV: CHILD ABUSE AND DAY CARE

Child abuse is a sensitive and difficult issue for children, parents, and day care providers as well as for professionals who work with victims and their families. The three chapters of Part IV are concerned with ensuring that parents, caregivers, and health care professionals are able to help abused children recover trust and the capacity for positive interactions with adults and peers. In Chapter 12, Robert Kelly describes the oscillation of public opinion from indifference to hysteria regarding the incidence of sexual abuse in day care, and reminds us that although abuse does occur in day care settings, it is more likely to occur at home. The author reports on a recent study examining the impact of day care sexual abuse on the community, family, and child, and offers suggestions for prevention, detection, and intervention.

In Chapter 13, Martin Glasser presents criteria for detecting abuse and a step-by-step guide to assessment, intervention, and rehabilitation. The author's emphasis is on early detection and helping parents to recognize signs of distress in children.

Chapter 14, by Catherine Ayoub, Penelope Grace, and Carolyn Newberger, is addressed to professional caregivers, who must be able to identify and respond appropriately to suspected parental abuse of children. The authors explore the complex societal, economic, and familial variables that can contribute to abuse. Because day care providers can play a crucial role in child rehabilitation, the authors provide a comprehensive description of signs and symptoms of emotional, physical, and sexual maltreatment and suggest guidelines for caregiver intervention in cases of suspected abuse. Clinical vignettes are used to illustrate the importance of a mental health care consultant in working with abused children and their families in day care settings.

PART V: NATIONAL POLICY AND DAY CARE

The two chapters in Part V provide a survey of the legislative and policy issues surrounding child care in the context of the current lack of uniform national quality standards, funding, and regulation. Before the early 1980s, the controversy over the role of the federal government in child care was represented by two opposing political viewpoints. The conservative view held that because child care responsibility rested with the family, the federal government should not participate in child care policy. On the other side, those in favor of federal action maintained that because of the changing structure of the American family and economy, there was an urgent need for a comprehensive national policy on child care. Although the current debate revolves around the extent and nature of governmental involvement, echoes of earlier arguments continue to be heard.

In Chapter 15, Congressman George Miller (D-CA) reviews the legislative history of federal child care programs in the United States and explains the need for a comprehensive national child care policy. Available, high-quality child care, the author believes, is not a luxury or a frill; it is an essential need. He concludes with important suggestions for future funding of child care.

Carol Stevenson presents a discussion of the current chaotic nature of child care regulation in Chapter 16. The questions of who will pay for child care, where it will be located, and how it will be regulated are critical, regardless of whether a uniform national policy emerges or the current diversity of facilities and options is simply enhanced.

The picture this volume draws of the issues surrounding child care today is intentionally as broad as possible. The contributors include research psychologists, politicians, pediatricians, and psychoanalysts, all brought together by their common interest in improving our understanding of the complex issues surrounding child care and by their desire to improve the care of children in our society. This volume's broad-spectrum approach is intended to make it maximally useful as a resource. It is the hope of all those who have contributed to this volume that it will be of real use to workers in the fields of mental health, child care, education, child care law, and health, and particularly to parents and their children.

Shahla S. Chehrazi, M.D.

Part I

Developmental Considerations and Day Care

Chapter 1

Psychological-Developmental Implications of Current Patterns of Early Child Care

Edward F. Zigler, Ph.D., and Johanna Freedman, M.Phil.

Two decades ago, the 1970 White House Conference on Children deemed a lack of affordable, good-quality child care to be the most serious problem facing children and families in the United States. The following year, Congress delivered the Child Development Act (S. 2007) to President Richard Nixon, calling for an expansion of day care facilities, increased federal day care subsidies to welfare recipients, and augmented tax deductions to families using day care. However, because of political pressures from day care opponents, President Richard vetoed the bill. Since then, the United States has come no closer to instituting major reforms to child care, and the situation has grown still more serious.

In this chapter we discuss how and why this problem evolved and define the problem in terms of the number of people affected by the lack of day care. In addition, we discuss the developmental concerns that surround the issue of day care, the issue of quality in day care, and the different day

3

care options currently available. Finally, we propose a possible solution to this problem—a solution that could carry the United States into the 21st century.

It is especially appropriate that this chapter should appear in a psychoanalytically oriented collection, because much of current child care theory and practice rests on the work of the psychoanalytic movement. The list of psychoanalysts who have contributed to our knowledge and understanding of the needs of children is a long and prestigious one. One such contributor is the renowned scientist Sally Provence. Her pioneering, family-oriented child care center, Children's House, was established on psychoanalytic principles, and, in the words of Albert Solnit (Provence and Naylor 1983, p. xi), this program is a perfect example of how "psychoanalytic theory has been adapted and refined for practical application." The center, open from 1967 to 1972, offered family health care, day care when needed, and a home visitor who provided general family support in the form of nutritional advice, assistance in finding better housing, job training, or education (Provence and Naylor 1983).

A second psychoanalyst who has greatly contributed to our understanding of child care theory is Gerald Caplan. He was instrumental in outlining the theoretical basis for family support programs and has provided both policymakers and families with a blueprint for what can and should be done to help families get involved (Caplan 1974). Two additional names that must be mentioned are Selma Fraiberg (1977) and Stanley Greenspan (Greenspan and Greenspan 1986). Their work in the area of early attachment has provided a sound social science basis for the current movement for infant care leave.

Finally, even the most select list of psychoanalytic thinkers would be incomplete without some mention of the work of Albert Solnit and Anna Freud (Goldstein et al. 1979). Their cogent demonstrations of children's need for stability and continuity of care have had a major impact on child custody decisions. Yet, despite this impressive body of work delineating the nature of the needs of children and their families, child care in this country continues to be inadequate in supply and mediocre in quality.

THE PROBLEM DEFINED

The social scene today is replete with books and media presentations with titles such as *The Child Care Crisis* (Maynard 1985) and *The Day Care Dilemma* (Blum 1983). This level of concern is appropriate, for some of the main determinants of parents' choice of child care are often more expedient than developmentally sound. Such factors include considerations of cost and proximity to home. High-quality child care can be prohibitively expensive, even for families with two wage-earning adults. On the private market, high-quality day care for infants and toddlers can cost up to $200 per child per week (Hewlett 1986). Costs for older children are generally lower, but even these fees are a financial strain on low- to moderate-income families. Many of these arrangements are less than optimal for children's development, and almost all of them induce stress and anxiety for parents (Kahn and Kamerman 1987).

A second factor that can lead busy parents to place their child in care that may be less than desirable is simple proximity to home (Endsley and Broadbard 1981; McCartney et al. 1982). In their attempt to accommodate inflexible schedules and demanding job requirements, some parents must place their children in homes that are merely convenient rather than carefully selected to meet their children's needs. It is not that these parents do not care for their children; many simply do not know what characterizes good care (Endsley and Broadbard 1981). Others fail to recognize that day care is not just a convenience that frees them to work but that what is being purchased is the child's daily environment for months and even years—an environment that will invariably affect their children's development.

These "methods" of choosing day care are a sign of a deeper malaise. For too long child care has been regarded as a private problem, to be resolved by individual families as best they can; government and corporate policies reflect past rather than present realities. Such policies still function as if every mother were a housewife, which is no longer the case. Fewer than 10% of all families have a mother at home full-time while the father supports the family (Schroeder 1988); the numbers of "traditional" and single-parent families being formed are now roughly equal (Moynihan 1987). Even in two-parent families, only one-fourth can survive comfortably without two wage earners (Hayes 1982). Yet parents receive little expert guidance and less practical support in their efforts to provide their children with appropriate care (Maynard 1985). As a result, the problem of child care in America has now reached such vast proportions that it strikes many as insoluble. It is not. The problem must be disaggregated into its con-stituent units, and each individual aspect of the problem must be ad-dressed, including parent education, availability of high-quality care, and cost. Recognizing the problem is an important first step. When the Child Development Act was vetoed almost two decades ago, the nation saw the dangers of the "sovietization" (Nelson 1982) of the American family as more serious than the problem of out-of-home care. Today, the depth of the need for day care is evident to everyone.

Some progress has been made recently in addressing the issue. Follow-ing the termination of the White House Conference on Children and the downgrading of the Children's Bureau (Zigler and Muenchow 1985), for many years there was no national podium from which to discuss family issues. Today there is the bipartisan House Select Committee on Children,

Youth, and Families chaired by Rep. George Miller (D-California) and the Senate Subcommittee on Children, Families, Drugs, and Alcoholism chaired by Sen. Christopher Dodd (D-Connecticut).

Unfortunately, there remains a dearth of leadership on this issue in the executive branch of government. Other than maintaining Head Start, which provides care for fewer than 20% of the eligible families (Zigler 1985), the Reagan administration failed to implement a single positive program dealing with the child care problem. However, it should be noted that although no programs have actually been implemented, the problem has received some attention; Secretary of Labor Ann McLaughlin did publish a lengthy summary of the child care situation (U.S. Department of Labor 1988). This initiative was a positive first step, but even there a sanguine attitude was evident. The problem demands more than simply another report; it demands action.

THE MAGNITUDE OF THE DAY CARE PROBLEM

Almost two-thirds of all school-age children and more than half of all preschoolers have mothers who work outside the home (Kahn and Kamerman 1987). Still more startling, approximately 50% of all mothers with infants aged under 1 year were in the work force in 1984 (U.S. Congress 1984). It is anticipated that by 1990, fully one-half the labor force will be comprised of women, and 80% of those women will be of childbearing age (Bates 1987). At some point during their work lives, 93% will become pregnant (U.S. Congress 1984). As a result, the need for child care will continue to grow.

Some claim that the solution to the child care problem is sending mothers home (Stephan 1988). It is not. The driving force behind the massive entrance of women, especially mothers, into the labor force is economic. A recent U.S. Bureau of Labor Statistics report stated that "women seem driven more than ever before into the market place to provide or supplement family income" (qtd. in Schroeder 1988, p. 327). This movement is in response to two major changes: the radical alteration of the American family as a consequence of recent increases in divorce and single parenthood, and the decline in median family income.

In 1940, there was one divorce for every six marriages; in 1980, that number had reached one for every two. Almost 25% of all families and more than 50% of all black families are headed by a single mother (Committee for Economic Development 1987). Roughly 90% of single-parent families are women (Bates 1987). If these women did not work, their median expected income was an appalling $4,607 in 1983; if they did, it was only $13,609 (see Table 1-1).

Table 1-1. Median annual income for families with children aged under 18 years, United States, 1983

Family characteristics	All	White	Black
Two parent families			
Mother in work force	$31,323	$31,661	$26,994
Mother not in work force	24,433	25,043	14,472
Female-headed families			
Mother in work force	13,609	13,382	10,055[a]
Mother not in work force	4,607	4,787	4,385[a]

[a]1984 annual income

Source. Women's Bureau, Special and Irregular Publications: Time of Change: 1983 Handbook on Women Workers. Women's Bureau Bulletin 298, Ser No 029-002-0065-7, 1984.

Prospects are only marginally better for married women. According to the most current data, 40% of married working women have husbands who earn less than $15,000 annually (Schroeder 1988). The median income for American families, adjusted for inflation, has fallen by an average of $300 per year over the past 11 years. This drop means the average American family has $3,300 less today than it did in 1975 for housing, education, food, and clothing. The report of the congressional Joint Economic Committee (U.S. Congress 1986) indicates that although the median family income in America fell 3.1% between 1973 and 1984, if mothers had not joined the work force to support their families, the drop in median income would have been 9.5%. It is clear that such a drastic decline in family income would have had immediate, concrete, and devastating effects on children and families. Instead, in the words of Rep. David Obey (D-Wisconsin), working wives and mothers have assumed a role that "carries with it both the anguish of worrying about children left in other's care and the fatigue and frustration of working longer hours, usually at lower pay than [that] given working men" (U.S. Congress 1986, p. 2). These women must work, and their children need care while they do so.

DAY CARE—A DEVELOPMENTAL APPROACH

The most important aspect of the child care problem is the impact of this care on the development of children. Recent research has focused on differences within the population of children enrolled in the day care setting and the quality of the care provided (Howes 1986; McCartney et al. 1985; Steinberg 1986). Specifically, researchers have found that the needs of children vary across ages; the needs of infants and toddlers are very different from those of preschoolers, and these in turn are different from those of school-age children. Any viable child care system, therefore, must be developmentally appropriate and must answer the needs of children at each stage of development.

It is most useful to distinguish among three developmental stages: from birth to about 2½ years, preschoolers up to age 5, and school-age children. Good-quality care is always essential, but the particulars that distinguish quality differ for these three age groups, as determined by the children's developmental needs.

Infant Day Care

Infant care is an area of special concern because it is a relatively new social form—so new that little research exists on children 10 or more years after they were enrolled in infant day care. It is clear, however, that some crucial developmental landmarks occur in infancy (Kolata 1984). Some of the most important new work on infancy, and arguably the most relevant to issues of day care, has been in the area of attachment. The work of Stern (1985) and others (e.g., Brazelton 1986) demonstrates the need for parents and infants to spend sufficient time with each other to grow "attuned" to one another. Family systems theory suggests that the birth of a new baby necessitates the adjustment of all family members to the presence of the new infant and to the consequent changes in family roles and family functioning (Belsky 1985; Goldberg and Easterbrooks 1984; Minuchin 1985). In a recent controversial review of placement in day care before 1 year of age, Belsky (1985) found cause for concern in a possible relation between insecurity of attachment, aggression, noncompliance, and social withdrawal in the preschool and early school years (see also Chapter 3, this volume). A number of researchers have taken issue with this finding, asserting that Belsky's review of the research was selective. These researchers argue that on measures of socioemotional adjustment, children who have attended high-quality, part-time day care are not different from children reared at home (Chess 1987; Phillips et al. 1987). What remains clear, however, is that low-quality child care can have a detrimental effect on the development of children.

The crucial socioemotional developmental task of infants during this period is the formation of secure attachments, and numerous studies have linked secure attachment in infancy with increased competence in preschool (Pastor 1981; Waters et al. 1979). Although infants do form multiple attachments and more than one caregiver can play a significant role in an infant's development, continuity of care is essential (Bretherton 1985; Parke 1981). It is indeed unfortunate that 60% of mothers in the work force are allowed virtually no leave from work and are therefore unable to spend time with their infants (Ad Hoc Day Care Coalition 1985). In addition, some concern has been expressed over the developmental preparedness of toddlers to engage in peer relations (Rutter 1982).

Preschoolers

Numerous studies have demonstrated that there is less cause for concern in the case of preschoolers. High-quality care seems to result in no adverse effects, and it can benefit children intellectually and socially, particularly in the case of low-income children (Howes 1983, 1985, 1986; McCartney et al. 1985; U.S. Congress 1984).

At this age, in the words of Rutter (1982, p. 25), "Children gain much from their peers and there is less exclusive reliance on adults for meeting their needs." Researchers have shown that the opportunity to interact with children of the same age is not only desirable but necessary for normal social development. Children who do not play with age-mates miss important social learning experiences and are at risk of becoming uncertain of themselves in interpersonal situations. Whereas children learn from their parents how to get along in one sort of social hierarchy, the family, it is from their interactions with peers that they learn how to interact with equals in a wide range of social situations (Hartup 1978; Mueller and Vandell 1979). With the increase in later marriage and reduced family size (U.S. Congress 1984), high-quality preschool may be a valuable avenue for peer socialization among preschoolers. In addition, excellent remedial programs for the disadvantaged have succeeded in spurring the developmental and cognitive growth of low-income 3- and 4-year-old children (Ambach 1986; Berrueta-Clement et al. 1984; Deutsch et al. 1983; Lazar and Darlington 1982; Pierson et al. 1984).

School-age Day Care

Although the fact receives little attention from either academic journals or the popular press, children over 6 years comprise greater than one-half the need for day care (Zigler and Muenchow 1985). In 1982, two to four million children returned each day to empty homes after school (School Age Child Care Project 1982). This largely unmet need for school-age day care has contributed to the growing number of "latchkey" or "self-care" children, that is, children who are not under adult supervision after school hours. Researchers are at odds concerning the consequences of self-care. Some have found no differences between self- and adult-care children on a variety of measures including locus of control, self-esteem, and social and interpersonal competence (Leischman 1980; Rodman et al. 1985). At least one worker has gone on record as believing that self-care contributes to independent functioning (Korchin, cited in Langway et al. 1981).

In contrast, other researchers have reported that self-care children tend to be more fearful (Long and Long 1983). Some researchers have warned of safety hazards to unattended children, and links have been found between self-care and juvenile delinquency (Zigler and Hall 1988). In testimony before Congress in 1984, a number of latchkey children spoke of being afraid of not knowing what to do in emergencies and of being sexually abused (U.S. Congress 1984). Work by Steinberg (1986), Ginter (1981), and others has helped resolve the source of some of these contradictory findings. As these researchers cogently pointed out, not all self-care situations are alike, nor are all children. A 14-year-old who returns home promptly after school, telephones an adult, and arranges to engage in appropriate activities until an adult returns is unlike a 7-year-old youngster from a ghetto who is either left alone in a small apartment or spends afternoons on street corners. These researchers have stressed that it is essential to identify the salient characteristics of each child's situation, the child's developmental needs, and how variations within the latchkey population affect relevant outcome measures such as children's fears, the dangers to which they may be exposed, and the likelihood that they will engage in undesirable behavior that they would not engage in if adults were nearby. What remains clear, however, is that many children in need of supervision are not receiving it and that measures should be taken so that those children who need care will be adequately supervised.

CHILD CARE TODAY

There is an enormous range of day care settings in America, but most fall into one of three types: in-home care, family and group day care homes, and day care centers.

In-Home Care

According to U.S. Bureau of the Census (1982) figures for day care use, 26% of the children of working parents are in in-home care, a situation in which one caregiver comes to the child's home or one child is taken to the caregiver's home to receive individual care. Of this group, 6% are cared for by regular sitters, nannies, or housekeepers (Fallows 1985). The remainder are cared for by a patchwork of grandparents, fathers, other relatives, and neighbors. Although the children receive individual care in a familiar setting, there are disadvantages. In-home care is far more costly than other forms of care, because the entire salary of the caregiver is borne by the family of the one child cared for rather than shared with other families. In addition, such arrangements may be difficult to create and maintain.

Qualified caregivers are hard to find, and parents are often forced to rely on students or recent immigrants who may not share the family's values or speak its language (Fallows 1985). The informality of the arrangement poses other problems as well. First, parents can offer few benefits. In addition, changes in caregivers' school or work status may leave parents with no caregiver, and there is no backup in case of illness or other absences. In such cases, parents must struggle to make alternate arrangements or miss work to care for their children.

Family and Group Day Care Homes

Because parents view it as "homelike," the most popular arrangement for children in substitute care is the family (1 to 6 children) or group (6 to 12 children) day care home (Young and Zigler 1986). Both family and group day care operate in private homes in which the caregivers may or may not be related to the children. Of all children receiving supplemental care, 56% are in family day care (U.S. Bureau of the Census 1982), and over two-thirds of these children are between 3 and 5 years of age (U.S. Congress 1984). Despite the large numbers of children in such care, it is the arrangement least researched. In fact, although 44 states have regulations to guide the operation of family day care homes (Young and Zigler 1986), these regulations are largely ignored; more that 90% of family day care homes operate outside any regulatory system (Fosburg et al. 1981). In addition, only 14 states have specific regulations for group day care homes (Young and Zigler 1986).

As a result of the lack of regulation of such facilities, we know little about the quality of family day care in general. As a group, family day care can be characterized only by its heterogeneity. A study conducted by the National Council of Jewish Women (Keyserling 1972) examined day care facilities of this type and found that only 10% provided "superior" care, about half provided custodial care, and a shocking 11% provided care that was rated "poor." Settings were rated "poor" based on some or all of the following qualities: overcrowded, dirty, unstimulating and/or dangerous conditions, and day care providers who were more interested in increasing cash flow than in enhancing development. Some of these settings were so bad that they constituted neglectful or abusive environments. Most, however, fell somewhere between the two extremes by providing adequate care for basic needs only. Family day care tends to be relatively affordable, because the caregiver's overhead tends to be low, and it is generally conveniently located and the caregiver is flexible about drop-off and pickup times. Again, because of the lack of regulation and licensing, the possibility of finding some very bad family day care is quite high.

Day Care Centers

Approximately 18% of children in out-of-home care are enrolled in day care centers (Zigler and Hall 1988). The centers fall into two subcategories: for-profit centers, including large chains like Kinder-Care, and nonprofit centers, such as those run by churches, community centers, and employers. Little is yet known about how quality of care may differ between for-profit and nonprofit centers. Centers tend to be reliable and well equipped, and they may offer sliding fee scales. They may, however, fail to provide sufficient individual attention to particular children, and children who are easily overstimulated by large numbers of people may be overwhelmed. They may also be less flexible than other forms of care, given their heavier administrative responsibilities. Another potential problem associated with centers is arranging care when children fall ill, because most centers do not accept sick children on account of the dangers they pose to other children.

QUALITY OF CARE

Recent research has focused on differences within the population of children enrolled in day care settings and the quality of the care provided (Howes 1986, Chapter 2, this volume; McCartney et al. 1985; Steinberg 1986). Not surprisingly, all the evidence indicates that children develop better when they receive appropriate care. However, if the quality of care falls below a certain minimum, the development of the child is compromised. Unfortunately, just as there is no coherent set of national public policies about child care, there is no coherent federal debate about child care regulations. Instead, available child care services constitute an uncoordinated patchwork of programs, funded from a host of different sources, that serve fragments of the population in need of child care. Quality varies tremendously within every type of child care setting (Young and Zigler 1986).

Regulation of child care programs provides a mechanism for establishing a floor of quality below which children's safety is jeopardized (Morgan 1980). Licensing is the primary means of regulation, and it is controlled by the states. It offers a means of monitoring programs for compliance with health and fire codes as well as with additional guidelines established and enforced by state agencies responsible for child care. The states' guidelines are typically framed in terms of minimum standards that reflect a philosophy of preventing harm to children in child care, rather than providing high-quality, developmentally appropriate programming (Kendall and Walker 1984).

The need for regulations to protect children's safety in child care is widely accepted. Even critics of a strong government role in child care have asserted that children's health and safety should be safeguarded by some public regulatory body (Phillips and Zigler 1987). There is no controversy as to what minimum standards must be met to ensure that children's development is not impaired; in fact, the degree of consensus is surprising in a field usually fraught with conflict. Experts concur that staff-child ratio, group size, and staff training affect children's development (Ruopp and Travers 1982). The consensus dissipates, however, as discussions turn to whether the federal government should assume responsibility for this protective function.

Our nation has been struggling with the problem of standards for almost two decades. When the original Federal Interagency Day Care Regulations (FIDCRs) were established in 1968, they were ambiguous, vague, and largely impracticable (Nelson 1982). Subsequently, President Nixon advanced a sweeping welfare proposal, the Family Assistance Plan, which was to include a massive federal day care program; it was obvious, however, that such an extensive day care program could not be run effectively under guidelines as vague as the 1968 FIDCRs. Therefore, the Office of Child Development, under the direction of Edward Zigler, convened a day care conference of more than 1,000 parents, child care professionals, social scientists, and child advocates to discuss how to revise and make more concrete the 1968 FIDCRs (Nelson 1982). This task was completed by 1972; however, as before, decision makers in the Department of Health, Education, and Welfare (DHEW) were at odds over the federal government's role in promulgating standards. The Family Assistance Plan collapsed in 1972, and these standards became moot.

The 1972 standards were slightly revised in 1980 in an effort led by the Children's Defense Fund. These standards were endorsed by HEW Secretary Patricia Harris from the Carter administration after a lengthy analysis in the Department of Health and Human Services (DHHS) and were sent to Congress for consideration. Congress, however, took no action pending further cost studies, and the standards once again quietly vanished. The most recent effort to produce standards was precipitated by the urging of the DHHS in 1985.

The results can be described only as a travesty. Instead of the thoroughly researched, developmentally sound standards of 1980 simply being updated, the problem of child care quality was largely ignored. Instead, the focus was on sexual abuse, a relatively rare phenomenon in child care settings. The real problem is that so many children are receiving unregulated care or care regulated at such a low level as to compromise their development. Consequently, it is safe to say that the quality of care children are receiving can best be described as heterogeneous. More ominous, although increasing numbers of 3- to 5-year-olds are now attending preschool programs, divergence in child care patterns according to family income and parents' educational levels seems to be growing (Ambach 1986; U.S. Congress 1984). There is some danger that this trend may mark the emergence of a dual system of child care in which children of affluent and well-educated parents attend high-quality child care programs and children of low-income families are placed at even greater risk of poor developmental outcome by being forced into poor child care settings. The long-range implications are indeed disturbing; as these children become adults, the consequences to development of their different pathways will be manifest. One group will have received environmental nutrients that enhance optimal development. The other group, except for the rare invulnerable child, will experience the negative effects that result from poor care.

CONCLUSION: A PROPOSED SOLUTION

As has been suggested, any viable solution must address the question of quality. What kinds of care are appropriate for children at the different developmental stages?

Infants

If this fine-grained question is posed with regard to infants, the early work of a number of researchers represents a broad range of opinion. At one end of the spectrum is the view held by Clarke-Stewart (1982, p. 118), who believed that "in terms of cognitive gains or achievement of social competence, age of starting day-care does not seem to matter." At the opposite end of the spectrum is Fraiberg (1977), who warned against the dangers to children of changing caregivers, regimented day care homes, and inadequately staffed and equipped centers. She urged mothers to stay with their children to provide them with proper care and a stable human relationship.

A range of views exists between these two extremes. Through a review of the research on attachment and infant care, Gamble and Zigler (1986, p. 35) reached a number of tentative conclusions:

1) In families facing significant life stresses, substitute care during the first year increases the likelihood of insecure parent-child attachments; 2) an insecure attachment makes the,child more vulnerable to stress encountered later on; and 3) the best predictor of later pathology is a cumulative frequency of stressful life events coupled with an insecure attachment in infancy.

In conclusion, these researchers suggested the following:

Alternatives to infant day care should be made available to those working couples who would prefer to be with their infants during the first months of life. . . . The most attractive alternative to infant day care is a policy of paid infant care leaves during the first few months of [the] baby's life. (p. 40)

This opinion is far from unique. A committee of experts convened in 1983 by the Yale Bush Center in Child Development and Social Policy reached the conclusion that parents should receive a minimum of a 6-month leave of absence to care for a newborn or newly adopted infant. They concluded that this leave should include partial income replacement (75% of salary) for 3 months, up to a realistic maximum benefit (Zigler and Frank 1988). In fact, more than two-thirds of the nations of the world, including almost all industrialized nations, have some provisions for parents of infants to take paid, job-protected leaves of absence from the workplace for physical recovery from labor and birth and to care for their newborn infants (Kamerman 1988).

Preschoolers and School-age Children

For 3- to 5-year-olds and for school-age children, we propose a solution to the problem that makes use of an already existing institution—the neighborhood school. We need a school that provides care for every child in need of care. By making use of the neighborhood school we can create a system that could meet the needs of working parents, offer play and educational opportunities for children, strengthen community and family ties, and solve the child care crisis.

The most cost-effective way to provide universally available—again, not compulsory—care would be to create the "school of the 21st century." We advocate a return to the concept of the community school as a local center for all the social services required by the surrounding neighborhood. In this way, the neighborhood school building could be used for two purposes: formal education for 6- to 12-year-olds, and a second system that provides full-day, high-quality child care for 3- to 5-year-olds, early morning and after-school care for 6- to 12-year-olds, and full-time care for all children during vacations.

Such a program, although operating on school grounds, should not be staffed solely by teachers for two reasons. First, teachers are already overburdened with the task of educating our children; it would be unfair to ask them to take sole responsibility for on-site care as well. In addition, many elementary school teachers are not trained to work with very young children and their families. When we speak of on-site child care, we are not advocating early formal education. What we envision is a quality child care system that would be structured to meet the developmental needs of preschoolers, a place where they would go primarily for recreation and socialization, the real business of preschoolers. We propose, therefore, that teachers should have the option to participate in the before- and after-school program. The school-based child care program for 3- to 5-year-olds, on the other hand, should be headed by an early education specialist who would be assisted by child development associates, who are certified child caregivers.

On a larger scale, many aspects of the funding issue must be addressed. Currently, there are 13 model 21st-century schools operating within two school districts in Missouri. Administrators of these school districts found that because this system made use of an already existing resource (i.e., the neighborhood school building), the cost of implementing the program was kept to a minimum. This initial funding may come from one of three sources: charitable foundations, state governments, or the federal government. In Missouri, start-up funds were obtained from the Kansas City Association of Charitable Trusts and Foundations. The state of Connecticut, on the other hand, recently passed a bill that authorized $500,000 for start-up funds for creating and eventually evaluating demonstration schools to be placed in rural, urban, and suburban areas throughout Connecticut. Finally, at the federal level, a bill calling for $120 million for funding a minimum of 60 demonstration schools, at least one per state, has been introduced by Sen. Christopher Dodd (D-Connecticut) and Rep. Dale Kildee (D-Michigan). Beyond the initial funding, parents would be expected to pay for the maintenance of the program on a sliding fee scale.

This family-oriented, multiservice community school could meet the many different needs of children and their families by offering a variety of programs from which families could select. Three such outreach programs would include a family support system for parents of newborns, such as the Parents as First Teachers program currently operating in Missouri (Meyerhoff and White 1986; Vento and Winter 1986); support for family day care homes in the neighborhood; and information and referral services. In this way, the school could act as a provider of day care, but it would also be a training and referral agency for other day care workers in the area. The importance of such flexibility and variety in our changing society is obvious. The time has come to put into effect a high-quality day care system that will be available and affordable to all who need it. The well-being of our children, the future of our nation, depends on it.

REFERENCES

Ad Hoc Day Care Coalition: The Crisis in Infant and Toddler Child Care. Washington, DC, Ad Hoc Day Care Coalition, 1985

Ambach G: Should 4- and 5-year-olds be in school? Yes, optional public preschool is essential. The Christian Science Monitor, March 28, 1986, B7–B9

Bates TH: The changing family to the year 2000: planning for our children's future. Berkeley, CA, California Joint Publications, 1987

Belsky J: Experimenting with the family in the newborn period. Child Dev 56:407–414, 1985

Berrueta-Clement D, Schweinhart LO, Burnett WS, et al: Changed Lives: Effects of the Perry Preschool Program on Youths Through Age 19. Ypsilanti, MI, High/Scope Press, 1984

Blum PM: The Day-care Dilemma: Women and Children First. Lexington, MA, Lexington Books, 1983

Brazelton TB: Issues for working parents. Am J Orthopsychiatry 56:14–25, 1986

Bretherton I: Attachment theory: retrospect and prospect, in Growing Points in Attachment Theory and Research. Edited by Bretherton I, Waters E. Monographs of the Society for Research in Child Development 50(ser no 209):3–36, 1985

Caplan G: Support Systems and Community Mental Health. New York, Behavioral Publications, 1974

Chess S: Comments: infant day care: a cause for concern. Zero to Three 7:24–25, 1987

Clarke-Stewart A: Day Care. Cambridge, MA, Harvard University Press, 1982

Committee for Economic Development: Children in Need: Investment Strategies for the Educationally Disadvantaged. New York, Committee for Economic Development, 1987

Deutsch M, Deutsch C, Jordan T, et al: The IDS program: an experiment in early and sustained enrichment, in As the Twig Is Bent. Edited by the Consortium for Longitudinal Studies. Hillsdale, NJ, Erlbaum, 1983

Endsley R, Broadbard M: Quality Day Care: A Handbook of Choices for Parents and Caregivers. Englewood Cliffs, NJ, Spectrum, 1981

Fallows D: A Mother's Work. Boston, MA, Houghton Mifflin, 1985

Fosburg S, Singer J, Irwin N: Family day care in the United States: final report of the National Day Care Home Study, Vol 1. Washington DC, Department of Health and Human Services, Office of Human Development Services (OHDS), 80-30282, 1981

Fraiberg S: Every Child's Birthright: In Defense of Mothering. New York, Basic Books, 1977

Gamble TJ, Zigler E: Effects of infant day care: another look at the evidence. Am J Orthopsychiatry, 56:26–42, 1986

Ginter M: An exploratory study of the "latchkey child": children who care for themselves. Unpublished predissertation project, Yale University, New Haven, CT, 1981

Goldberg WA, Easterbrooks MA: Role of marital quality in toddler development. Developmental Psychology 20:504–514, 1984

Goldstein J, Freud A, Solnit A: Before the Best Interests of the Child. New York, Free Press, 1979

Greenspan S, Greenspan N: First Feelings. New York, Penguin, 1986

Hartup WW: Perspectives on child and family interaction: past, present and future, in Child Influences on Marital and Family Interactions: A Life-span Perspective. Edited by Lerner RM, Spanier GB. New York, Academic, 1978, pp 23–47

Hayes CD: Making Policies for Children: A Study of the Federal Process. Washington, DC, National Academy Press, 1982

Hewlett S: Lesser Life: The Myth of Women's Liberation in America. New York, William Morrow, 1986

Howes C: Care giver behavior in center and family day care. Journal of Applied Developmental Psychology 4:99–107, 1983

Howes C: Sharing fantasy: social pretend play in toddlers. Child Dev 56:1253–1258, 1985

Howes C: Current research on early day care. Review paper presented at The San Francisco Psychoanalytic Institute Seminar, "Infant and Toddler Care—Meeting the Needs of Parents and Children in a Changing Society," San Francisco, CA, September 1986

Kahn A, Kamerman D: Child Care: Facing the Hard Choices. Dover, MA, Auburn House, 1987

Kamerman SB: Maternity and parenting benefits: an international overview, in The Parental Leave Crisis: Toward a National Policy. Edited by Zigler E, Frank M. New Haven, CT, Yale University Press, 1988, pp 235–245

Kendall ED, Walker LH: Day care licensing: the eroding regulations. Child Care Quarterly 13(4):278–290, 1984

Keyserling M: Windows on Day Care. New York, National Council of Jewish Women, 1972

Kolata G: Studying learning in the womb. Science 225:302–303, 1984

Langway L, Abramson P, Foote D: The latchkey children. Newsweek, Feb 16, 1981, pp 96–97

Lazar I, Darlington R: Lasting Effects of Early Education: A Report From the Consortium for Longitudinal Studies. Monographs of the Society for Research in Child Development, Vol 47, 1982

Leischman K: When kids are home alone: how mothers make sure they're safe. Working Mothers 3:21–25, 1980

Long T, Long L: Latchkey Children. Urbana, IL, ERIC Clearinghouse on Elementary and Early Childhood Education, 1983. Prepared with funding from the National Institute of Education, U.S. Department of Education, contract number 400-78-0008.

Maynard F: The Child Care Crisis. Markham, Ontario, Viking, 1985

McCartney K, Scarr S, Phillips D, et al: Environmental differences among day care centers and their effects on children's development, in Day Care: Scientific and Social Policy Issues. Edited by Zigler E, Gordon E. Dover, MA, Auburn House, 1982, pp 126–152

McCartney K, Scarr S, Phillips D, et al: Day care as intervention: comparisons of varying quality programs. Journal of Applied Developmental Psychology 6:247–260, 1985

Meyerhoff MK, White BL: New parents as teachers. Educ Leadership, 1986, pp 42–46

Minuchin S: Families and individual development: provocations from the field of family therapy. Child Dev 56:289–302, 1985

Morgan G: Federal day care requirements: one more round. Day Care and Early Education 8(2):26–30, 1980

Moynihan DPC: The Family Security Act of 1987. Letter to New York. Washington, DC, U.S. Senate, 70521-3201, May 26, 1987

Mueller E, Vandell D: Infant-infant interaction, in Handbook of Infant Development. Edited by Osofsky JD. New York, John Wiley, 1979, pp 591–623

Nelson C: The politics of federal day care regulation, in Day Care: Scientific and Social Policy Issues. Edited by Zigler E, Gordon E. Dover, MA, Arbor House, 1982, pp 267–307

Parke R: Fathers. Cambridge, MA, Harvard University Press, 1981

Pastor DC: The quality of mother-infant attachment and its relationship to toddler's initial sociability with peers. Developmental Psychology 17:326–335, 1981

Phillips D, Zigler E: The checkered history of federal day care regulation, in Review of Research in Education, Vol 14. Edited by Rothkopf E. Washington, DC, American Educational Research Association, 1987

Phillips D, McCartney L, Scarr S, et al: Selective review of infant day care research: a cause for concern. Zero to Three 7(3):18–21, 1987

Pierson D, Tivnan D, Walker T: A school based program from infancy to kindergarten for children and their parents. Personnel and Guidance Journal 4:448–455, 1984

Provence S, Naylor A: Working with Disadvantaged Parents and Their Children. New Haven, CT, Yale University Press, 1983

Rodman H, Pratto DJ, Nelson RS: Child care arrangements and children's functioning: a comparison of self-care and adult-care children. Developmental Psychology 21:413–418, 1985

Ruopp R, Travers J: Janus faces day care: perspectives on quality and cost, in Day Care: Scientific and Social Policy Issues. Edited by Zigler E, Gordon E. Dover, MA, Auburn House, 1982, pp 72–102

Rutter M: Socio-emotional consequences of day care for preschool children, in Day Care: Scientific and Social Policy Issues. Edited by Zigler E, Gordon E. Dover, MA, Auburn House, 1982, pp 3–33

School Age Child Care Project: School-age child care, in Day Care: Scientific and Social Policy Issues. Edited by Zigler E, Gordon E. Dover, MA, Auburn House, 1982, pp 457–476

Schroeder P: Parental leave: the need for a federal policy, in Infant Care and Infant Care Leaves. Edited by Zigler E, Frank M. New Haven, CT, Yale University Press, 1988, pp 326–333

Steinberg L: Latchkey children and susceptibility to peer pressure: an ecological analysis. Developmental Psychology 22:433–439, 1986

Stephan S: Child Day Care: Federal Policy Issues and Legislation (order code IB87193). Washington, DC, Congressional Research Service, 1988

Stern D: The Interpersonal World of the Infant: A View from Psychoanalysis and Developmental Psychology. New York, Basic Books, 1985

U.S. Bureau of the Census: Current Population Reports. Series P-23, No 129. Washington DC, U.S. Bureau of the Census, 1982

U.S. Congress, House Select Committee on Children, Youth, and Families: Families and Child Care: Improving the Options. Washington, DC, U.S. Government Printing Office, 1984

U.S. Congress (99th, Second Session). Joint Economic Committee: Working Mothers Are Preserving Family Living Standards: A Staff Study. Washington, DC, Joint Economic Committee, 1986

U.S. Department of Labor: Child Care: A Workforce Issue. Report of the Secretary's Task Force. Washington DC, U.S. Government Printing Office, 1988

Vento VA, Winter M: Beginning at the beginning: Missouri's Parents as First Teachers program. Community Education Journal 14:6–8, 1986

Waters E, Wippman J, Sroufe LA: Attachment, positive effect and competence in the peer group: two studies in construct validation. Child Dev 50:821–829, 1979

Women's Bureau, Special and Irregular Publications: Time of Change: 1983 Handbook on Women Workers. Women's Bureau Bulletin 298, Ser No 029-002-0065-7, 1984

Young KT, Zigler E: Infant and toddler day care: regulations and policy implications. Am J Orthopsychiatry 56:43–55, 1986

Zigler E: Assessing Head Start at 20: an invited commentary. Am J Orthopsychiatry 55:603–609, 1985

Zigler E, Frank M (eds): Parental Leave Crisis: Toward a National Policy. New Haven, CT, Yale University Press, 1988

Zigler E, Hall N: Day care and its effects on children: an overview for pediatric health professionals. Journal of Developmental and Behavioral Pediatrics 9:38–46, 1988

Zigler E, Muenchow S: A room of their own: a proposal to renovate the Children's Bureau. Am Psychol 40:953–959, 1985

Chapter 2

Current Research on Early Day Care

Carollee Howes, Ph.D.

This chapter is a review of psychological research on infant and toddler child care, which is defined here as any type of care by nonfamily members: for example, in-home care by nannies, babysitters, and housekeepers, as well as out-of-home care in family day care homes or centers. The optimal development of children who enter child care as infants or toddlers is a concern shared by parents and by mental health and child care professionals. Such development is also increasingly a matter of public policy, for approximately one-half of mothers of infants are in the paid labor force. Few of these women can choose not to use early child care. Mothers, for the most part, are in the work force because of economic pressures. The need to establish a career makes early child care a necessity for many women, especially given the lack of a cohesive national policy on parental leaves.

The interpretation of psychological research on infant and toddler child care has recently been the topic of controversy in the scholarly literature (see, e.g., Belsky 1986, Chapter 3, this volume; Clarke-Stewart 1988; Phillips et al. 1987a, 1987b; Richters and Zahn-Waxler 1988; Thompson 1988) as well as in the popular press. Part of the controversy concerns the framing of the question. If the question is whether or not infants should be in child care at all, then the only research that must be reviewed is those

21

studies that compare family care with nonfamily care. If the question is what aspects or parameters of child care facilitate more optimal long-term development, then we must examine both the quality of care provided to the child within child care and the interactions between the family and child care systems.

SHOULD INFANTS BE IN CHILD CARE?; SHOULD MOTHERS WORK?: THE ISSUE OF MATERNAL ATTACHMENT

In an attachment theory framework, children's early experiences with caregiving adults provide the first basis for children's internal working models of the self and the self in relation to others (see Barglow et al. 1987; Howes 1987b; Sroufe 1988; Thompson 1988; and Vaughn et al. 1985 for further elaborations of the implications of attachment theory for child care). Thus, the child who experiences sensitivity and warmth from a caregiver comes to believe that he or she is lovable and initiates future relationships from this secure base. A reasonably large number of empirical studies suggest that under conditions of continuity of care over time, early security of maternal attachment predicts a wide range of later positive socioemotional functioning (for reviews see Bretherton 1985; Lamb et al. 1985; Sroufe 1983).

If we are asking whether infants should be in child care, then the security of the child's attachment to the mother becomes the focus of concern. Three recent reviews (Belsky 1986, Chapter 3, this volume; Clarke-Stewart 1988) have concluded that when a child is enrolled in nonmaternal child care before his or her first birthday, the child has an increased risk of avoidance of the mother following separation and of insecure attachment as measured in the Ainsworth Strange Situation (Ainsworth et al. 1978).

[The Strange Situation is a brief laboratory procedure, consisting of a standard series of eight episodes: 1) parent and child are ushered into the room with an observer; 2) parent and child are alone; 3) a stranger enters; 4) parent leaves; 5) parent returns, stranger leaves; 6) parent leaves again; 7) stranger returns; 8) parent returns. Each episode except the first is 3 minutes long, unless the child becomes unduly distressed at the parent's absence, in which case the parent returns immediately. The reunion episodes are critical to the assessment of quality of attachment. Avoidant children (Group A) show little or no reaction to the parent's leaving and show active avoidance of the parent in the reunion episodes. Secure children (Group B) may or may not show distress upon separation but are distinguished by positive greeting or proximity seeking upon reunion. Another group of insecure children (Group C—resistant) are distinguished by high distress on separation and combining proximity seeking with resistant, angry behavior upon reunion.]

These reviews differ in assessing the magnitude of the risk associated with infant child care. They also differ in their interpretation of the meaning of the Strange Situation for children enrolled in child care and, therefore, experiencing daily separations similar to those assessed in the Strange Situation. Belsky (1986) argued that there is a significant and important risk associated with infant care when mothers are working more than 20 hours per week during the infant's first year of life. Clarke-Stewart argued that there is approximately 9% increased risk of insecure maternal attachment associated with early maternal employment, that the methods of assessment may be inappropriate for children of working mothers, and that a recommendation that mothers stay home is unlikely to ensure an infant's secure development. Clarke-Stewart called for increased research to understand the dynamics of maternal employment, child care, and child development.

Three other reviews suggest that there is no increased risk of insecure attachment associated with infant child care (McCartney and Phillips 1988; Richters and Zahn-Waxler 1988; Thompson 1988). These reviews of the association between maternal attachment security and child care enrollment concur with Clarke-Stewart's suggestion that focusing on insecure maternal attachment is too narrow a perspective.

There is a consensus among researchers that we need to know more about the family's alternatives to child care in order to understand relations between child care and maternal attachment security. Is a child not in child care because the mother is not working? What are the effects of marital stress or maternal depression? Is a child enrolled in child care because of a difficult parent-child relationship or because of inadequate home-based caregiving? Or was the decision to use child care made by sensitive, competent, financially secure parents who were striving for a balance between their work and family lives? Beyond these larger concerns we know little about the day-to-day experiences of infants and their parents when infants are enrolled in child care. Does the child experience an available, sensitive, and affectionate parent when he or she is not in child care, or a tired, stressed, and unavailable parent? In other words, is it the nature of women's work outside the home and the general lack of support for family life in our society that promote insecure maternal-child attachments, or is it child care?

The literature on child care and maternal attachment has tended to assume that only the maternal attachment is significant for the child's future social and emotional development. However, when mothers go to work and infants go to child care, the infant acquires at least one other significant caregiver: the child care provider. Attachment theory suggests that infants can form simultaneous multiple attachments and that these attachments are not necessarily concordant (Bretherton 1985). That is, all of the child's attachments do not necessarily take the same form. Three studies of American infants in child care (Colin 1986; Howes et al. 1988; Krentz 1988) and one study of Israeli children cared for by metapelets (caregivers) (Sagi et al. 1985) found that infants do not necessarily form the same type of attachment relationship to alternative caregivers as they do to their mothers. A child may be secure with the mother and insecure with the caregiver, or vice versa. Only one study (Howes et al. 1988) has examined the consequences of nonconcordant attachments for future social relationships, and it has done so only for toddlers. In this study, toddlers with two secure attachments were most socially competent with peers, whereas toddlers with two insecure attachments were the least competent. Toddlers who had one secure and one insecure attachment were intermediate in their social competence with peers. Future longitudinal research is needed to examine the possible compensatory effects of one secure attachment, but this study suggests that examining only maternal attachment is insufficient when attempting to predict future socioemotional development as a consequence of child care.

HOW WE CAN FACILITATE DEVELOPMENT IN CHILD CARE: ASPECTS OF OPTIMAL CHILD CARE

We now turn to the question of what aspects of child care facilitate more optimal long-term development of infants. Three aspects emerge as important:

- The stability of the child care (whether the infant is cared for by the same person and within the same peer group)
- The quality of the child care arrangement, particularly the adult-child ratio, staff training, and developmentally appropriate programming
- The interaction between family characteristics and child care (whether the family is having a difficult time parenting associated with unstable, low-quality child care)

Two additional aspects often cited by mental health professionals emerge as less important: the age the child entered child care and the type of child care arrangement. Evidence supports the argument that age of entry and type of child care are important only as they interact with the stability and quality of the child care arrangement and with the particular family characteristics.

Stability

The stability of the child care arrangement is defined in the research literature in several ways. In studies conducted primarily in child care centers, stability is defined as the regularity or permanence of the child care teacher. Cummings (1980) reported that when infants and toddlers arrived at child care, they were more emotionally positive when left with a stable caregiver than with an irregular one. Rubenstein and Howes (1979) reported that toddlers engaged in social interaction more with the head teacher in the classroom than with the assistant teachers or volunteers. These studies highlight the importance to the child of a stable, trustworthy caregiver. They also provide evidence that contradicts the myth that because only the parental attachment relationship is important to the child, the child does not discriminate between, or care about, the alternative caregivers.

As infant and toddler child care has become more widespread, the definition of stability has changed. Increasingly, infants and toddlers experience multiple child care arrangements before the age of 2. The following vignette illustrates this point:

> When James was born, his parents initially selected in-home care. They had three different experiences with in-home caregivers; two did not fit into their family life, and a third left to handle her own family crisis. Next the parents decided to move James to a neighborhood family day care home. Unfortunately, this provider moved away with her husband, who had accepted a job out of state, and so James was taken to a second family day care home. All the children in this home were much older or much younger than James, and so when his name came up on the waiting list of the child care center where his parents had listed him before he was born, his parents entered him there. Thus, through a series of rational decisions forced on the parents by the reality of child care, James experienced six different child care arrangements.

In several studies the number of different child care arrangements has been used to assess the influences of stability of care. Three studies have examined relations between attachment to parents and the stability of child care arrangements. Children from a highly stressed, low-income sample who had experienced multiple child care arrangements were reported to have a higher proportion of insecure maternal attachments (Vaughn et al. 1980). In one middle-class sample, the number of different child care arrangements bore no relation to the quality of the maternal attachment relationship (Benn 1985). In another study using a middle-class sample, insecure maternal attachment relationships were associated with low stability of child care, while secure attachments were not (Suwalsky et al. 1986). Almost all of the infants with insecure attachments had experienced multiple caregiving arrangements, whereas infants with secure attachments were equally likely to have experienced unstable and stable arrangements. These findings suggest two competing hypotheses: 1) infants who are left in multiple child care arrangements may become unable to trust any adult caregiver, or 2) multiple child care arrangements may mark a lack of maternal sensitivity that is associated with insecure attachment relationships.

In two other studies using middle-class samples, the number of changes in child care arrangements was associated with indices of child competence. The first, a study of children enrolled in family day care homes, found that a greater number of different child care arrangements was associated with less competent play with objects, adults, and peers (Howes and Stewart 1987). The second study assessed the influence of the number of different child care arrangements prior to entering a prekindergarten program on first-grade children's adjustment to school and their sociometric status with peers (Howes 1988). In other words, the influence of the number of child care changes children had experienced as infants and toddlers was examined after 3 years in a stable school setting. Children who had experienced more child care changes had greater trouble adjusting to school and were less popular with their peers.

These results suggest that optimal short-term and long-term development of the child are negatively influenced by changes in child care. The earlier the child enters child care, the more likely the child is to experience changes. In-home care and family day care arrangements are more likely than a center child care situation to be associated with changes in child care arrangements.

The reverse picture is that children who enter center-based child care as infants and toddlers and remain with the same peer group and center do experience optimal child development. One commonly used marker of optimal development of the preschool child is the ability both to form reciprocated friendships with peers and to be sociable and accepted by peers. Sociability and peer acceptance are measured by sociometric status, a peer rating of popularity. In a study of 329 children who entered center-based child care as infants, toddlers, or preschoolers, children who experienced the most stable child care arrangements—remaining in the same centers and with the same peer group—were most likely to have long-term reciprocal friendships, to have higher sociometric ratings, and to engage in competent social interactions with their peers (Howes 1987a). Furthermore, children who lost their reciprocated friendships because their friends left the child care center were less socially competent 1 year later than those children who did not lose their friends.

A series of recent studies has documented that toddlers in child care do form stable, reciprocated friendships with their peers and that they engage in relatively sophisticated forms of social pretend play—or the sharing of fantasy—within these intimate relationships (Howes 1983b, 1985). These experiences function to benefit the children emotionally as well as to increase their social-cognitive competence (Howes 1983b). Studies of victims of child abuse illustrate this point. Abused toddlers enrolled in a child care program were observed to form friendships and to engage in relatively competent social interactions with their abused and non-maltreated peers (Howes 1984; Howes and Espinosa 1985). Abused children who received child care interventions were also reported to be more socially competent with peers than were abused children who received no direct intervention, although in both groups the parents were enrolled in therapy (Howes and Espinosa 1985). Therefore, intimate relations with peers, even in toddlers, may buffer emotional stressors, including the daily separation from parents experienced by all child care children and, perhaps, the more severe stress of abuse.

The studies demonstrating positive socioemotional outcomes in children who are enrolled in child care as infants and toddlers are encouraging. They suggest that if child care is stable and (as will be discussed) of high quality, children emerge socially competent and capable of sustaining positive and intimate friendship relations with peers. The discussion thus far has been limited to children who enter child care as infants or toddlers; however, Clarke-Stewart (1984) found a similar pattern of outcomes in her studies of children who entered child care as 2- and 3-year-olds.

Quality of Child Care

Stability of care. The stability of child care arrangements has also been used as a marker to indicate child care quality within child care centers. In this case, stability is defined in terms of staff turnover. In the only empirical study to use stability of caregivers as a quality indicator, high-quality centers were defined as those in which children had one or two primary caregivers over a year-long period; low-quality centers were defined as those in which children had three or more primary caregivers (Howes and Olenick 1986). Caregiver turnover in child care, which approaches 50% a year in some areas of California (Howes et al. 1986), for example, is an extremely serious matter. The low salaries and nonexistent benefits that most child care workers endure mean that many well-trained and otherwise dedicated caregivers cannot afford to work in child care.

Ratio and group size. Other important indices of quality in center and family day care homes are the adult-child ratio, the size of the group, and the training of the caregiver. All of these state licensing standards are regularly disregarded by child care centers and family day care homes.

Adult-child ratio and the number of children in the group are most closely associated with the quality of the caregiver-child interaction. When there are more than about 3 children per adult caregiver, or where there are more than about 8 to 10 infants and toddlers in a group, the caregivers tend to become managers rather than loving and playful providers (Howes 1983a; Howes and Rubenstein 1985; Ruopp et al. 1979). Children are moved from activity to activity rather than given the individualized attention so needed by infants and toddlers. A quiet and undemanding child may be unnoticed, whereas a reactive or irritable child may become stigmatized as the one who makes things harder for the caregivers.

An aspect of child care quality related to the adult-child ratio and the number of children in the group, yet less often discussed in terms of child care quality, is the number of adults present in the child care arrangement. A series of studies by Rubenstein and Howes (1979; Rubenstein et al. 1982) suggested that a second caregiving adult—another mother or another child care caregiver—reduces the amount of irritability and restrictiveness the adult expresses to the children. Also, a second adult in a child care facility should reduce the chances for child abuse.

Differences in adult-child interaction found in early studies comparing center child care with that in family day care homes probably reflected the dimension of the isolated caregiver. These studies suggested that adult-child interaction in family day care homes was more individualized—in both positive and less positive ways—than adult-child interaction in center care. Family day caregivers were more likely than center caregivers both to interact verbally with and to restrict and reprimand the children in their care; on the other hand, center caregivers tended to engage in more play with the children (Cochran 1977; Golden et al. 1978; Howes and Rubenstein 1985).

California now licenses what are called large family day care homes. These facilities care for up to 12 children and have at least two caregivers. The distinction between family day care homes and center child care arrangements appears to be disappearing. Large family day care homes function much as small day care centers do. One study suggested that adults in large family day care homes may engage in more frequent playful interactions with the children in their care than do adults in small family day care homes (Howes and Stewart 1987).

Training. As noted earlier, the training of center child care workers is regulated by state licensing. Caregivers must have some college training in child development, and a sizable proportion of caregivers have master's degrees (National Association for the Education of Young Children 1985). Despite the increased need for child care providers in the past few years, however, there are fewer child care providers being trained and more trained caregivers leaving the field. The lack of trained staff is now approaching the crisis point, for centers find it increasingly difficult to retain and replace teachers. Family day care providers do not have to have any training in child development to be licensed. The range of training for child care varies greatly by geographic area, and training levels are generally assumed to be low, although this point is difficult to document.

Several research studies have linked the training of the caregiver to the child's experiences within child care. For both center and family child care, formal training in child development is linked to greater social stimulation, responsivity, and cognitive and language stimulation; less adult negative affect; fewer restrictions; and less child apathy (Howes 1983a; Ruopp et al. 1979; Stallings and Porter 1980).

Without training, the caregiver has only his or her own experience of being mothered and, in many cases, of caring for his or her own children. With training, the caregiver can separate developmental issues from individual irritants. For example, the toddler's "No!" can be seen as an expression of autonomy rather than noncompliance. The trained caregiver is also more likely to be objective in dealing with the children's individual differences in temperament and style. Finally, the trained caregiver is likely to have more resources to handle the inevitable tensions that arise in dealing with parental anxieties.

Eleven studies during the 1980s compared child outcomes for children enrolled in high-quality versus low-quality child care settings. Infants, toddlers, and preschoolers appeared more socially and cognitively competent if they had been enrolled in high-quality as opposed to low-quality child care (Anderson et al. 1981; Goelman and Pence 1987; Haskin 1985; Howes 1988; Howes and Olenick 1986; Howes and Stewart 1987; Kontos and Fiene 1986; McCartney 1984; McCartney et al. 1982; Phillips and McCartney 1986; Vandell and Powers 1983). Similar results were reported whether the type of care compared was center care or family day care homes.

The Howes and Olenick (1986) child care study was motivated by a number of earlier studies suggesting that early entry into child care was associated with later aggressive or noncompliant behavior, particularly upon formal school entry (e.g., Haskin 1985; Macrea and Herbert-Jackson 1976; Moore 1975; Rubenstein et al. 1981; Schwartz et al. 1974). In the Howes and Olenick study, researchers compared three samples of families: families with toddlers enrolled in high-quality center care, families with toddlers enrolled in low-quality center care, and families with no child care experience. Families were interviewed regarding child-rearing practices and attitudes; parent-child interaction around compliance and control issues was observed at home; the children enrolled in child care were observed in their centers; and the child and the mother were seen in a laboratory session designed to measure self-regulation and compliance. Children enrolled in high-quality centers were better able to regulate their own behavior than children with no child care experience or children enrolled in low-quality child care. Children enrolled in low-quality centers were more likely to throw tantrums or otherwise resist performing tasks. Therefore, noncompliance and aggression as long-term outcomes of infant and toddler child care appeared to be mediated by the quality of the child care.

Family Characteristics

The Howes and Olenick (1986) study discussed above also illustrates the interaction between family characteristics and quality of child care. Although all families in the study were middle class and all centers had similar tuitions, families whose lives were more stressful were more likely to enroll their children in a low-quality center than in a high-quality center. Families whose lives are stressful may not have the resources to complete the process of finding and selecting high-quality child care. On the other hand, families might have become more stressed without the support of high-quality child care.

Furthermore, families with children enrolled in low-quality child care were observed at home to be less involved and invested in their children's compliance than were families with children in high-quality child care or families with no child care experience. These associations between child care quality, family stress, and child-rearing practices were replicated with a family day care sample (Howes and Stewart 1987). In this study. high-quality family day care was associated with families that reported being in frequent contact with friends and relatives, feeling supported by them, and having nurturing child-rearing attitudes. Low-quality family day care was associated with stress, poor maternal role satisfaction, and restrictive child-rearing attitudes.

In both the center and the family day care home studies, children's behavior could be best predicted and explained by examining both child care quality and family characteristics. Studies of preschool children (e.g., Kontos and Fiene 1986; Phillips et al. 1987a) reported similar associations between child care quality, family characteristics, and the child's optimal development. As a result of these studies, which attempted to examine and integrate family and child care influences on children's development, it has become more complicated to present information on the effects of child care on child development. To assess the influence of infant and toddler care on optimal development, it is also necessary to examine the influence of families on optimal development.

Relations between family and child care are only beginning to be researched and understood. Many questions remain unanswered. For example, the interaction between parents and child care providers has historically been tense (Gipps 1982; Zigler and Turner 1982). Parents may experience the anxieties associated with separation from their child. Child care providers may be ideologically opposed to a woman leaving her children or resentful of the higher pay and more prestigious status of the mother's career. The parents and the child care provider may feel that only they really understand the baby. The infant benefits most from the cooperative and supportive relationship between child care providers and parents. However, the factors influencing a harmonious, as opposed to a tense, caregiver-parent relationship are unknown.

Another area of the family–child care relation in which further research is needed is the potential compensatory or detrimental effects of child care when internal family relations are less than optimal. In California, for example, children at risk for child abuse are eligible for state-supported child care services. These services are justified as a chance for the potentially abusing parent to have time away from the child. What is the effect of child care on the child at risk for abuse? There are at least two plausible hypotheses. One is that the child with an insecure attachment relationship to his or her parents, such as the potentially abused child, may be further stressed by early separation from parents. In this case, infant or toddler child care would have a detrimental influence on optimal development. An alternative prediction is that the very young child with an insecure parental attachment relationship might be able to form an alternative and more secure attachment relationship with a child care provider. This alternative attachment relationship may provide the child with more secure models of self and other than do models derived from the parental attachment. In this case, child care would enhance the child's development. Further research is needed to test these competing hypotheses.

CONCLUSIONS

The influences of early child care on the development of children are complex and multidimensional. Further research is needed to examine the interactions between variations within both child care and families and the multiple interactions between these two major sources of influence. A few conclusions are warranted. First, the age at which the child begins child care and the type of child care arrangement selected are less important than the stability of the child care, the quality of the type of child care arrangement, and the interactions between child care providers and the family. Second, in general, stable child care is associated with optimal child development. In assessing the stability of child care, the number of different child care arrangements experienced by the child and the turnover rate of caregivers must be considered. Third, high-quality child care is also associated with optimal child development. Aspects of high-quality child care include having a sufficient number of adults to care for the children, limiting group size, and training the caregivers adequately. Finally, the development of the child can be understood only by examining family characteristics as well as child care characteristics.

REFERENCES

Ainsworth MDS, Blehar M, Waters E, et al: Patterns of Attachment. Hillsdale, NJ, Erlbaum, 1978

Anderson C, Nagle R, Roberts W, et al: Attachment to substitute caregivers as a function of center quality and caregiver involvement. Child Dev 52:53–81, 1981

Barglow P, Vaughn B, Molitor N: Effects of maternal absence due to employment on the quality of infant-mother attachment in a low-risk sample. Child Dev 58:945–954, 1987

Belsky J: Infant day care: cause for concern? Zero to Three 6:1–7, 1986

Benn R: Factors associated with security of attachment in dual career families. Paper presented to the biennial meeting of the Society for Research in Child Development, Toronto, April 1985

Bretherton I: Attachment theory: retrospect and prospect, in Growing Points in Attachment Theory and Research. Edited by Bretherton I, Waters E. Monographs of the Society for Research in Child Development 50(ser no 209):3–36, 1985

Clarke-Stewart A: Day care: a new context for research and development, in Minnesota Symposium on Child Psychology. Edited by Collins A. Hillsdale, NJ, Erlbaum, 1984, pp 214–253

Clarke-Stewart A: The "effects" of infant day care reconsidered: risks for parents, children, and researchers. Early Childhood Research Quarterly 3:293–318, 1988

Cochran M: A comparison of group day and family child rearing patterns in Sweden. Child Dev 48:702–707, 1977

Colin V: Hierarchies and patterns of infants' attachments to employed mothers and alternative caregivers. Paper presented at the International Conference on Infant Studies, Los Angeles, April 1986

Cummings E: Caregiver stability and daycare. Developmental Psychology 16:31–37, 1980

Gipps C: Nursery nurses and nursery teachers, II: their attitudes toward preschool children and their parent. J Child Psychol Psychiatry 23:255–265, 1982

Goelman H, Pence A: Some aspects of the relationship between family structure and child language development in three types of daycare, in Annual Advances in Applied Developmental Psychology, Vol 3: Continuity and Discontinuity of Experience in Child Care. Edited by Peters D, Kontos S. Norwood, NJ, Ablex, 1987

Golden M, Rosenbluth L, Grossi M, et al: The New York City Infant Day Care Study. New York, Medical and Health Research Association of New York City, 1978

Haskin R: Public school aggression among children with varying day care experiences. Child Dev 56:698–703, 1985

Howes C: Caregiver behavior in center and family day care. Journal of Applied Developmental Psychology 3:99–107, 1983a

Howes C: Patterns of friendship. Child Dev 54:1041–1053, 1983b

Howes C: Social interactions and patterns of friendship in normal and emotionally disturbed children, in Friendships in Normal and Handicapped Children. Edited by Field T. Norwood, NJ, Ablex, 1984, pp 163–186

Howes C: Sharing fantasy: social pretend play in toddlers. Child Dev 56:1253–1258, 1985

Howes C: Social competence with peers in young children: developmental sequences. Developmental Review 7:252–272, 1987a

Howes C: Social competency with peers: contributions from child care. Early Childhood Research Quarterly 2:155–168, 1987b

Howes C: Relationships between early child care and schooling. Developmental Psychology 24:53–57, 1988

Howes C, Espinosa M: The consequences of child abuse for the formation of relationships with peers. International Journal of Child Abuse and Neglect 9:397–404, 1985

Howes C, Olenick M: Family and child care influences on toddler compliance. Child Dev 57:202–216, 1986

Howes C, Rubenstein J: Determinants of toddler's experience in daycare. Child Care Quarterly 14:140–151, 1985

Howes C, Stewart P: Child's play with adults, toys, and peers: an examination of family and child care influences. Developmental Psychology 23:423–430, 1987

Howes C, Whitebook M, Pettygrove W: Variation in the recruitment and retention of qualified staff. Final report to the California Policy Seminar, 1986

Howes C, Rodning C, Galluzzo DC, et al: Attachment and child care: relationships with mother and caregiver. Early Childhood Research Quarterly 3:403–416, 1988

Kontos S, Fiene R: Predictors of quality and children's development in day care, in Predictors of Quality in Day Care. Edited by Phillips D. Washington, DC, National Association for the Education of Young Children, 1986, pp 314–324

Krentz S: Qualitative differences between mother-child and caregiver-child attachments and infants in family day care. Paper presented at the biennial meeting of the Society for Research in Child Development, Detroit, April 1983

Lamb ME, Thompson RA, Gardner W, et al: Infant-Mother Attachment: The Origins and Developmental Significance of Individual Differences in Strange Situation Behavior. Hillsdale, NJ, Erlbaum, 1985

Macrea J, Herbert-Jackson E: Are the behavioral effects of infant daycare program specific? Developmental Psychology 12:269–270, 1976

McCartney K: Effect of quality day care environment on children's language development. Developmental Psychology 20:244–280, 1984

McCartney K, Phillips D: Motherhood and child care, in The Different Faces of Motherhood. Edited by Birns B, Hay D. New York, Plenum, 1988, pp 157–183

McCartney K, Scarr S, Phillips D, et al: Environmental differences among day care centers and their effects on children's levels of intellectual language and social development, in Day Care: Scientific and Social Policy Issues. Edited by Zigler E, Gordon E. Dover, MA, Auburn House, 1982, pp 126–151

Moore T: Exclusive early mothering and its alternatives: the outcomes to adolescence. Scand J Psychol 16:255–272, 1975

National Association for the Education of Young Children: In Whose Hands?: A Demographic Fact Sheet on Child Care Providers. Washington, DC, National Association for the Education of Young Children, 1985

Phillips D, McCartney K: Child care quality: its influence on children's socioemotional development, in Predictors of Quality in Day Care, Edited by Phillips D. Washington, DC, National Association for the Education of Young Children, 1986, pp 287–312

Phillips D. McCartney K, Scarr S: Child-care quality and children's social development. Developmental Psychology 23:537–544, 1987a

Phillips D, McCartney K, Scarr S, et al: Selective review of infant day care research: a cause for concern. Zero to Three 7:18-21, 1987

Richters JE, Zahn-Waxler C: The infant day care controversy in perspective: current status and future directions. Early Childhood Research Quarterly 3:273–282, 1988

Rubenstein J, Howes C: Caregiving and infant behavior in daycare and homes. Developmental Psychology 15:1–24, 1979

Rubenstein J, Howes C, Boyle P: A two year follow up of infants in community based day care. J Child Psychol Psychiatry 22:209–218, 1981

Rubenstein B, Howes C, Pederson F: Second order effects on mother-toddler interaction. Infant Behavior and Development 2:185–194, 1982

Ruopp R, Travers J, Glantz F, et al: Children at the Center: Final Report of the National Daycare Study. Cambridge, MA, ABT Associates, l979

Sagi A, Lamb ME, Lewkowicz K, et al: Security of infant-mother, -father, and -metapelet attachments among Kibbutz-reared Israeli children, in Growing Points in Attachment Theory and Research. Edited by Bretherton I, Waters E. Monographs of the Society for Research in Child Development 50(ser no 209):257–275, 1985

Schwartz C, Strickland R, Krolick G: Infant day care: behavioral effects at preschool age. Developmental Psychology 10:502–610, 1974

Sroufe LA: Infant-caregiver attachment and patterns of adaptation in preschool: the roots of maladaptation and competence, in Minnesota Symposium in Child Psychology, Vol 16. Edited by Perlmutter M. Hillsdale, NJ, Erlbaum, 1983, pp 41–81

Sroufe LA: A developmental perspective on day care. Early Childhood Research Quarterly 3:283–292, 1988

Stallings J, Porter A: National Daycare Home Study. Palo Alto, CA, American Research International, 1980

Suwalsky J, Zaslow M, Klein R, et al: Continuity of substitute care in relation to infant-mother attachment. Paper presented at the annual meeting of the American Psychological Association, Washington, DC, August 1986

Thompson RA: The effects of infant day care through the prism of attachment theory: a critical appraisal. Early Childhood Research Quarterly 3:273–282, 1988

Vandell D, Powers C: Daycare quality and children's free play activities. Am J Orthopsychiatry 53:293–300, 1983

Vaughn B, Gove F, Egeland B: The relationship between out of home care and quality of infant-mother attachment in an economically deprived population. Child Dev 51:1203–1214, 1980

Vaughn B, Deane K, Waters E: The impact of out-of-home care on child-mother attachment quality: another look at some enduring questions, in Growing Points in Attachment Theory and Research. Edited by Bretherton I, Waters E. Monographs of the Society for Research in Child Development 50(ser no 209):110–123, 1985

Zigler E, Turner P: Parents and day care workers: a failed partnership? in Day Care: Scientific and Social Policy Issues. Edited by Zigler E, Gordon E. Dover, MA, Auburn House, 1982, pp 174–182

Chapter 3

Developmental Risks Associated With Infant Day Care: Attachment Insecurity, Noncompliance, and Aggression?

Jay Belsky, Ph.D.

During the 1980s, a dramatic change took place in child-rearing practices in the United States. Although it is not news that most American women are in the labor market and that almost 60% of mothers with children under 6 years of age are working, what is surprising is the rapid growth in the employment of mothers with infants. By 1985, 48% of mothers with infants aged less than 1 year were working, with virtually 75% of them employed full-time (Hofferth and Phillips 1987). Not only does this rate of employment reflect an increase of more than 50% in 10 years, but, as of

Work on this chapter was supported by a grant from the National Institute of Child Health and Human Development (R01-HD-15496) and by an NIMH Research Scientist Development Award (K02-MH-00486).

1987, it had increased still further, to 51.9% (Collins 1987). The change has been so rapid and the recording of such maternal employment figures so recent that when Hofferth and Phillips (1987) projected rates of maternal employment and child care demand through 1995, they had insufficient information to make forecasts about mothers with infants aged less than 1 year.

Systematic scrutiny of rates of maternal employment over the past decades reveals that what has changed is the amount of time mothers remain at home with their young children before reentering the labor market. Whereas fewer than one-third of mothers returned to their jobs before their infants' first birthday in the mid-1970s, today the majority of such mothers do so (Collins 1987). The reasons for this shift in child-rearing arrangements are varied and range from the economic to the ideological to, perhaps, the scientific. At the same time that child development researchers were reporting that adverse consequences did not inevitably arise when young children and even infants were cared for in day care centers—and under some conditions actually thrived in such settings (see Belsky and Steinberg 1978 for a review)—the nation was strapped with an inflation rate that would reach 20% before subsiding in this country's steepest recession since the Great Depression. Whereas in the late 1970s mothers entered the labor force for the additional income necessary to maintain middle-class living standards, by the early 1980s they did so in many cases to make up for the lost earning power of their unemployed and underemployed spouses. By the late 1980s, when the economy had become increasingly service oriented and was in the midst of the longest period of economic expansion in postwar history, business and industry had become so dependent on female labor that women were virtually expected to reenter the labor force soon after bearing a child.

As demand for child care grew, in direct response to these pressures on mothers to work and the coincident ideology of the women's movement, only the most modest response to the increasing demand for affordable child care was observed in both the private and public spheres. While the media were communicating that psychologists had given day care "the green light" and research was revealing that such confidence depended on the provision of quality care (for a review, see Belsky 1984 and Phillips 1988), state and federal child care standards often were not being promulgated, were going unenforced, or were actually being weakened (Martinez 1989). As the interval between childbirth and reemployment lessened, insightful members of the scientific and public policy community awakened to the fact that American parents, unlike their counterparts in virtually all other Western industrialized nations except South Africa, had no protection from job loss if they took more than the briefest maternity leave (Kamerman and Kahn 1978; Zigler and Frank 1988). In fact, in place of a parental leave policy were state-by-state regulations for infant day care that actually sanctioned what in many instances could only be regarded as conditions for child neglect (e.g., staff-child ratios of 1 to 8 [Young and Zigler 1986]).

Infant day care (i.e., extensive nonparental care during the first year of life) needs to be understood in the foregoing context. Although I argue that there is sufficient evidence to regard infant day care in its present forms as a risk factor for the development of insecure infant-parent attachment, noncompliance, and aggression, it does not inherently follow that infant day care is harmful. The research literature provides repeated indications that extensive nonparental care initiated in the first year of life and the maternal employment situation and family ecology associated with such a rearing niche are only probabilistically associated with the aforementioned patterns of behavioral development.

Many, perhaps even most, children growing up in nonparental child care arrangements beginning in their first year are probably not affected by them in any manner that is overwhelmingly apparent to the casual observer or even evident given the current sensitivity of our measurement instruments. Among those who are "affected" to the extent that they contribute to the child-rearing group differences that studies of central tendencies have persistently revealed, it remains unclear exactly where the causes of the differences are to be found. They may emanate from family processes that lead some families to rely on infant day care, or at least day care of varying quality. They may be the result of coping with repeated separations, insensitive caregivers, stressful family experiences, or (more probably) the combination of these and other factors. Because of the limited state of our knowledge, I am unable to say with any confidence what accounts for the differences between children who do and do not experience extensive nonparental care in the first year of life. Fortunately, things are changing, so that soon it should be possible to detail empirically under what conditions, for which children, and via what processes infant day care, broadly defined, poses a risk or an opportunity for the developing child.

Is There a Risk Factor?

In this chapter I consider evidence that suggests, for reasons that are by no means clear, that extensive nonparental care initiated in the first year of life is associated with heightened risk of insecure infant-parent attachment relationships in infancy and elevated levels of noncompliance/disobedience and aggression in the toddler through the elementary school years. I attempt to summarize and extend recent reviews of the research evidence that have generated a great deal of media attention, mostly because of the controversy they have engendered among the community of empirically oriented developmental psychologists (Belsky 1986a, 1986b, 1986c, 1987, 1988; Clarke-Stewart 1988; Phillips et al. 1987b; Richters and Zahn-Waxler 1988; Thompson 1988). Not every study implicates extensive infant day care experience as a correlate of insecurity, noncompliance, or aggression. Yet current research designs offer little insight into whether extensive day care is a cause or merely a correlate of such developmental outcomes or what the factors are that mediate or moderate the relation. At best I will highlight an ecological niche in which a variety of important factors such as reasons for using day care, quality of day care, infant characteristics, and family processes are interrelated. These processes have to be disentangled so that a more precise statement can be made about the conditions under which risk associated with infant day care in some studies is and is not realized.

The reason for our limited state of knowledge is that most investigations of infant day care have been of the between-group rather than the within-group variety; that is, most inquiries have involved comparisons of children with and without infant day care experience rather than variations in the nature and quality of care. This situation contrasts markedly with that concerning day care for older children in which child developmentalists, after carrying out between-group studies, moved on to within-group investigations to identify the conditions under which children thrive in day care—or what I have elsewhere termed "the second wave" of day care research (Belsky 1984).

In view of all that remains unknown and in light of the conditions of maternal employment and infant day care already mentioned (e.g., parental leave, care quality), let me state now what I shall eventually conclude. Although in the research I see evidence for risks associated with infant day care, the data do not lead me to conclude that infant day care is bad for babies or that only mothers can care for babies. This is because the risks that I discern in the research literature can be understood only when considered in light of the ecology of current infant day care. Central to this ecology is the fact that quality care provided in stable arrangements is often beyond the economic means of many families. In addition, parents in general and mothers in particular do not have the freedom to remain at home with their young infants because of concerns of job loss or the option to work part-time during the infant's first year with assurances that they can return to work full-time thereafter. Even though infant day care is a risk factor for the development of insecure infant-parent relationships, noncompliance, and aggression, it will not be appropriate to draw the inference that infant day care causes these problematic behavioral patterns or is bad for babies until the foregoing ecological conditions change or until more refined research is conducted.

To some readers such reasoning may seem illogical, but only if the concept of risk factor is misunderstood. To say that X (i.e., infant day care) is a risk factor for the development of Y (insecure attachment, noncompliance, aggression) does not mean that X causes Y or, especially, that X alone is responsible for the development of Y. Rather, it means that X is probabilistically associated with Y and that, in concert with other sources of risk, the relation between X and Y will be strengthened. This latter point is most important. For example, in the case of the relation between infant day care and insecure infant-parent attachment, it means that although groups of children in a particular study vary in terms of infant day care experience, they do not necessarily differ in attachment security when only child care experience is considered. It may well be the case, as with risk factors for many known behavioral and medical problems, that an empirically discernible relation between the putative risk factor and the problem emerges only in interaction with other risk factors. Thus, the failure of one or another study to discern differences between groups of children—in the face of substantial evidence to the contrary—does not disconfirm the notion that such experience is a risk factor for the development of insecure infant-parent attachments and subsequent aggression and noncompliance. The question to be addressed, then, is whether there is sufficient evidence consistent with the contention that infant day care is probabilistically associated with elevated rates of attachment insecurity, noncompliance, and aggression.

Before initiating my review of the research evidence, I wish to make one final comment, which pertains to the definition of the term "infant day care" as it is used in this chapter. Throughout the preceding paragraphs, the terms "infant day care" and "nonparental care" have been used interchangeably. The reason is that those highly visible day care centers that most people associate with the term "day care" serve only a small minority of those children in the first year of life whose mothers are employed. The large majority (78%) of babies whose parents are employed receive their care in private homes, either their own or that of someone else, and are cared for by relatives, neighbors, or fellow community members (Hofferth and Phillips 1987).

It would be ideal to distinguish types of arrangements when considering the developmental correlates of infant day care, but unfortunately the available evidence does not permit such discrimination. In fact, in many investigations the day care arrangement per se goes unspecified, because all that is known is that as a result of employment, a mother is not providing care for her child during her hours on the job. Even though equating day care and maternal employment during the preschool years is problematic—because many children experience group care even when their mothers are not employed (e.g., nursery school)—this situation is decidedly not the case for infants, except perhaps in rare and unusual circumstances. Thus, it must be recognized that studies of maternal employment in the first year and studies of day care are sampling the same population, even if they are labeled differently.

INFANT DAY CARE AND SOCIOEMOTIONAL DEVELOPMENT

The central focus of the chapter is on socioemotional development, for such development is the arena of psychological functioning that has most interested researchers studying day care, principally because it has led many to be concerned with infant day care (e.g., Fraiberg 1977). In particular, the emotional tie between infant and mother conceptualized in terms of the attachment relationship has figured prominently in most day care research—basically because it has figured so prominently in most writings concerning infant socioemotional development (Ainsworth 1973; Bowlby 1973; Sroufe 1979). The attention devoted to the infant-mother attachment bond in this chapter is not meant to imply a lack of concern for, or interest in, the child's other relationships in and out of the family; rather, it is dictated by its central place in the day care literature and by the belief that a special focus on the infant-mother relationship is ecologically and developmentally appropriate. Not only do most American infants today, whether in day care or not, establish their first attachments with their mothers, but a wealth of empirical data now documents the utility of 12- to 18-month evaluations of the security of the infant-mother attachment relationship in forecasting individual differences in child development during the preschool and early school years (for reviews, see Bretherton 1985, Lamb et al. 1984, and Sroufe 1985).

Earlier it was noted that two waves of day care research can be identified: one involving between-group comparisons, the other within-group analyses. The so-called second wave of research on infant day care, which focuses on variations in care conditions as they relate to developmental outcomes of infants in day care, has been relatively recent (e.g., Howes and Stewart 1987; Howes, Chapter 2, this volume). Consideration of the research that has been undertaken on nonparental care initiated in the first year of life suggests that it may be more accurate to speak of this most recent wave of inquiry as the "third wave" of infant day care research. Whereas the 1980s witnessed a series of between-group investigations of children growing up in families routinely using nonparental care, this work actually followed an earlier wave of inquiry that involved comparisons of children growing up in high-quality, university-based, research-oriented day care centers with age-mates being reared under more traditional conditions. In large measure it was because the first wave of investigation found little evidence of deleterious consequences of such care that research on variation in care in the first year of life was not extensively pursued. Only as a result of findings emerging from studies of infants growing up in nonparental care arrangements more representative of those routinely available to families around the country, which were also of the between-group variety (the second wave), did impetus emerge to initiate within-group investigations of infant day care (the third wave).

First I touch briefly in this chapter on the first wave of university-based investigations, providing a short critique and summary. Then I turn to the second wave of inquiry, which was principally responsible for altering my own opinion of the nature of the evidence pertaining to the developmental correlates of day care. This work involves comparisons of groups of children with and without extensive infant day care experience. Finally, I discuss issues pertaining to the recently initiated third wave of inquiry to underscore unresolved issues and the need to consider the conditions under which risks and benefits are associated with extensive infant day care experience.

THE EARLY STUDIES

With the exception of the very first published study regarding day care and attachment, which used home observation and interview techniques (Caldwell et al. 1970), most of the early investigations of this topic employed experimental, laboratory-based paradigms developed by research scientists for studying normative processes of infant development. As a consequence, particular attention was paid to the degree to which infants became distressed upon separation from mother or following exposure to a strange adult. What was never clear in the initial day care research was whether it was considered developmentally advantageous or problematic for the child to display greater or lesser stranger wariness and/or separation distress. As it turned out, most investigations of infant day care that focused on such affective responses discerned no differences between home-reared and day care–reared infants (Cochran 1977; Hock 1980; Kagan et al. 1976, 1978; Saunders 1972). Nevertheless, several indicated that either day care infants (Cummings 1980; Ricciuti 1974) or home-reared infants (Doyle and Somers 1978) were somewhat more likely to become distressed. Still another indicated that the degree of upset was related in a curvilinear fashion to nonmaternal child care experience (Jacobsen and Wille 1984).

A second procedure focused on children's willingness to move away from their mothers. This research produced more consistent findings indicating that infants and toddlers with early experience in university-affiliated infant centers were more willing to leave their mothers' sides to approach unfamiliar children or a strange adult (Finkelstein and Wilson 1977; Kagan et al. 1976, 1978; Ricciuti 1974). Even though such evidence suggested to the investigators that young children with early care experience were less apprehensive and more ready to engage novel social agents, other interpretations are conceivable (e.g., the infants were less closely attached to their mothers). But the major problem with these or other interpretations, like those concerning variation in stranger wariness and separation protest, is their speculative nature, given that no evidence exists that documents the developmental significance of inclinations to move away from or remain physically close to the mother.

Although Clarke-Stewart (1988) has contested this last point by noting that it is well established that as children grow older they increasingly distance themselves from their parents, a problem arises, in my view, in her developmental reasoning. It does not simply follow that just because a developing agent is normatively more likely to display a behavior pattern at a later point in development than at an earlier point that the earlier emergence of such behavior (i.e., distance from mother) provides evidence of advanced—in the positive sense of the word—development. Consider, for instance, the implications of going through the pubescent growth spurt at age 8 (in third grade) or of a 12-year-old drinking alcohol or driving an automobile. To equate precocity with a developmental advantage in the absence of evidence is illogical and potentially risky.

The issue of the *meaning* of behavior raised by this discussion is one that eventually became central to scientists interested in understanding the characteristics, consequences, and determinants of individual differences in the infant-mother attachment relationship (Masters and Wellman 1974; Waters 1978). In fact, lack of confidence in the validity of any number of potential indices of attachment resulted in a great deal of basic research being carried out, all of which was unconcerned with day care but which nevertheless produced a means of discriminating secure from insecure relationships and, thereby, of enhancing day care research. In the years that followed the publication of the initial day care attachment studies, basic research on infant development revealed that it was not so much crying upon separation or even willingness to approach an unfamiliar other that reliably indexed individual differences in the security of the infant-mother attachment relationship. Rather it was the behavior the infant or toddler directed or failed to direct *to the mother upon reunion following separation* that was significant. Studies by Waters (1978) and others at the University of Minnesota (Matas et al. 1978; Waters and Sroufe 1983) convincingly demonstrated that the behavior of secure infants was characterized by their tendency to greet the mother positively following separation and approach (especially if distressed) and to be comforted by her (when upset by separation). Babies whose relationships were insecure tended to engage in one of two quite different behavior patterns. Those whose relationships were labeled insecure-avoidant actively avoided psychological contact with the mother, moving away from her, aborting approaches to her, or averting gaze so as not to make eye contact with her. On the other hand, those infants whose relationships were labeled insecure-resistant actively resisted contact with the mother by pushing away, even after seeking such contact, and were likely to cry in an angry, petulant manner or angrily push away a toy the mother offered.

Evidence of the validity of these distinctions comes from a large number of follow-up studies, conducted by a variety of investigators across the country, which indicate that infants who avoid and/or resist the mother to such an extent that they can be classified as anxiously attached generally appear less competent as they grow older. Such infants have been found as toddlers and preschoolers to be less empathic, less compliant, and less cooperative, and to exhibit more negative affect and less self-control (e.g., Egeland 1983; Joffee 1981; LaFreniere and Sroufe 1985; Londerville and Main 1981; Main 1973; Main and Weston 1981; Maslin and Bates 1982). These infants have also been found, as 5- and 6-year-olds, to be more at risk for developing behavior problems (for boys only, see Erickson et al. 1985 and Lewis et al. 1984; for failure to replicate, see Bates et al. 1985).

The point here is not that every study indicates that reunion behaviors in the Strange Situation (Ainsworth et al. 1978) and the attachment classifications derived from them discriminate children's subsequent functioning in other settings. Rather, the point is that incontestable patterns are evident in the literature regarding the future functioning of children with secure versus insecure infant attachment relationships. The implication is that the initial day care research concerned with infant-mother attachment was misguided given its focus on infant behaviors that ultimately proved to be insensitive indicators of the affective quality of the attachment bond (i.e., separation distress, stranger wariness, approach to novel social agents).

LATER STUDIES

Since 1980 and the emergence of evidence validating the focus on infant reunion behavior as a "window" on individual differences in the security of the infant-mother attachment bond, a number of studies of maternal employment and infant day care have been reported. These studies have all been of community-based as opposed to university-based nonmaternal care. I restrict myself in this discussion to only those investigations that have relied on formal classifications of attachment security derived from Strange Situation assessments. I do not discuss findings obtained via alternative methodologies, principally because measurements such as parental Q-sorts have not yet been validated and because of space limitations. It would be misleading, however, not to acknowledge that in the few instances in which these potentially unreliable and invalid assessments have been employed they have yet to reveal consistent differences between groups of children with and without infant day care experience (Clarke-Stewart 1988).

Infant Day Care and Attachment Security

In studying a large sample of infants from economically impoverished families, Vaughn and his colleagues (1980) were the first to report an association between routine nonparental care in the first year of life and the security of the infant-mother attachment. In particular, these researchers discovered that infants whose mothers had returned to work in their child's first year, but not thereafter, were significantly more likely to be classified as anxious-avoidant in the Strange Situation. Several features of this investigation merit special attention, for they have inclined some reviewers of the research evidence to make light of this finding (see Hoffman 1983; McCartney and Phillips 1988; Rubenstein 1985). First, these researchers did not discover that infants who began out-of-home care in their first year were more likely to be insecure in their attachments to their mothers; they were only more likely to express their insecurity in an avoidant as opposed to resistant manner. Second, because the sample was economically at risk and the care provided appeared to be of poor quality and unstable in terms of changing arrangements, questions can be raised about the generalizability of the results.

By 1988, five separate investigations had compared groups of children from nonrisk families who relied on a variety of nonparental care arrangements as a result of maternal employment in the first year of life with children from similar families without such care experience (Barglow et al. 1987; Belsky and Rovine 1988; Chase-Lansdale and Owen 1987; Jacobsen and Wille 1984; Owen and Cox 1989). Even though each investigation did not discern a reliable association between infant day care experience/maternal employment and attachment security, a remarkably robust statistical association emerged when the data were compiled for a single aggregate analysis (Belsky and Rovine 1988). Specifically, when the 491 cases studied were combined, the rate of insecurity was 40% among those infants who averaged 20 or more hours per week of nonmaternal care in their first year. The corresponding figure for infants with less care per week or none at all was 26%, a difference reliable at the $P < .0005$ level.

Several features of these investigations are worth noting. First, in at least one study, which itself discerned the association between extensive nonparental care and attachment insecurity, all infants came from affluent homes and were being cared for on a one-to-one basis by nannies—the arrangement presupposed by many to be ideal (Barglow et al. 1987). In a second investigation, it was discovered that among the infants with extensive nonmaternal care experience who were being cared for by their fathers ($n = 7$), 100% of these infants established secure attachments to their mothers (Belsky and Rovine 1988). In fact, when these infants were deleted from the data analysis to determine the rate of insecurity among infants with extensive *nonparental* care rather than *nonmaternal* care, the rate of insecurity climbed from 43% to 49%—a figure virtually identical to that reported by Barglow and his colleagues (1987), whose research design was the only one to explicitly exclude paternal care from consideration. Finally, and perhaps most importantly, when a secondary analysis was conducted using subjects from the single study (Chase-Lansdale and Owen 1987) that failed to reveal a statistically reliable association between infant-mother attachment insecurity and extensive infant day care experience, it was discovered that timing of enrollment in the research process was significant. Among infants whose families were recruited into the research process *prior* to their birth, a far higher rate of insecurity was discerned in the case of those with full-time working mothers than of those infants with full-time working mothers who were recruited at the end of the infants' first year of life (60% versus 17%). In fact, when data on infant-mother and infant-father attachment security were combined and examined as a function of timing of enrollment, the differential rates of insecurity among prenatally and postnatally recruited families with full-time working mothers was remarkably robust ($P < .005$) (Belsky and Rovine 1988).

It is noteworthy that the preceding comparisons were conducted to test a hypothesis advanced by reviewers of the Chase-Lansdale and Owen (1987) manuscript when it was initially submitted for publication. Without even knowing that in the Chase-Lansdale and Owen data set there existed subsamples of families recruited into the research process at different points in time, reviewers expressed puzzlement about why the findings from this study diverged from those of other investigations that involved similar samples (particularly Barglow et al. 1987; Belsky and Rovine 1988). In fact, reviewers were led to wonder whether enrollment timing was indeed significant, because in the latter investigations families had been recruited prenatally into studies of infant and family development, not late in the first year of day care or maternal employment. Can it be, therefore, that enrollment of families into research studies (particularly investigations of day care/maternal employment) late in the first year results in systematically biased samples in which children in day care who have established insecure infant-parent attachment relationships are under-represented? The fact that it apparently can renders quite problematic the interpretation of findings that reveal no differences and derive from studies of families recruited postnatally. The preceding evidence pertaining to father care when mothers work also suggests that research that fails to distinguish nonparental care from nonmaternal care may also underestimate the degree of association between infant day care and attachment insecurity. For these reasons I take issue with Clarke-Stewart's (1989) recent compilation of more than 1,200 cases to examine the relation between infant day care and attachment security, although even in her analysis a statistically robust association emerges that is consistent with the above-mentioned findings.

In the short time since attention was first drawn to the association between extensive nonparental care in the first year and elevated rates of attachment security as measured in the Strange Situation, three additional investigations with research designs that include comparison groups were reported at the 1988 International Conference of Infant Studies in Washington, D.C. In a presentation by Rodning (1988) regarding two of the samples—one of maritally intact, middle-class families rearing healthy babies; the other of economically impoverished, single mothers rearing at-risk premature infants—it was observed that within each sample no association between extensive infant day care experience (i.e., >20 hours per week of maternal employment) and attachment security was discerned. My reanalysis of the data (while I was serving as discussant of the paper) revealed, however, that when the two samples were combined to enhance statistical power, a robust association emerged between any maternal employment (full- or part-time) and increased risk of insecure infant-mother attachment as measured in the Strange Situation (48% versus 26%, $P < .005$) (Belsky 1988).

Although concerns may be raised about combining such different samples for aggregate analysis, the findings of my reanalysis underscore the risk of embracing the null hypothesis (i.e., groups do not differ) when sample sizes are such that statistical power may be too limited to discern a difference if one does exist. This problem is most certain with the third sample, in which comparisons were made between a group of 23 infants with extensive infant day care experience and a group of 23 infants without such experience (O'Connor and Sigman 1988). B. Vaughn (personal communication, August 1987) has noted that with samples of fewer than 150 it is difficult to discern differences even when they do exist, because of the lack of sensitivity of the statistical tests that can be conducted with a variable (e.g., attachment security) that is scored categorically (e.g., secure versus insecure-avoidant vs. secure versus insecure-resistant). In addition, he has noted a lack of sensitivity for such variables (again, for example, attachment security) for which it is normatively expected that two-thirds to three-quarters of a sample will receive classifications of security.

Critiques of Attachment Findings

In recent critiques of my writings highlighting the statistical association between extensive infant day care experience and insecure infant-parent attachment, several issues have been raised about the significance and meaning of the findings. These merit consideration (Clarke-Stewart 1988; Richters and Zahn-Waxler 1988; Thompson 1988). First and foremost is the concern that the association is a function of maternal and/or family processes and may have little to do with nonparental care per se. More specifically, it has been suggested—not unreasonably—that certain parents or families that use extensive nonparental care may be more likely to rear insecure infants irrespective of their utilization of infant day care arrangements. Thus, it is proposed that infants who develop insecure infant-mother relationships when in day care may be likely to do so even if not in day care. Because of the absence of random assignment of children to care conditions in studies of the relation between infant day care and attachment, and because of recent evidence indicating that the quality of care is systematically associated with characteristics of parents and features of families (e.g., Howes and Stewart 1987; Phillips et al. 1987a), this possibility cannot be discounted.

It seems likely, nevertheless, that care experiences can contribute to the development of insecure relationships over and above family processes, or at least in interaction with them. For example, it seems reasonable to speculate that extensive time away from the infant, coupled with time together at the end of the day that is characterized by infant and parent exhaustion and multiple demands on parental time (e.g., baby care, meal preparation), can undermine the parent's capacity to read and respond to the infant's signals in a manner conducive to developing a secure relationship (Ainsworth et al. 1978). For parents who are well resourced psychologically and materially, the likelihood of this eventuality may be lessened, for they may be better able to establish and maintain the kinds of interaction patterns presumed to foster a secure attachment simply because they are less stressed. Indirect support for this hypothesis can be found in several studies indicating that the risk of insecure infant-mother attachments among infants with extensive infant day care experience is particularly pronounced where mothers are not psychologically integrated (Benn 1986), are lacking in sensitivity to the affect of others (Belsky and Rovine 1988), or are overcontrolling of impulses (Barglow and Vaughn 1987).

Also consistent with this line of reasoning are research findings that show that risk of insecurity is elevated among infants with extensive day care experience when marital relations are more troubled and family relations are less cohesive (Ainslie 1987; Belsky and Rovine 1988). Just as a risk factor framework suggests, then, the likelihood of developing insecure attachment relationships becomes more pronounced when multiple risks characterize the family and child care systems.

A second major criticism that has been wielded against my observation and interpretation of the association between extensive infant day care experience and increased risk of insecure infant-parent attachment is based on the supposition that the Strange Situation is experienced differently by infants with and without routine nonparental care experience. Because the elevated rates of insecure attachments found to be associated with extensive nonparental care initiated in the first year are disproportionately a function of insecure-avoidant as opposed to insecure-resistant classifications, the following argument has been advanced. First, infants with multiple separation experiences are less stressed by the Strange Situation. This fact, in concert with the infants' separation experiences, results in infants with extensive day care experience being more independent of their parents and thus maintaining more distance from their mothers in the Strange Situation. Second, this independent behavior is inaccurately appraised as avoidance, which results in misclassification of insecure-avoidant attachment relationships.

Until research is reported documenting the validity of this critique, I remain unconvinced that the problems thought to plague the utilization of the Strange Situation in day care research are as serious as some suggest. First, a large body of data is available that indicates that infants in full-time day care are just as stressed by the Strange Situation (as indexed by their distress on separation from their mother) as are more traditionally reared infants (e.g., Jacobsen and Wille 1984; Kagan et al. 1978; Ricciuti 1974). Second, in a study of infants with varying child care histories, Sroufe and colleagues (1983) found that infants classified as secure behaved in the most instrumentally independent manner as preschoolers, whereas infants classified as insecure-avoidant behaved in a more dependent manner in the preschool classroom. These findings run contrary to a precocious-independence interpretation of avoidance behavior. Finally, recent studies that compared both maternal personality and marital relations with infants in extensive nonparental care who do and do not establish secure attachments to their mothers suggest rather strongly that the Strange Situation accurately measures attachment security in just the group of subjects critics consider it to mismeasure. After all, if utilization of this assessment procedure resulted in the misclassification of such infants, one would not expect to find, as mentioned previously, that infants in day care who are classified as insecure have mothers who are less psychologically integrated (Benn 1986), less interpersonally sensitive (Belsky and Rovine 1988), more overcontrolling of impulses and desires (Barglow and Vaughn 1987), less positive about their marriages (Belsky and Rovine 1988), and in families with less cohesive and more conflicted relationships (Ainslie 1987).

The preceding discussion is not intended to imply that the Strange Situation methodology may not present an equivalent psychological experience for infants with varying rearing histories. As well, it may not result in the erroneous classification of infants with day care experience as insecure, and particularly as insecure-avoidant. Rather, the discussion is intended to convey that there is sufficient evidence at the present time to question seriously such propositions. My concerns do not rest exclusively on findings emanating from studies using the Strange Situation to evaluate attachment security. In fact, it is the attachment data in concert with findings pertaining to the behavioral functioning of older children with infant day care histories that lead me to think about infant day care in risk-factor terms. Either set of data on its own is insufficient, in my opinion, to raise concerns about an issue as sensitive as nonparental care in the first year of life. Only when considered collectively do the data form a pattern that is hard to discount, even when limitations in any finding, study, or set of findings are identified.

THE SOCIAL BEHAVIOR OF DAY CARE INFANTS AT OLDER AGES

Several investigations of the developmental sequelae of insecure attachment in general, and insecure-avoidant attachment in particular, provide evidence that children with such relationship histories (as measured in the Strange Situation) exhibit more behavioral difficulties in the years following infancy than do other children. These children are more noncompliant, aggressive, and socially withdrawn, and evince behavior problems more generally during the toddler through early elementary school years than do age-mates with histories of secure attachment relationships (Erickson et al. 1985; Main and Weston 1982; Maslin and Bates 1982; Sroufe 1983). Although not every investigation of the developmental correlates of attachment security has revealed such disconcerting "consequences" of infant-mother attachment insecurity (Lamb et al. 1985), to my knowledge it has never been shown that infants with secure attachment histories display these behavioral patterns to a significantly greater extent than do their counterparts with insecure relationship histories. Without presuming that such potentially problematic development outcomes are "caused" by early attachment insecurity, or at least are not susceptible to subsequent influence, the evidence seems to take on added meaning. What if these apparent correlates of insecure attachment also emerged as correlates of extensive infant day care experience in studies of older children who vary in terms of their exposure to routine nonparental care in their first year of life? In fact, for almost 15 years research findings have persistently emerged indicating that nonparental care initiated in the first year is associated with many of the same behavior patterns that have been found to be associated with insecure attachment. Specific studies are discussed in the following paragraphs, as are findings inconsistent with this conclusion.

The first longitudinal follow-up of children with extensive infant day care experience, this time in a high-quality, university-based center, revealed such early experience to be associated with disquieting patterns of behavior (Schwarz et al. 1974). Observations made on a group of children following 4 months of experience in a new preschool program indicated that 3- and 4-year-olds from impoverished backgrounds with infant care histories were more aggressive (both physically and verbally) with adults and peers, less cooperative with grown-ups, and more motorically active than a comparison group for whom the preschool represented the first supplementary care experience. An additional difference between groups, significant at the 10% level only, indicated greater tolerance for frustration on the part of home-reared children (as reflected in the ability to accept failure and to be interrupted).

All data did not point in the direction of negative effects of early day care, however, for another observational study of apparently the same sample indicated that the children with prior group rearing were more social with age-mates (Lay and Meyer 1973). Moreover, an unpublished conference presentation assessing the frequencies of behaviors (in contrast to more global ratings) indicated that even though children with infant day care experience spent more time in high-activity areas and less time in focused-task areas, and exhibited more negative behaviors (especially girls) than late-entry children, over time the difference in negative behavior between groups diminished and eventually disappeared (Meyer 1979). In fact, a recent longitudinal follow-up of this sample of children whose families received not only extensive day care support beginning in infancy but also home-based family interventions suggests that this comprehensive service system resulted, over the long term, in boys being significantly less likely to be involved with the juvenile justice system as 13- to 16-year-olds (Lally et al., in press). Although there is reason to be concerned about sample attrition and thus about whether these findings are entirely representative of the children initially enrolled in the study, these results certainly mitigate some of the concerns raised by the preschool findings reported on the entire sample.

In a variety of respects the findings regarding children first enrolled in an experimental infant center at Syracuse University are much like those subsequently reported in the literature. Consider for instance, Rubenstein and Howes's (1983) comparison of a small sample of middle-class, 3½-year-old children who had been enrolled in one of five community-based infant-toddler centers toward the end of their first year with age-mates who had been continuously reared at home by their mothers. Even though groups reared at home and in day care did not differ on the total score derived from Richman and Graham's (1971) behavior problem inventory (which was completed by mothers), a subscale analysis did reveal significant differences on 3 of 12 component ratings: children with infant day care experience were rated as having more fears, being more active (e.g., Schwarz et al. 1974), and throwing more frequent and intense temper tantrums. In fact, observations of children's behavior during a boring task revealed children with infant day care histories to be less compliant with maternal directives than home-reared children (compare to Schwarz et al. 1974 findings of less cooperation with adults). Lest compliance on a boring task be dismissed as an invalid measure—as Clarke-Stewart (1989) has implied—it should be noted that Rubenstein and Howes (1983) found compliance in this situation to be associated with the overall score on the behavior problems checklist. That is, these researchers found that those children who displayed more compliance were rated as having significantly fewer behavior problems. The observational data along with the maternal report data led Rubenstein and Howes (1983, p. 34) to conclude that

> noncompliance in this study reflected a more *anxious or angry* child. It should be emphasized that noncompliance and temper tantrums are more characteristic of two-year-old rather than three-year-old behavior. Thus, we are considering the differences in the day care children to reflect a delay in the negotiation of an age-appropriate developmental issue. At this point it is unclear whether this delay has any significant long term implications. (emphasis added)

That it may have significant long-term effects is suggested by Haskins (1985). This study monitored social behavior of lower-class kindergartners, first graders, and second graders who had been reared on a full-time basis at the Frank Porter Graham Child Development Center, affiliated with the University of North Carolina, throughout their first 4 years of life. Ratings made by school teachers at the end of each school year indicated that children who received center-based care in the first year of life, in contrast to those receiving such care any time thereafter were

> more likely to use the aggressive acts hit, kick, and push than children in the control group. Second, they were more likely to threaten, swear, and argue.

Third, they demonstrated those propensities in several school settings—the playground, the hallway, the lunchroom, and the classroom. Fourth, teachers were more likely to rate these children as having aggressiveness as a serious deficit in social behavior. Fifth, teachers viewed these children as less likely to use such strategies as walking away or discussion to avoid or extract themselves from situations that could lead to aggression. (Haskins 1985, p. 700)

Lest these findings be dismissed as biased teacher reports, it should be noted not only that teachers were likely to rate the children with infant day care experience as more intelligent, but also that observations of their behavior in the classroom by observers blind to rearing conditions revealed them to be more aggressive (L. Feagans, personal communication, April 1986). Like Meyer (1979) in his follow-up study of the more aggressive 3- and 4-year-olds from the Syracuse infant center, Haskins (1985, p. 701), too, discerned a trend suggesting "that the excess aggressiveness of children in the experimental group appears to diminish" across time. Nevertheless, Haskins found that at the end of the second grade, significant differences remained between child care groups on several measures of aggression.

Clarke-Stewart (1989) and others are inclined to attribute the Haskins (1985) findings to the particular curriculum of the center rather than to the first-year, full-time entry into day care because of some evidence that when the preschool curriculum was changed, aggression declined (Finkelstein 1982). At this point it is difficult to be certain whether extensive care initiated in the first year of life or the preschool curriculum—or even the interaction of the two factors—was responsible for heightened aggression. To be noted, however, is the fact that just because the level of aggression decreased with curriculum modification in preschool does not mean the curriculum was solely responsible for the children's aggressiveness. It is possible that there is something about the developmental consequence of extensive care initiated in the first year that makes children susceptible to aggression if the context affords such behavior. Furthermore, there is nothing in the theory of attachment or the risk factor concept to suggest that amelioration with intervention (i.e., curriculum change) is not possible. Indeed, most conceptualizations of risk factors explicitly acknowledge the significance of protective factors for reducing the likelihood that problems associated with specific risk factors will be realized (Belsky 1984; Rutter and Garmezy 1983; Sroufe and Rutter 1984). Finally, it must be noted that even after curriculum change in preschool, the children who began care on a full-time basis early in their first year received higher scores as kindergartners on a teacher-reported measure of "hostility" than did other children (Bryant 1988).

The pattern of differences between children with varying infant care experiences that are evident after the first 2 years of life and generate clear cause for concern, yet appear to dissipate over time, is evident in other studies. Consider the results of the comprehensive testing of a large number of 2-year-olds (aged 24–30 months) on the island of Bermuda. These results enabled Schwarz and his colleagues (1981; Schwarz 1983) to compare the functioning of children with varying child care histories. Those children

> who experienced predominantly center group care in the first two years of life, at two years of age were found to have poorer communication skills than children cared for at home, according to the mothers' own report and ratings by our testers. During the assessment, which occurred in the home, center group care infants were rated by teachers as more apathetic, less attentive, and less socially responsive. They were judged by testers to be more deviant than children cared for at home. (Scwharz 1983, p. 2)

Several features of this study are noteworthy. The first is that these group differences held principally for black children and emerged even after controlling for a host of important background variables (i.e., mother's IQ, parents' education, and occupational prestige). Second, within-group variation in quality and extent of care appeared extremely influential in explaining the differences in the Bermudan sample, for performance was poorest for those children who experienced long hours of care in large groups with more limited staff-child ratios. Finally, and possibly most important, the differences between center-care and home-care children diminished over time, so that by 4 years of age it seemed to be the children reared in family day care homes or by sitters in their third and fourth years of life, rather than those reared in centers in their first 2 years, who performed most problematically (Schwarz 1983).

Although these longer term findings mitigate to some extent the concern raised about center rearing in the first years of life, at least as experienced by most Bermudan infants, another report by this same research group using a larger number of 3- to 5-year-olds rekindled concern. Specifically, McCartney and her colleagues (1982, p. 148), reporting on a sample of some 156 children, found that even though age of entry in center care exerted no apparent effect on intelligence and language development, it did adversely affect emotional development: "Children who began group care in infancy were rated as more maladjusted than those who were cared for by sitters or in family day care homes for the early years and who began center care at later ages." That is, these children were judged by caregivers to be more anxious, aggressive, and hyperactive—patterns of behavior remarkably consistent with those observed by Schwarz and his colleagues (1974), Haskins (1985), and Rubenstein and Howes (1983).

Although it is not clear whether the differences associated with infant care disappeared over time or whether—if they did disappear—they should be regarded as unimportant, it remains the case that not all studies point to their eventual disappearance. Consider a retrospective investigation of some 191 middle-class 9- and 10-year-olds (Barton and Schwarz 1981). Even though teacher ratings did not distinguish between children with varying degrees of out-of-home care prior to kindergarten, peer ratings indicated, even after controlling for both parents' education, that children who entered day care in early infancy to 18 months were viewed as most misbehaving. In addition, children who experienced supplementary care in their first year were "most likely to be labeled troublemakers" (p. 7). Similar results emerged when the variable of interest was "likelihood to cry," with those entering day care on a full- or part-time basis prior to 18 months rated most highly on this behavior. These early day care entrants also appeared susceptible to internalizing behaviors such as withdrawal, for they were most often characterized as loners. In sum, the results of this study indicate that children who entered day care before 1 year of age were characterized by age-mates (when they were 9–10 years old) "as more likely to misbehave ... as more likely to cry when frustrated and more likely to spend time alone than children in other care settings" (Barton and Schwarz 1981, p. 12).

These findings take on special meaning in view of a recent analysis of data collected on middle-class, white children enrolled in seven suburban elementary schools in Dallas, Texas. This study was undertaken to address the ongoing debate about the "effects" of infant day care. In this investigation Vandell and Corasaniti (1988) examined parent, teacher, peer, and self-reports as well as school achievement and conduct grades of 236 third graders who varied in their child care histories. Five types of child care histories were distinguishable on the basis of maternal reports: at home with mother until kindergarten ($n = 37$); began part-time care (<30 hours/week) after the first year ($n = 119$); began part-time care during infancy and continued at this level until public school ($n = 18$); stayed with mother during the first year and began full-time care (>30 hours/week) sometime thereafter ($n = 20$); and began full-time care in the first year ($n = 42$). Results revealed, after controlling for family socioeconomic status and concurrent (i.e., third-grade) afterschool care arrangements, that "extensive child care during the first year was associated with negative outcomes" (p. 22). Children who began full-time care as infants were rated by parents and teachers as being less compliant and having poorer peer relationships than children who began full-time care later. That is, when these children were first graders, the ones who began child care on a full-time basis in infancy also had poorer academic and work habit grades. When compared with all children except those who began full-time care after infancy, those children who began full-time care in infancy also rated themselves less positively, received poorer conduct and academic grades in first through third grades, and received more negative evaluations from peers. Thus, whether one considers information obtained from school records or from teacher, parent, peer, or self-reports, the third graders in the Dallas school district under study who performed among the most poorly were those who began full-time nonmaternal care in their first year of life.

As was the case with respect to the association between infant day care and attachment, not all studies of social development in the postinfancy years discern reliable differences between children with varying infant care experiences. Perhaps most noteworthy in view of the Vandell and Corasaniti (1988) findings are those of a prospective, longitudinal study that followed children from age 1 into second grade. This study discerned virtually no relation between part- and full-time maternal employment initiated in infancy or thereafter on repeated measurements of cognitive functioning, academic achievement, temperament, social competence, and behavioral problems/adjustment (Gottfried et al. 1989). How are we to reconcile such divergent findings?

In general, prospective studies are usually of greater value than retrospective inquiries, if only because of the potential inaccuracy of, in the case of the Vandell and Corasaniti (1988) research, maternal recall of employment history and the child's day care experience. On the other hand, it must be acknowledged that Vandell and Corasaniti (1988) studied third graders in an entire school district rather than a select sample of highly motivated families willing to participate in an extensive 6-year longitudinal study. This issue of sampling seems of particular concern given the earlier reported findings that families that enroll in studies at the end of the infant's first year—as in the Gottfried et al. (1989) inquiry—might be unrepresentative of households in which mothers work full-time, particularly when infant-parent relationships are not developing well. Although there is no way of knowing whether such biased sampling occurred in the Gottfried investigation, its possibility should not be precluded.

It is not just the case, however, that some studies fail to discern differences in compliance and aggression between children with and without extensive day care experience in their first year. In fact, in some research, children with first-year care experiences actually seem more socially skilled or well adjusted. In this regard, consider Ramey and Campbell's (1979) finding that children from their high-quality, university-based center appeared more socially confident during testing throughout the first and second year of life than those without infant care experience (Ramey et al. 1982). Note, however, that in a similar study, Fowler and Khan (1974/1975) discerned no group differences. Another investigation that pointed toward positive effects of infant day care involved a comparison of

2-year-olds using the same rating scales employed by Schwarz and his colleagues (1974), which had shown day care infants to be more aggressive and uncooperative at age 4. In this study of 16 children, it was observed that those who began care in the first year scored higher on ability to get along with others than children whose care began around 2 years of age, and also that these two groups were equivalent with respect to cooperation with adults, aggression, and tolerance of frustration (MaCrae and Herbert-Jackson 1975).

Although MaCrae and Herbert-Jackson (1975) interpreted their findings as a failure to replicate those of Schwarz and his colleagues (1974), an issue can be raised—namely, the fact that all the children in the former investigation were 2 years younger than those participating in the latter study might actually indicate that the differences discerned by Schwarz and his colleagues (1974) may take time to emerge. Certainly Haskins' (1985) findings regarding heightened aggression in the first 3 years of public schooling of children with infant care experience are consistent with this possibility, since Ramey and Campbell (1979) actually found that these eventually more aggressive children seemed more confident when tested at 6, 12, 18, and 24 months of age. Could it be, then, that studying the Schwarz subjects at 2 years of age would have revealed few differences (in fact, it did—see Caldwell et al. 1970), whereas studying the MaCrae and Herbert-Jackson subjects at age 4 would have revealed more pronounced differences between groups? Might there be a need, then, to consider manifest and latent effects?

That there might is suggested by a follow-up study of the same sample of Minnesota children on which an association between insecure-avoidant attachment and nonmaternal care in the first year was first chronicled (Farber and Egeland 1982). This investigation is the only one that has examined infant-mother attachment at the end of the first year with a focus on reunion behavior and also has examined subsequent development—specifically, children's functioning when confronted with a challenging problem. Although Farber and Egeland (1982, p. 120) concluded that for their 2-year-old subjects "the effects of out-of-home care were no longer striking" and that "the cumulative adverse effects of out-of-home care were minimal," careful scrutiny of the data lead a more cautious reader to a different conclusion. Not only did toddlers whose mothers began working prior to their infants' first birthdays display significantly less enthusiasm than children without early experience in day care, but, in addition, these day care–reared infants tended to be less compliant in following their mothers' instructions and less persistent in dealing with a difficult problem, and displayed more negative affect.

A more thorough analysis of these data by Vaughn and his colleagues (1985) revealed, moreover, that although 2-year-olds with insecure attachment histories seemed less competent, irrespective of their infant-care experiences, those with first-year experience in nonmaternal care who had been classified as securely attached to their mothers at 18 months "showed a deterioration in the quality of adaptation over the period from 18–24 months" (p. 133). This deterioration rendered formerly secure children indistinguishable from formerly insecure children. Thus, it was only formerly secure infants without early care experience who displayed the competencies that might be expected on the basis of their histories of secure attachment relationships. When considered in developmental perspective, these data raise the possibility that one consequence of early care may be heightened vulnerability to subsequent stress, irrespective of early attachment history.

More than anything else, these data highlight the need to look for subtle and complex effects of nonmaternal care initiated in the first year. They also underscore the need to think developmentally about enduring effects. We have seen on several occasions that potentially deleterious consequences of early care may dissipate over time; in the reanalysis of the Farber and Egeland (1982) data we see that potential "sleeper effects" may emerge even for children who initially seem to be developing well. Not only must we consider, then, those nonmaternal care experiences that intervene between early day care and follow-up assessments of the "effects" of such care, but also exactly which assessments are made at what time. Can it be that the diminishing of some effects reflects the fact that some assessments used at one developmental period are inappropriate at a later time, rather than a true disappearance? Or can it be that even when manifest effects disappear, latent vulnerabilities remain?

CONCLUSIONS

Open-minded consideration of all the research evidence summarized in this chapter indicates that a variety of behavioral patterns—which, when collectively considered, would seem to be a source of concern—have all too persistently been found to be associated with extensive nonparental care initiated in the first year of life. Evidence seems to support the conclusion that, on average, extensive nonparental care initiated in the first year is a risk factor for developments such as insecure attachment to the mother, noncompliance, aggressiveness, and possibly withdrawn behavior. Nevertheless, by no means has every investigation that has focused on day care experience in the first year revealed such findings.

To conclude that such early child care experience is a risk factor does not mean—nor should it be read to imply—that each child with such a rearing history will develop an insecure attachment relationship or be disobedient and aggressive. Nor does it mean that infant day care experience is the necessary or sole cause of these patterns of behavior. Rather, it means that extensive nonparental care initiated in the first year is, to a statistically significant extent, probabilistically associated with insecure attachment, aggression, and noncompliance. What remains strikingly unclear at present are the reasons why the associations discerned in this review emerge so persistently in the research literature. One theoretically plausible account is that the separations invariably involved in routine nonparental care foster doubt and mistrust in the developing infant about the emotional and physical availability of the mother, resulting in an insecure attachment relationship. Such insecurity may be responsible for subsequent noncompliance and aggression, perhaps because the child is less susceptible to socialization by adult standards. Conceivably, too, these later developments emerge because the insecure-avoidant characteristics that the children are most likely to manifest as infants reflect a deep-seated anger and hostility that is expressed with age-mates and nonparental adults.

It must be acknowledged, however, that only a single investigation (Vaughn et al. 1985) has measured attachment security in infancy and subsequent socioemotional functioning with day care–reared infants, and in that study aggression and noncompliance were not the principal foci because of the youthfulness of the children at the point of longitudinal follow-up. In addition, a wide variety of explanations for the assembled evidence is possible. Consider, for example, the prospect that the data actually reflect a process of self-selection into infant day care, whereby families predisposed to rear insecure, noncompliant, or aggressive children are most likely to utilize nonparental care arrangements on a full-time basis beginning in the infant's first year of life. Indeed, it might well be that children from such families would display the behavior patterns under consideration even if they were home in the care of their parents on a full-time basis.

Another alternative to be considered, attractive especially to proponents of quality day care (e.g., Phillips et al. 1987b), is that it is not the timing of entry into or the extent of nonparental care that carries the risk, but rather the quality of day care that the child (and family) experiences. In considering this explanation, the issue of self-selection must once again be acknowledged, for evidence clearly indicates that quality of care is by no means "randomly assigned"; that is, families with the greatest economic and psychological resources usually obtain higher quality care (Howes and Olenick 1986; Phillips et al. 1987a). Thus, to the extent that quality of care is implicated as mediating the relation between extensive infant day care and insecurity, noncompliance, and aggression, the prospect must be entertained that family factors rather than child care processes are actually responsible for any discerned empirical associations.

My own suspicion is that the final explanation will involve both child care and family processes. It seems quite reasonable to speculate that the process of separation and the time parents spend apart from the infant may undermine their capacity to get to know and understand the child as well as they might otherwise. As a result, the sensitive, responsive patterns of parent-infant interaction considered to foster attachment security may be less likely to take place between parent and infant. This scenario seems particularly reasonable if the time that full-time working parents spend with their infant is at the end of the day when they (and the infant) are tired and many household and, perhaps, occupational tasks compete for their time and attention. With interactional patterns not as well synchronized and relationships not as well established as they may otherwise be, families with infants in day care on a full-time basis beginning in the first year may enter the so-called terrible twos with both parent and child less skilled in relating to one another. In consequence, power struggles over issues of autonomy and compliance may be exacerbated, and conceivably it may be such family processes, affected as they are by early day care experience, that may be responsible for the noncompliance and aggression discerned at older ages, rather than events going on in day care per se.

What should be most apparent in light of the preceding discussion is that even though evidence links extensive early infant day care with what I regard as disconcerting patterns of behavior—particularly when it is recognized that more than 50% of mothers of infants under 1 year of age are employed—it is by no means clear why these links obtain. The empirical testing of the explanations represents the research agenda of the next wave of day care research. Like many others (Clarke-Stewart 1988; Hoffman 1983; Phillips et al. 1987b; Richters and Zahn-Waxler 1988; Thompson 1988), I believe that a multiplicity of factors must be considered to explain fully when risks (and benefits) ensue. Unlike critics of my analysis, however, I suspect that first-year entry and extent of care will be included in this list of factors.

The most recent evidence consistent with this viewpoint emerges from a longitudinal follow-up of children with varying quality of day care experience in their second and third years of life. Even though Howes (1990) discovered that quality of toddler care was an indisputably better predictor of toddler, preschooler, and kindergartner functioning than age of entry into day care, rather consistently the evidence also indicated that it was children in poorer quality care in the toddler years whose full-time nonparental care was initiated in the first year who were developing most poorly. In other words, there was an interaction between quality of care and age of entry into care, just as a risk-factor model would suggest (i.e., risk increases as risk factors increase).

That the effects of poor-quality care were most notable among the children who began care in their first year suggests not only that babies may be particularly vulnerable to nonparental care that is not of high quality, but also that first-year care should not be regarded as inherently risky. In other words, it is inappropriate to conclude that only mothers can care for babies or that infant day care is inherently bad. Perhaps the most convincing evidence on this point comes from a recent longitudinal investigation of Swedish children with varying day care experience. Andersson (1989) found that 8-year-olds who began day care in their first year were, in some respects, more competent than age-mates whose care began thereafter. What must be acknowledged, of course, is that the ecology of day care in Sweden contrasts markedly to the ecology of day care in the United States. Not only are Swedish parents given paid leaves (now up to a year) so that they can remain at home with their infants while their jobs are protected, but Swedish child care providers also receive extensive, government-supported training and work in centers that are very well equipped and funded by American standards.

When I conclude, then, that infant day care is a risk factor, it must be recognized that I am speaking of the state of care as it is routinely available in the United States today and the circumstances surrounding parental utilization of these arrangements. Not only do we not know why insecurity, aggression, and noncompliance turn up with such frequency as correlates of extensive nonparental care initiated in the first year, but we also do not know whether if circumstances in this country were different, the correlates of infant day care would also be different. The Swedish data suggest rather strongly that they would. For this reason I draw three policy-relevant conclusions from my reading of the empirical evidence. First, parents need the option to remain at home with their infants for, at the very least, the first several months of the child's life without fear of job loss. Second, parents need the option to work on a part-time basis in the infant's first year with assurances that their jobs will revert to full-time thereafter. Finally, in the absence of either of these options, and given the economic conditions of some families even if these options were available, parents need affordable, high-quality care for their infants and toddlers.

REFERENCES

Ainslie R: The social ecology of day care children with secure and insecure maternal attachment. Paper presented at the annual meeting of the American Psychological Association. New York, August 1987

Ainsworth MDS: The development of infant-mother attachment, in Review of Child Development Research, Vol 3. Edited by Caldwell BM, Ricciuti HN. Chicago, IL, University of Chicago Press, 1973, pp 1–94

Ainsworth MDS, Blehar M, Waters E, et al: Patterns of Attachment. Hillsdale, NJ, Erlbaum, 1978

Andersson B: Effects of public day care: a longitudinal study. Child Dev 60:857–866, 1989

Barglow P, Vaughn B: Psychological and demographic variables associated with attachment security for infants of working mothers. Paper presented at the annual meeting of the American Psychological Association, New York, August 1987

Barglow P, Vaughn B, Molitor N: Effects of maternal absence due to employment on the quality of infant-mother attachment in a low-risk sample. Child Dev 58:945–954, 1987

Barton M, Schwarz J: Day care in the middle class: effects in elementary school. Paper presented at the annual meeting of the American Psychological Association, Los Angeles, August 1981

Bates J, Maslin C, Frankel K: Attachment security, mother-child interaction, and temperament as predictors of behavior problem ratings at age three years, in Growing Points in Attachment Theory and Research. Edited by Bretherton I, Waters E. Monographs of the Society for Research in Child Development 50 (ser no 209):167–193, 1985

Belsky J: The determinants of parenting: a process model. Child Dev 55:83–96, 1984

Belsky J: Infant day care: a cause for concern? Zero to Three 6:1–7, 1986a

Belsky J: Infant day care: a continuing cause for concern. Paper presented at the International Conference on Infant Studies, Washington, DC, April 1986b

Belsky J: Two waves of day care research: developmental effects and conditions of quality, in The Child and the Day Care Setting. Edited by Ainslie R. New York, Praeger, 1986c

Belsky J: Risks remain. Zero to Three 7:22–24, 1987

Belsky J: The "effects" of infant day care reconsidered. Early Childhood Research Quarterly 3:235–273, 1988

Belsky J, Rovine M: Nonmaternal care in the first year of life and infant-parent attachment security. Child Dev 59:157–167, 1988

Belsky J, Steinberg LD: The effects of day care: a critical review. Child Dev 49:929–949, 1978

Benn R: Factors promoting secure attachment relationships between employed mothers and their sons. Child Dev 57:1224–1231, 1986

Bowlby J: Attachment and Loss, Vol 2: Separation. New York, Basic Books, 1973

Bretherton I: Attachment theory: retrospect and prospect, in Growing Points in Attachment Theory and Research. Edited by Bretherton I, Waters E. Monographs of the Society for Research in Child Development 50 (ser no 209):3–36, 1985

Bryant D: Comments to workshop on the policy implications of child care. Panel on Child Care Policy, Committee on Child Development Research and Public Policy, National Academy of Sciences, Washington, DC, 1988

Caldwell BM, Wright CM, Honig AS, et al: Infant care and attachment. Am J Orthopsychiatry 40:397–412, 1970

Chase-Lansdale L, Owen MT: Maternal employment in a family context: effects on infant-mother and infant-father attachments. Child Dev 58:1505–1512, 1987

Clarke-Stewart KA: The "effects" of infant day care reconsidered: risks for parents, children, and researchers. Early Childhood Research Quarterly 3:293–318, 1988

Clarke-Stewart KA: Infant day care: maligned or malignant? Am Psychol 44:266–273, 1989

Cochran M: A comparison of group day and family childrearing patterns in Sweden. Child Dev 48:702–707, 1977

Collins G: Day care for infants: debate turns to long term effects. New York Times, Nov 25, 1987, sec 1

Cummings EM: Caregiver stability and day care. Developmental Psychology 16:31–37, 1980

Doyle A, Somers K: The effects of group and family day care on infant attachment behaviors. Canadian Journal of Behavioral Science 10:38–45, 1978

Egeland B: Comments on Kopp, Krakow, and Vaughn's chapter, in Minnesota Symposium in Child Psychology, Vol 16. Edited by Perlmutter M. Hillsdale, NJ, Erlbaum, 1983

Erickson M, Sroufe A, Egeland B: The relationship between quality of attachment and behavior problems in preschool in a high-risk sample, in Growing Points in Attachment Theory and Research. Edited by Bretherton I, Waters E. Monographs of the Society for Research in Child Development 50(ser no 209):147–166

Farber EA, Egeland B: Developmental consequences of out-of-home care for infants in a low income population, in Day Care: Scientific and Social Policy Issues. Edited by Zigler E, Gordon E. Dover, MA, Auburn House, 1982, pp 102–125

Finkelstein N: Aggression: is it stimulated by day care? Young Children 37:3–12, 1982

Finkelstein N, Wilson K: The influence of day care on social behaviors towards peers and adults. Paper presented at the biennial meeting of the Society for Research in Child Development, New Orleans, April 1977

Fowler W, Khan N: The development of a prototype infant and child day care center in metropolitan Toronto, Ontario. Ontario Institute for Studies in Education, Year III Progress Report, December 1974; Year IV Progress Report, 1974/1975

Fraiberg S: Every Child's Birthright: In Defense of Mothering. New York, Basic Books, 1977

Gottfried AE, Gottfried AW, Bathhurst K: Maternal employment, family environment, and children's development: infancy through the school years, in Maternal Employment and Children's Development: Longitudinal Research. Edited by Gottfried AE, Gottfried AW. New York, Plenum, 1989

Haskins R: Public school aggression among children with varying day-care experience. Child Dev 56:689–703, 1985

Hock E: Working and nonworking mothers and their infants: a comparative study of maternal caregiving characteristics and infant social behavior. Merrill-Palmer Quarterly 26:79–101, 1980

Hofferth S, Phillips D: Child care in the United States, 1970–1995. Journal of Marriage and the Family 49:559–571, 1987

Hoffman L: Maternal employment and the young child, in Minnesota Symposium on Child Psychiatry, Vol 16. Edited by Perlmutter M. Hillsdale, NJ, Erlbaum, 1983, pp 101–127

Howes C: Can the age of entry and the quality of infant child care predict behaviors in kindergarten? Developmental Psychology 26:292–303, 1990

Howes C, Olenick M: Family and child care influences on toddler's compliance. Child Dev 59:202–216, 1986

Howes C, Stewart P: Children's play with adults and peers: an examination of family and child care influences. Developmental Psychology 23:423–430, 1987

Jacobsen J, Wille D: Influence of attachment and separation experience on separation distress at 18 months. Developmental Psychology 20:477–484, 1984

Joffee L: The quality of mother-infant attachment and its relationship to compliance with maternal commands and prohibitions. Paper presented at the biennial meeting of the Society for Research in Child Development, Boston, MA, April 1981

Kagan J, Kearsley R, Zelazo P: The effects of infant day care on psychological development. Paper presented at the annual meeting of the American Association for the Advancement of Science, Boston, MA, May 1976

Kagan J, Kearsley R, Zelazo P: Infancy: Its Place in Human Development. Cambridge, MA, Harvard University Press, 1978

Kamerman S, Kahn A: Family Policy: Government and Families in 14 Countries. New York, Columbia University Press, 1978

LaFreniere P, Sroufe LA: Profiles of peer competence in the preschool: interrelations between measures, influence of social ecology and relation to attachment history. Developmental Psychology 21:56–68, 1985

Lally J, Margione P, Honig A: The Syracuse University family development research program: long-range impact of early intervention with low-income children and their families, in Parent Education in Early Childhood Intervention. Edited by Powell D. Hillsdale, NJ, Erlbaum (in press)

Lamb ME, Thompson RA, Gardner W, et al: Security of infantile attachment as assessed in the "Strange Situation": its study and biological interpretation. Behavioral and Brain Sciences 7:127–147, 1984

Lamb ME, Thompson RA, Gardner W, et al: Infant-Mother Attachment: The Origins and Developmental Significance of Individual Differences in Strange Situation Behavior. Hillsdale, NJ, Erlbaum, 1985

Lay M, Meyer W: Teacher/Child Behaviors in an Open Environment Day Care Program. Syracuse, NY, Syracuse University Children's Center, 1973

Lewis M, Feiring C, McGuffog C, et al: Predicting psychopathology in six-year-olds from early social relations. Child Dev 55:123–136, 1984

Londerville S, Main M: Security, compliance, and maternal training methods in the second year of life. Developmental Psychology 17:289–299, 1981

MaCrae JW, Herbert-Jackson E: Are behavioral effects of infant day care programs specific? Developmental Psychology 12:269–270, 1975

Main M: Play, exploration, and competence as related to child-adult attachment. Unpublished doctoral dissertation, Johns Hopkins University, Baltimore, MD, 1973

Main M, Weston DR: The quality of the toddler's relationship to mother and to father: related to conflict behavior and the readiness to establish new relationships. Child Dev 52:932–940, 1981

Main M, Weston DR: Avoidance of the attachment figure in infancy: description and interpretation, in The Place of Attachment in Human Behavior. Edited by Parkes C, Stevenson-Hinde J. New York, Basic Books, 1982

Martinez S: Child care and federal policy, in Caring for Children. Edited by Lande J, Scarr S. Hillsdale, NJ, Erlbaum, 1989, pp 111–124

Maslin L, Bates J: Anxious attachment as a predictor of disharmony in the mother-toddler relationship. Paper presented at the International Conference on Infant Studies, Austin, TX, April 1982

Masters J, Wellman H: Human infant attachment: a procedural critique. Psychol Bull 81:218–237, 1974

Matas L, Arend RA, Sroufe LA: Continuity of adaptation in the second year: the relationship between quality of attachment and later competence. Child Dev 49:547–556, 1978

McCartney K, Phillips D: Motherhood and child care, in The Different Faces of Motherhood. Edited by Birns B, Hay D. New York, Plenum, 1988, pp 157–183

McCartney K, Scarr S, Phillips D, et al: Environmental differences among day care centers and their effects on children's development, in Day Care: Scientific and Social Policy Issues. Edited by Zigler E, Gordon E. Dover, MA, Auburn House, 1982, pp 126–151

Meyer W: Developmental effects of infant day care: an empirical study. Paper presented at the annual meeting of the American Educational Research Association, San Francisco, CA, April 1979

O'Connor S, Sigman M: Maternal work status in relation to infant-mother attachment. Paper presented at the International Conference on Infant Studies, Washington, DC, April 1988

Owen M, Cox M: Maternal employment and the transition to parenthood, in Maternal Employment and Children's Development: Longitudinal Studies. Edited by Gottfried AE, Gottfried AW. New York, Plenum, 1989

Phillips D: Quality in Child Care: What Does Research Tell Us? Washington, DC, National Association for the Education of Young Children, 1988

Phillips D, McCartney D, Scarr S: The effect of quality of day care environment upon children's social and emotional development. Developmental Psychology 23:537–543, 1987a

Phillips D, McCartney D, Scarr S, et al: Selective review of infant day care research: a cause for concern. Zero to Three 7:18–21, 1987b

Ramey C, Campbell FA: Contemporary education for disadvantaged children. School Review 87:171–189, 1979

Ramey C, McPhee D, Yeates K: Preventing developmental retardation: a general systems model, in Facilitating Infant and Early Childhood Development. Edited by Bond L, Joffee J. Primary Prevention of Psychopathology, Vol 6. Hanover, NH, University Press of New England, 1982

Ricciuti HN: Fear and the development of social attachments in the first year of life, in The Origins of Fear. Edited by Lewis M, Rosenblum LA. New York, John Wiley, 1974, pp 73–106

Richman N, Graham P: A behavioral screening questionnaire for use with three year old children. J Child Psychol Psychiatry 12:5–33, 1971

Richters J, Zahn-Waxler C: The infant day care controversy in perspective: current status and future directions. Childhood Research Quarterly 3:319–336, 1988

Rodning C: Part-time working mothers: a closer look. Paper presented at the International Conference on Infant Studies, Washington, DC, 1988

Rubenstein J: The effects of maternal employment on young children. Applied Developmental Psychology 2:99–128, April 1985

Rubenstein J, Howes C: Adaptation to toddler day care, in Advances in Early Education and Day Care. Edited by Kilmer S. Greenwich, CT, JAI Press, 1983, pp 39–62

Rutter M, Garmezy N: Developmental psychopathology, in Handbook of Child Psychology, Vol 4: Socialization, Personality, and Social Development. Edited by Hetherington EM. New York, John Wiley, 1983, pp 775–912

Saunders M: Some aspects of the effects of day care on infants' emotional and personality development. Unpublished doctoral dissertation, Chapel Hill, NC, University of North Carolina, 1972

Schwarz JC: Effects of group day care in the first two years. Paper presented at the biennial meeting of the Society for Research in Child Development, Detroit, MI, April 1983

Schwarz JC, Strickland RG, Krolick G: Infant day care: behavioral effects at preschool age. Developmental Psychology 10:502–506, 1974

Schwarz JC, Scarr S, Caparulo B, et al: Center, sitter. and home day care before age two: a report on the first Bermuda Infant Care Study. Paper presented at the annual meeting of the American Psychological Association. Los Angeles, August 1981

Sroufe LA: The coherence of individual development. Am Psychol 34:834–841, 1979

Sroufe LA: Infant-caregiver attachment and patterns of adaptation in preschool: the roots of maladaption and competence, in Minnesota Symposium in Child Psychology, Vol 16. Edited by Perlmutter M. Hillsdale, NJ, Erlbaum, 1983, pp 41–83

Sroufe LA: Attachment classification from the perspective of infant-caregiver relationships and infant temperament. Child Dev 56:1–14, 1985

Sroufe LA, Rutter M: The domain of developmental psychopathology. Child Dev 55:17–29, 1984

Sroufe LA, Fox N, Pancake V: Attachment and dependency in developmental perspective. Child Dev 54:1615–1627, 1983

Thompson R: The effects of infant day care through the prism of attachment theory: a critical appraisal. Early Childhood Research Quarterly 3:273–282, 1988

Vandell D, Corasaniti M: Variations in early child care: do they predict subsequent social, emotional and cognitive development? Paper presented at the International Conference on Infant Studies, Washington, DC, April 1988

Vaughn B, Gove FL, Egeland B: The relationship between out-of-home care and the quality of infant-mother attachment in an economically disadvantaged population. Child Dev 51:971–975, 1980

Vaughn B, Deane K, Waters E: The impact of out-of-home care on child-mother attachment quality: another look at some enduring questions, in Growing Points in Attachment Theory and Research. Edited by Bretherton I, Waters E. Monographs for Research in Child Development 50(ser no 209):110–135, 1985

Waters E: The reliability and stability of individual differences in infant-mother attachment. Child Dev 49:483–494, 1978

Waters E, Sroufe LA: Social competence as a developmental construct. Developmental Review 3:79–87, 1983

Young K, Zigler E: Infant and toddler day care: regulations and policy implications. Am J Orthopsychiatry 56:43–55, 1986

Zigler E, Frank M: The Parental Leave Crisis: Toward a National Policy. New Haven, CT, Yale University Press, 1988

Chapter 4

Early Day Care From an Infant Mental Health Perspective

Alicia F. Lieberman, Ph.D.

Clinical assessments of the effects of day care have clearly been influenced by the changing understanding of infant development. A similar trend can be discerned in the recent research on day care in infancy. The debate among researchers centers primarily on the correct interpretation of research findings that infants placed in day care tend, as a group, to show a higher incidence of behaviors suggesting anxious attachment to the mother than does a comparison group. Some interpret these findings as an alarming early indication of possible harm to the child's mental health. Others point to methodological flaws in the research, call attention to other studies showing positive developmental correlates of early day care, and question the meaning attributed to the behaviors in question (for contrasting reviews of the data, see Belsky 1986; Phillips et al. 1987; Thompson 1987). It is worth highlighting, in this context, that in the 1970s the concern was over the possible deleterious effects of day care for 3-year-olds (e.g., Blehar 1974; Caldwell et al. 1970). Currently, the focus has shifted primarily to day care beginning before 2 years of age (see Belsky, Chapter 3; Howes, Chapter 2, this volume), reflecting the growing scientific interest in the first year of life and in toddlerhood.

Perhaps the most striking feature of the recurrent controversy over the effects of day care is the emotional intensity with which divergent views are held. Given that implicit in one's position on day care are one's values about mothering, the intensity of the controversy is hardly surprising, but it is seldom addressed directly. The question being asked is often not whether day care is good or bad, but whether a mother who places her child in day care is good or bad (Rossi 1968). The possible answers have emotional implications for everybody—not only for the populations studied, but also for the very clinicians, researchers, sociologists, historians, and politicians searching for answers.

The United States is no longer a traditional society in which change is slow and gradual and child-rearing practices can be passed on from one generation to the next without need for revision. On the contrary, immigration, industrialization, and changing family patterns have created a rapidly changing society in which the demands of the marketplace often place the needs of parents and children in direct conflict. The traditional middle-class model of a mother who stays home with her children is still upheld by many as the desirable norm, but increasing numbers of people are unable or unwilling to follow this model and are searching for socially sanctioned alternatives such as day care.

In this climate, there are no solutions without conflict because there is no social consensus regarding the validity of each individual choice. The emotionality of the debate on day care is fueled by the fact that those who study its effects are not immune from having to make real-life decisions that involve difficult compromises among compelling priorities. Each of us hears the echo of the phantom question: Have I done well by my child? This unavoidable personal correlate does not permit a completely unbiased appraisal of the relationship between day care and infant mental health. The reflections that follow are presented with this caveat in mind.

DAY CARE AND INFANT MENTAL HEALTH

In the controversy over the effects of day care there is a tendency to overlook the fact that day care attendance is not in itself a psychological variable. Day care is a multiform activity that may carry very different psychological implications depending on the individual child's developmental status, temperament, and personality, his or her previous experience with separation, the quality of the parent-child relationship, the meaning of day care for parents and how this meaning is conveyed to and perceived by the child, the quality of the caregiver-child relationship, the opportunities for developmentally appropriate play and exploration, the continuity between home care and day care, and a host of other variables. From a clinical perspective, the child's subjective experience in the context of these factors is paramount to understanding the mental health implications of day care attendance. In contrast, research on group findings, although of interest in pointing to general trends, is of necessity insensitive to the individual differences that, to the clinician, represent the very essence of the issue at hand.

Models of the Infant's Experience

Although the child's subjective experience is pivotal, we are hampered by the fact that we have only indirect access to it. In this context, Stern (1985) argued that two models are necessary to understand the development of the infant's sense of self: the "observed infant" and the "clinical infant." The observed infant is the picture that emerges from the naturalistic observations and research findings yielded by developmental psychology. The clinical infant, in contrast, is the joint creation of a patient remembering his or her past and a therapist with a theory about infant experience. This infant is reconstructed on the basis of the patient's memories and of the therapist's theoretically based interpretations. In Stern's view, both approaches are indispensable: "The clinical infant breathes subjective life into the observed infant, while the observed infant points toward the general theories upon which one can build the informed subjective life of the clinical infant" (p. 14).

This approach can be useful for addressing the child's day care experience. Different conceptions of this experience emerge depending on the model of the infant one derives from the wealth of clinical data and research findings. Two general models seem to be prevalent. One model highlights the centrality of the experience of separation anxiety and object loss; the second emphasizes the infant's adaptiveness in self-regulation and social interactions.

An anxiety-based model. The first model has its historical origins in Freud's (1926/1971, p. 166) clinical discussion of anxiety and his postulation that the ultimate danger situation is a "recognized, remembered, expected situation of helplessness." This situation is associated with the mother's absence because she is perceived, through experience, to be the person who satisfies all the child's needs. Anxiety is the child's response to the danger of losing the love object, whereas pain or mourning (grief) is the response to the actual loss. When faced with such experiences, the child mobilizes psychological processes (defenses) to cope with anxiety and pain.

The most influential current elaborations on Freud's theory of anxiety are the work on separation-individuation (Mahler et al. 1975) and attachment theory (Ainsworth 1969; Ainsworth et al. 1978; Bowlby 1969, 1973). Although quite different in their description of the developmental process, the two theories share an emphasis on the primacy of the mother-child unit as the cornerstone of the child's object relations and sense of self, on the psychological centrality of anxiety in shaping the child's development, and on the pathogenic effects of premature separations.

For Mahler and her colleagues (1975, p. 3), the normal separation-individuation process involves the "child's achievement of separate functioning in the presence of, and with the emotional availability of the mother." Every step of the maturational process is seen as presenting the child with situations that entail minimal threats of object loss that must be negotiated and mastered. These developmentally appropriate challenges occur in the context of the child's readiness for independent functioning and consequent pleasure in it. The mother's phase-appropriate sensitivity in being supportively available but not overprotective is seen as the necessary matrix for the child's successful completion of the separation process and the full attainment of individuality. Deviations in this optimal availability, whether through longer separations than considered appropriate for the child's developmental phase or through deficiencies in the mother's responsiveness, are conducive to concomitant disturbances in the developmental process.

In attachment theory, the intense bond between a mother and child is seen as mediated by behaviors that promote proximity and contact, and this bond is postulated to serve a specific biological function—that of protection from predators. The protection from physical dangers has psychological correlates as well: "The knowledge that an attachment figure is available and responsive provides a strong and pervasive feeling of security" (Bowlby 1982, p. 668). In contrast, the knowledge that the attachment figure is not available triggers strong anxiety and distress as well as intense efforts to restore proximity and contact. Separation reactions were seen by Bowlby (1969, 1973) as adaptive responses that evolve to forestall the increased risk to survival posed by a child's separation from the mother.

Bowlby (1973) was in basic agreement with Freud's view that anxiety is a response to the danger of losing the love object, grief and mourning are the responses to the actual loss, and defenses are the psychological mechanisms employed to cope with anxiety and pain. The different models of motivation held by psychoanalytic theory and by attachment theory, however, lead to divergent accounts of the psychological underpinnings of separation anxiety. Freud (1926/1971) interpreted the child's fear of being alone and fear of strangers as fears of unknown dangers and, hence, as neurotic anxiety. This anxiety translates into fear of losing the love object and fear of the helplessness that would ensue, fears based both on reality and on unconscious sexual or aggressive fantasies. Neurosis was considered a universal childhood condition because all children experience fear of these unknown dangers, but they ordinarily grow out of their neuroses as they learn to appraise the unrealistic foundation of their fears. In this theoretical framework, separation anxiety represents the key to the problem of understanding neurotic anxiety.

On the other hand, working within a theoretical framework in which the attachment system is seen as having the distinct biological function of promoting survival, Bowlby (1973) reached quite different conclusions regarding the meaning of separation anxiety. He considers the mother's actual presence a "natural clue" to safety. Her absence is by implication a natural clue to danger, and the child's resulting distress, far from being neurotic, is interpreted as an adaptive mechanism that increases the chance of survival by signaling the mother to return. The link to psychopathology is established when the child is forced to cope prematurely with the prolonged physical or psychological unavailability of the attachment figure or with threats that he or she will become unavailable. This premature mobilization of defenses involves a process of detachment from the attachment figure in order to cope with the anger and grief caused by the mother's actual or anticipated loss.

In this view, the significance of separation experience for the onset of psychiatric conditions lies in the premature onset of detachment in childhood. Bowlby (1973, p. 73) was so impressed by the intensity and pervasiveness of early responses to separation that he likened the effects of separation from the mother to the effects of smoking or radiation: "Although the effects of small doses appear negligible, they are cumulative. The safest dose is a zero dose."

The model of the infant that emerges from these anxiety-centered approaches is one that highlights the psychological primacy of one person (usually the mother) as the preferred attachment figure in a hierarchy of attachment relationships (Bowlby 1969) and as a "beacon of orientation in the world of reality" (Mahler et al. 1975, p. 7). In this view, the mother-child relationship is seen as the prototype of all later love relationships (Freud 1938), and the infant is considered to be uniquely vulnerable to disruptions and discontinuities in the attachment relationship (Bowlby 1973, 1982). The implications of this model for thinking about the effects of day care attendance are straightforward. The lengthy daily separation from the mother may be in itself a risk factor for the infant's mental health because it creates a situation that repeatedly renders the mother unavailable for prolonged periods, mobilizes separation distress, and predisposes the child to the early onset of detachment reactions (Belsky 1986; Blehar 1974).

A competence-based model. An alternative model of the infant is one that stresses the extraordinary impetus toward self-organization and learning that characterizes the neonate and becomes increasingly differentiated in the course of development (e.g., Brazelton 1980; Emde 1981; Stern 1985).

The foundations for this model can be traced to White's (1959) seminal treatment of competence as an intrinsic motivational mechanism. The recent burgeoning of documentation about the self-directed capabilities of the infant have brought new life to this early work and spearheaded an integration of clinical and research contributions (Emde 1980a, 1980b; Greenspan 1981; Lichtenberg 1983; Stern 1985).

The evidence for the coherence, differentiation, and self-directedness of the infant's early experience is so voluminous that a comprehensive review is beyond the scope of this chapter. The reader is referred to Stern (1985) and Emde (1987) for scholarly updates of this topic. Some highlights follow: neonates can discriminate the mother's voice from another woman's voice reading the same material (DeCasper and Fifer 1980) and can discriminate the smell of their own mother's milk from the smell of other nursing women (MacFarlane 1975); they reliably imitate the facial expressions of an adult who smiles, frowns, or shows surprise (Field et al. 1982); they scan faces differently than they scan inanimate patterns, moving their eyes more freely rather than focusing on single features (Donee 1973) and vocalizing more (Brazelton et al. 1974). By 2 months of age, the infant is capable of detecting regularity, and on this basis he or she develops expectancies and acts on them. Haith (1980), for example, reported that at this age an infant begins to show anticipatory eye movements in response to the pattern of presentation of interesting pictures, indicating that he or she is acting on subjective predictions of what will happen next.

These accomplishments indicate that the infant has a well-developed capacity for storing perceptual events in memory and using them to organize experience (Stern 1985). This ability accelerates rapidly: by 5–7 months, infants can recognize the photograph of a stranger's face that has been shown to them only once, for less than a minute, and a full week earlier. Other research shows that infants at this age can also recall a week later the conditions that elicited a specific affective experience (Nachman and Stern 1983).

Such evidence prompted Emde (1983) to postulate an affective core to the prerepresentational self, and Stern (1985) described the continuity of cognitive and affective experience that contributes to the infant's sense of self-coherence. This affective continuity takes place in an interpersonal context in which social interaction serves to regulate, support, expand, and refine or, less optimally, undermine and restrict the infant's organization of his or her experience.

The view of an actively discriminating and self-organizing infant with an affectively continuous core self has implications for the place assigned to the mother-child relationship in the child's cognitive, social, and emotional landscape. Because of the infant's capacity to discriminate, abstract, generalize, and remember, he or she is engaged from the beginning in forming and elaborating personal representations. These representations are based on expectations developed by the infant in the course of interactions with all the members of his or her social world, not only with the mother. Although the mother or primary caregiver remains at the center of the child's emotional life, this person is not its only inhabitant.

Stern (1985) developed the concept of *representations of interactions that have been generalized* (RIGs) to describe this process. He argued that RIGs are formed gradually when a specific interactive episode with another (e.g., a peek-a-boo game) is repeated in similar fashion again and again. The specific meaning associated with the first episode becomes enriched and modified with each slightly different repetition, until the episode is remembered not as an individual event but as a generalized experience of all such similar events.

Stern argued that RIGs are formed gradually in the course of interactions with anyone who changes the child's self-experience, not only in relation to the mother. Moreover, these memories are retrievable even in the absence of the social partner. In other words, interactive experiences become internalized even in the first few months of life. The infant can evoke these experiences either when alone or, for purposes of comparison with previous experience, when interacting with a social companion. In this sense, the infant is seldom subjectively alone: he or she is "accompanied by evoked companions, drawn from several RIGs, who operate at various levels of activation and awareness" (Stern 1985, p. 118). The subjective experience of always being with another (the sense of "we-go" postulated by Klein [1967]) provides the formulation of the sense of trust.

The implications of this view for thinking about the effects of day care are profound. The infant is less exclusively dependent on the mother-child relationship and need not be psychologically undone by time-limited separations from her. If the experiences with a substitute caregiver are predictable and conducive to an increased organization and differentiation of experience, the infant will begin forming expectations and memories associated with this person and with the alternative caregiving situation. These internal structures will alter the infant's sense of self but not necessarily undermine his or her sense of trust. The infant will also be able to evoke memories of the absent mother in moments of need and use these memories as bridges to her until she returns. The infant's sense of self, even in the first few months, will not collapse in the mother's absence. In this view, then, the infant is seen as having more well-developed psychological mechanisms for coping adaptively with separation and its resulting distress than in the anxiety-based model.

An integrated model. Both models have significant contributions to make to our understanding of the infant's subjective experience. The anxiety-based model highlights our awareness of and empathy for the "dark" side of the infant's emotional life—the unspoken but deeply felt fear and acute distress that he or she is capable of experiencing. The competence-based model restores a sense of optimism and balance by reminding us of the developmental importance of the positive emotions (joy, surprise, interest) as independent incentives for social interaction, exploration, and learning (Emde 1987). Our appreciation of the infant's subjective experience becomes more richly multidimensional when the full range and intensity of affective possibilities are made part of the model.

From the integrated model perspective, we can more thoroughly explore the likely subjective experiences awaiting an infant who enters day care. We can be respectful of the realness of the separation distress and of the psychological accommodations the infant must make to adapt to it. We can also be confident that the infant possesses psychological mechanisms that will allow him or her not only to develop defensive responses to the situation but also to create new and adaptive pathways in the development of the self and of social relationships.

As mentioned earlier, the specific characteristics of the infant's environment and social relations—both in the home and elsewhere—are highly instrumental in shaping his or her experience. Just as every attachment relationship is unique, every relationship with another caregiver acquires specific affective nuances that become a part of the infant's affective domain.

In optimal conditions, the supplemental caregivers become cherished figures in their own right and provide the cognitive and affective nourishment that will enable the child to continue the work of learning and organizing experience even in the mother's absence. In these circumstances, the distress of the separation will be experienced and reexperienced episodically in the course of the day, but it will be amenable to modulation and relief because there are opportunities available for the experience of joy, interest, and curiosity. It is even conceivable, and often actually the case, that the alternative care setting might supply more affective availability, predictability, and cognitive challenges and have more opportunities for empathic connections than the home setting or, more specifically, the mother-child interaction. This argument has long been advanced by advocates of day care as a remedial approach to children from deprived or disadvantaged backgrounds (e.g., Bronfenbrenner 1974; Caldwell 1971; Zigler 1976).

At the other end of the quality spectrum, alternative caregiving can be dismally lacking in every feature that is conducive to adequate development. The figures cited in *Windows on Day Care* (Keyserling 1972), the comprehensive 1972 survey of the quality of day care, showed that 50% of the licensed centers visited were rated as "poor," a little more than one-third were considered "fair," and only 15% were judged to be "good." The standard for rating was not unduly strict. Individual appraisals of the centers rated "poor" described them as "abominable," "barren," and "re-pulsive," and centers that provided custodial care received a rating of only "fair" (Keyserling 1972). Although the survey was conducted 15 years ago, the conditions are unlikely to have improved. As Rothman (1973, p. 14) noted, there is "a long and disheartening tradition in this country of legitimating new institutions which, in the course of one generation, decline into custodial places, or worse." There is little hope that such places can provide young infants with the opportunities they need for healthy development.

The evidence of the poor quality of much of the day care actually available is a sobering reminder that we cannot be complacent about the mental health implications of day care attendance. However, it is important not to confuse poor quality with attendance per se. One could contend, in the light of present knowledge, that the infant is far better equipped developmentally to adjust to day care than is day care to respond to the infant's developmental needs. If so, it is our adult failure to create adequate institutions, rather than the infant's supposed lack of appropriate psy-chological resources, that is most urgently in need of examination.

Models For Day Care

What, then, is a clinician's proper position regarding the effects of day care on an infant's mental health? The following reflections represent a personal approach that has evolved in the course of assessing and treating infants and parents with a variety of daily routines and caregiving arrange-ments.

Out-of-home care is a child-rearing choice that needs to be considered in the context of the family values, psychodynamics, and external cir-cumstances. Particular approaches to child-rearing and parenting prac-tices cannot be advocated on the basis of abstract notions of what is right and what is wrong. The available evidence does not warrant a wholesale professional position for or against day care; it does warrant a sober exploration of the benefits and the psychological demands of attendance for individual families.

A good fit between the parents' individual needs and wishes and the choice of child care is essential if the child is to have a comfortable place in the family's emotional constellation. When asked about child care choices, a clinician needs to extend to this question the traditional thera-peutic stance of unbiased exploration, without imbuing the issue with the therapist's personal values. Consequences of different modes of child care for the parents and for the child need to be explored with no preconceived solutions in mind other than finding a course of action that feels right to the family and enhancing the parents' recognition of the compromises that each choice will involve for them and for the child.

The most difficult component in this clinical approach is how to speak to the child's experience in a manner that does not become a projection of the therapist's own conflicts and values. Here again, the traditional therapeutic stance should prove useful. The clinician needs to become acquainted with the growing body of knowledge about infancy and with the prevailing theoretical models of the infant; to be aware of his or her personal preferences, biases, and conflicts; to be informed about the specific programs being considered by the parents in order to assess their quality; and to use this knowledge in a flexible manner that is responsive to the subjective experience of the different family members.

Most of the major developmental milestones are progressively achieved while the young child is in day care: for example, the transition from the bottle to solid foods and from being fed to eating by himself or herself; learning to walk; toilet training; and, perhaps less concrete but equally important, learning about objects through play, learning about the environment through exploration, and learning about human relations and trust/mistrust through repeated interactions with other children and adults. All these events occur in the daily course of day care in undramatic but profound ways.

Underlying and buttressing these developmental achievements are the child's minute-to-minute subjective experiences as he or she encounters, makes sense of, and negotiates the interface between the self and the external world. In this process, the child finds out which signals work and which do not in securing what he or she wants and also with whom different approaches may work best or not at all. The child must also learn to manage his or her anxiety, anger, and frustration when the satisfaction of needs and wishes is not immediately forthcoming.

The concept of "optimal frustration" is useful in thinking about the child's successful management of anxiety. Tolpin (1971) suggested that the internalization of new psychological structures takes place when the love object or attachment figure no longer performs a particular function for the child. The child's psyche "does not resign itself" (p. 317) to this loss, but if the loss is phase appropriate and hence tolerable, the child makes up for it by taking over the function and observing it through internalization. The resulting psychic structures gradually enable the child to satisfy some of his or her own needs, deriving increasing independence from the need-satisfying object. The mother's availability and the child's closeness to the mother serve to alleviate the child's anxiety response to the phase-appropriate loss, modulating it so that it becomes tolerable and conducive to internalization rather than to disorganization.

CONCLUSIONS

For many, perhaps most, children, day-long separations from the mother in day care intensify anxiety responses beyond an optimally tolerable degree. These children's resources to cope with separation may be strained. Such children need assistance both from the parent and from the caregiver in converting acute anxiety into manageable anxiety. Provence and colleagues (1977), in their classic work on "the challenge of day care," documented the daily fluctuations of separation anxiety experienced by children and offered exquisitely sensitive ways of helping children in modulating it. And Kalmanson (Chapter 9, this volume) discusses some of the overt and hidden manifestations of separation anxiety both in infants and in their parents and offers helpful suggestions to understand and address these difficulties.

These contributions make the most important point about a clinical perspective on day care. Out-of-home care may elicit a heavier than optimal anxiety reaction in children, but the unavoidable experience of anxiety can be used as an opportunity for psychological growth when managed with patience and sensitivity by the important people in the child's life. For the vast majority of parents, life circumstances are such that they cannot screen out all external conditions that may exacerbate some anxiety experiences for their children. Day care may be one of those conditions. It behooves the clinician to serve as an ally to the child and to the parents in trying to prevent or fend off avoidable anxiety-arousing situations and in helping them to cope as adaptively as possible with those situations they cannot avoid.

REFERENCES

Ainsworth MDS: Object relations, dependency and attachment: a theoretical review of the infant-mother relationship. Child Dev 40:969–1025, 1969

Ainsworth MDS, Blehar MD, Waters E, et al: The Strange Situation: Observing Patterns of Attachment. Hillsdale, NJ, Erlbaum, 1978

Belsky J: Infant day care: a cause for concern? Zero to Three 5:1–7, 1986

Blehar M: Anxious attachment and defensive reactions associated with day care. Child Dev 45:683–692, 1974

Bowlby J: Attachment and Loss, Vol 1: Attachment. New York, Basic Books, 1969

Bowlby J: Attachment and Loss, Vol 2: Separation. New York, Basic Books, 1973

Bowlby J: Attachment and loss: retrospect and prospect. Am J Orthopsychiatry 52:664–678, 1982

Brazelton TB: New knowledge about the infant from current research: implications for psychoanalysis. Paper presented at the annual meeting of the American Psychoanalytic Association, San Francisco, CA, 1980

Brazelton TB, Koslowski B, Main M: The origins of reciprocity: the early mother-infant interaction, in The Effects of the Infant on Its Caregiver. Edited by Lewis M, Rosenblum LA. New York, John Wiley, 1974, pp 49–76

Bronfenbrenner U: Is early intervention effective? in Handbook of Evaluation Research, Vol 2. Edited by Guttentag M, Struening EL. Beverly Hills, CA, Sage Publications, 1975, pp 519–603

Caldwell BM: Impact of interest in early cognitive stimulation, in Perspectives in Child Psychopathology. Edited by Rie HE. Chicago, IL, Aldine-Atherton, 1971, pp 293–334

Caldwell BM, Wright CM, Honig AS, et al: Infant day care and attachment. Am J Orthopsychiatry 40:397–412, 1970

DeCasper AJ, Fifer WP: Of human bonding: newborns prefer their mothers' voices. Science 208:1174–1176, 1980

Donee LH: Infants' development scanning patterns of face and non-face stimuli under various auditory conditions. Paper presented at the annual meeting of the Society for Research, in Child Development, Philadelphia, PA, March 1973

Emde RN: Toward a psychoanalytic theory of affect, I: the organizational model and its propositions, in The Course of Life, Vol. 1: Infancy and Early Childhood. Edited by Greenspan SI, Pollock GH. Washington, DC, National Institute of Mental Health, 1980a, pp 63–84

Emde RN: Toward a psychoanalytic theory of affect, II: emerging models of emotional development in infancy, in The Course of Life, Vol 1: Infancy and Early Childhood. Edited by Greenspan SI, Pollock GH. Washington, DC, National Institute of Mental Health, 1980b, pp 85–112

Emde RN: Changing models of infancy and the nature of early development: remodeling the foundation. J Am Psychoanal Assoc 29:179–219, 1981

Emde RN: The prerepresentational self and its affective core. Psychoanal Study Child 38:165–192, 1983

Emde RN: Affective core of the self: motivational structures from infancy. Paper presented at the continuing education seminar The World of Self and Other: The Impact of New Infant Research on Treatment of Adults, Beverly Hills, CA, 1987

Field TM, Woodson R, Greenberg R, et al: Discrimination and imitation of facial expression by neonates. Science 218:179–181, 1982

Freud S: An Outline of Psychoanalysis. London, Hogarth Press, 1938

Freud S: Inhibitions, symptoms and anxiety (1926), in The Standard Edition of the Complete Psychological Works of Sigmund Freud, Vol 20. Translated and edited by Strachey J. London, Hogarth Press, 1971, pp 75–175

Greenspan SI: Psychopathology and Adaptation in Infancy and Early Childhood. New York, International Universities Press, 1981

Haith MM: Rules Newborns Look By. Hillsdale, NJ, Erlbaum, 1980

Keyserling MD: Windows on Day Care. New York, National Council of Jewish Women, 1972

Klein GS: Peremptory Ideation: Structure and Force in Motivated Ideas. Psychological Issues, Vol 5 (No 2–3). New York, International Universities Press, 1967, pp 80–128

Lichtenberg JD: Psychoanalysis and Infant Research. Hillsdale, NJ, Erlbaum, 1983

Lieberman AF: Psychology and day care. Social Research 45:416–451, 1978

MacFarlane J: Olfaction in the development of social preferences in the human neonate, in Parent-Infant Interaction. Edited by Hoper M. Amsterdam, Elsevier, 1975, pp 103–118

Mahler MS, Pine F, Bergman A: The Psychological Birth of the Human Infant: Symbiosis and Individuation. New York, Basic Books, 1975

Nachman P, Stern DN: Recall memory for emotional experience in pre-linguistic infants. Paper presented at the National Clinical Infancy Fellows Conference, Yale University, New Haven, CT, 1983

Phillips D, McCartney K, Scarr S, et al: Selective review of infant day care research: a cause for concern. Zero to Three 3:18–21, 1987

Provence S, Naylor A, Patterson J: The Challenge of Day Care. New Haven, CT, Yale University Press, 1977

Rossi AS: Transition to parenthood. Journal of Marriage and the Family 30:26–39, 1968

Rothman SM: Other people's children: the day care experience in America. The Public Interest 30:11–27, 1973

Stern DN: Interpersonal World of the Infant. New York, Basic Books, 1985

Thompson RA: Attachment theory and day care research. Zero to Three 2:19–20, 1987

Tolpin M: On the beginnings of a cohesive self. Psychoanal Study Child 26:316–352, 1971

White RW: Motivation reconsidered: the concept of competence. Psychol Rev 66:297–333, 1959

Zigler EF: Head Start: not a program but an evolving concept, in Early Childhood Education: It's an Art! It's a Science. Edited by Andrews JD. Washington, DC, National Association for the Education of Young Children, 1976

Chapter 5

Effects of Day Care: Implications of Current Knowledge

Steven A. Frankel, M.D.

Since about 1970, attempts have been made to assess the effects of the experience of day care on children. Efforts to refine criteria and control for socioeconomic status, quality of day care, and the length of exposure to day care, although currently only partially successful, have resulted in progressively more useful data. However, most of these efforts have been dedicated to measuring short-term effects. Some data are available on the outcome through 5 or 6 years following initial day care exposure, but only one longitudinal study (Moore 1975) has measured effects beyond this point. At present, then, to discern long-term outcome, one must extrapolate from research in related areas, for example, the persistence of distortions in attachment or other psychopathology over time. One can also use what is known from developmental theory to make inferences. In short, little is known about the long-term effects of day care. In this chapter, therefore, in exploring this issue I will consider existing research on day care and related areas as well as developmental theory.

RESEARCH CRITERIA

Translating from the frame of reference of one theoretical persuasion to that of another may be problematic. The psychodynamic perspective invokes intrapsychic correlates, whereas most of the research on day care uses behavioral criteria and measures of attachment. For example, if children who have been exposed to a particular type of substitute care are judged to be especially aggressive, has some facet of their capacity for interpersonal relatedness also been affected? If so, will this deviation show up as a measure of impaired attachment, or will it be more subtle or specific and require the kinds of formulations that psychoanalysts use to describe the vicissitudes of internalized aspects of relationships? Are these deviations best understood as a defense against or an expression of some vulnerability? Will they persist over time or will they fade?

In general, one would like to know about the effect of day care on the child's developing personality, on his or her current and future relationships, on his or her competence, capacity, and willingness to achieve—at first in school and later perhaps in a job—and whether overt psychopathology is eventually associated with exposure to day care. Specifically, the types of issues psychoanalytically oriented workers are likely to target include object relations (quality, consistency), the creation of specific areas of psychological vulnerability, and maladaptive defenses that may become incorporated into a child's character. In addition, there is the possibility of qualitative shifts in the child's developing personality and the intrapsychic correlates of these shifts.

Measurements commonly used in attachment and nonpsychodynamic research include the child's attachment to his or her mother and other caretakers; the child's socialization, including interest in people and preferences for peers versus adults; the frequency and types of interactions that occur among children and between children and adults; and influence on those interactions exerted by factors such as type and quality of day care. Assertiveness, aggression, and defiance versus passivity and compliance have been measured. Finally, tests of intelligence and developmental status have been used together with measures of the child's success in and attitude toward school.

RESEARCH LIMITATIONS

Unfortunately, the research literature on day care subjects suffers from a number of limitations. Almost all studies have at best a limited longitudinal component. Only one study (Moore 1975) has followed children through adolescence. Most studies are limited to children no older than preschool age. Critical factors such as age of entry into day care, length of day, and overall length of exposure to day care are frequently left within a fairly broad range and often are not assessed independently of one another.

In addition, characteristics of families tend to be neglected. This situation is striking, since disruption within the family (Bryant et al. 1980; Hock 1980; Vaughn et al. 1980) and a mother's satisfaction with her role (including her job) (Hock 1980; Hoffman 1979; Wallston 1973), as well as the child's history of stressful life events including family disruption (Werner and Smith 1982), seem to be highly correlated with the outcome for children. Characteristics that may distinguish one day care center from another, such as staff-child ratio, program characteristics, and stability of a child's placement, are important variables that are often neglected (Phillips et al. 1987). Most studies were originally done at university centers, which are distinctly more sophisticated than the typical day care center. It may frequently be difficult to relate findings from studies because the criteria they used may differ so widely: for example, differences in settings, age of children, and socioeconomic status.

Beyond these limitations, the studies frequently are deficient in research design. For example, control groups are difficult to define. It has been demonstrated that families who seek day care tend to be different from those that do not (Belsky and Steinberg 1978). Consequently, a valid control group cannot be taken from the general population. At the same time, it is difficult to assign subjects randomly between day care centers and home, although in one study (Peters 1973) this task was achieved and in two others (Cochran 1977; Ramey and Mills 1977) a control group was taken from the waiting lists for the day care centers studied. Again, the instruments used may yield data that may not be easy to correlate with "functional" outcomes.

Other difficulties include the fact that although child care centers are most frequently studied, in 1985 only about 10% of children under 3 years of age in day care were in these types of facilities (Kamerman 1986). Home and family care were used far more frequently. Finally, several factors may compound outcome, including stress at home and the use of poor quality day care.

Also refer to Belsky (Chapter 3, this volume) and Howes (Chapter 2, this volume) for current reviews of the research on the effects of day care on children.

SUMMARY OF RESEARCH

The research findings are ambiguous, but they seem to point in the direction of attachment disturbances being *potentially* associated with early entry into day care. The effect on social development is more equivocal in spite of a tentative association with heightened aggressivity and a tendency for the child to be more oriented toward peers and less oriented toward adults. Intelligence measures do not seem to be affected except in low socioeconomic populations, in which the effect is salutary. In contrast to those children who seem to be negatively affected, more than half do not show attachment disturbances. Judging from the literature, in addition to early entry, the emphasis needs to be placed on stability of the day care arrangements, quality of care, and stressful family circumstances. The last seems to be tied to negative effects on attachment and social outcomes.

The relevance of these findings to long-term outcome is highly conjectural. There has been only one long-term study (Moore 1975). Children who had experienced a minimum of 25 hours away from their mothers for at least 12 months before age 5 were compared at several points between ages 6 and 17 to those who remained exclusively with their mothers. Moore found that boys in the child care group seemed more fearless, aggressive, and nonconforming, whereas boys who received exclusive mothering were more "fastidious and conforming." The findings for girls were less clear. However, this study was poorly controlled, and in it a variety of care situations were combined. Obviously, there is a need for both long-term longitudinal studies and for more research on the predictive value of measures of attachment in infancy and childhood.

CONTRIBUTIONS OF DEVELOPMENTAL THEORIES

Both psychoanalytic and attachment theories are concerned with the critical nature of the relationship between mother and child and the potential consequences when that bond is disrupted or impaired.

Attachment Theory

Attachment theory regards the unique and specific attachment the child develops with the mother between about 6 months and 3 years of age as predicated on the biological need to ensure survival. Attachment behaviors have as their objective the promotion of proximity and contact. The loss of the mother, whether absolute or relative, has major consequences that lead to a specific sequence of reactions that Bowlby (1961, 1980, 1982) called protest, despair, and detachment. These stages of response presumably are analogous to the stages of the mourning process that occurs later in life. Bowlby (1969) derived this framework from his review of studies of the responses of children separated from their mothers. These studies ranged from children who were institutionalized (e.g., Burlingham and Freud 1944) to children who were separated for a matter of weeks (Robertson and Robertson 1971).

Repeated and prolonged separation may result in distortions in the quality of the child's attachments. Ainsworth and her colleagues (1978), utilizing the Strange Situation procedure, identified two primary types of deviant attachment behavior, which they labeled "anxious-avoidant" and "anxious-resistant." (See Belsky, Chapter 3, this volume, for a description of the Strange Situation procedure.) Many of the studies of the impact of day care utilize the Strange Situation technique for assessment. To establish the relevance of findings derived from the Strange Situation technique, it is necessary to know how stable these categorizations are and whether they are predictive of deviations in development over time. Vaughn and his colleagues (1979, 1980) and Thompson et al. (1982, 1983) demonstrated that approximately half of the children in their studies changed category toward both the development of and the resolution of attachment deviations. Further, changes in attachment, both positive and negative, were correlated with analogous changes in family circumstances (Thompson et al. 1982; Waters 1983). On the other hand, Sroufe et al. (1983) showed significant continuity between measures of insecurity at 12–18 months and assessments made during preschool. Lewis and his colleagues (1984) were able to use Strange Situation designations to predict psychopathology in 6-year-olds, especially males, with some success.

In brief, children who seemed insecure as infants continued to seem insecure and socially less competent by the time they reached preschool age. Sroufe and colleagues (1983, p. 1625) saw these findings as consistent with the "developmental/organizational perspective," which holds that "a secure attachment relationship in infancy provides the foundation for later autonomous functioning." In addition, Ainsworth and her colleagues (1978) delineated associations between a child's attachment category and the responsiveness of the mothering the child received.

In presenting both this theoretical position and the data that underscore it, it is necessary, however, to emphasize its lack of precision. First, attachment category can change dramatically over 3 to 4 years. Second, the change seems to be predicated on situational factors. Finally, to have confidence in the perpetuation of these categories, it is necessary to know both the family and personal circumstances of the child over the course of time as well as the impact of interventions such as day care. At best, these data seem to underscore the relationship between attachment and social behavior, and they sound an optimistic note for the persistence of secure attachment over time, providing circumstances conspire.

This point of view raises the questions of the extent to which the mother-child relationship is exclusive in helping a child to regulate anxiety and whether other relationships can serve an analogous purpose. (Note that here and throughout this chapter, "mother-child relationship" is used as a shorthand for the relationship between the child and the primary early figures in his or her life.) Schaffer and Emerson (1964), Schaffer (1977), and Rutter (1981) all took the position that the child forms a multitude of bonds that are selective and provide comfort and security. In fact, Schaffer (1977, p. 103) took the position that "the person the child chooses to become attached to depends on the adult's behavior and interaction—on subtle qualities like sensitivity, responsiveness, emotional involvement, and probable others we know little about." These researchers would agree, however, that among these attachments there is a hierarchy with the mother most frequently at the top.

These notions are consistent with the observation that children are impressively malleable. Tizard and Hodges (1978) demonstrated that children who had been institutionalized since infancy formed strong and selective attachments when adopted at a mean age of 3 years. A number of other studies underscore this possibility (Kadushin 1970) and relate a problematic outcome to the quality of care rather than solely to the effect of change in caregivers (Yarrow and Klein 1980). The developmental framework established by both Thomas and Chess (1980) and Kagan (1984) is in accordance with these findings and emphasizes the repeated and renewed potentialities children have for adaptation. In effect, if day care acted as a source of destabilization, these studies would tend to underscore the potential for those effects to be counteracted, providing a child's personal circumstances were facilitating. The emphasis is on handicapping developments, within either the child's life or the child's family.

In fact, studies of children's vulnerability over time tend to emphasize the lack of predictability and the potential for shifts to occur in development (Anthony and Cohler 1987). This position acknowledges the findings that situations in a child's environment or family such as parental psychopathology or family disruption can increase a child's vulnerability (Brown et al. 1985; Rutter 1982, 1984a, 1984b; Siefer and Sameroff 1987; Sroufe 1979; Sroufe et al. 1983). The question needs to be asked whether day care exacerbates or ameliorates these conditions.

Overall, the evidence seems to support the notion that day care should function as a nondisruptive system in a child's life as long as the child's developmental needs for proximity and contact with his or her primary caregivers are respected. In part, these needs appear to be age specific and reach their peak at around 18 months, declining by about 3 years. Whether the child will be flexible and able to use the child care situation comfortably appears to be a function of the child's resilience, background, and family circumstances. In addition, a maximum safe level of exposure probably exists. This idea is reinforced by recent research that suggests that extensive placement in day care in the first year of life may be associated with greater insecure-avoidant attachment (see Belsky, Chapter 3, this volume). In contrast, although there is some indication that deviant attachment may tend to persist, there is a good deal of evidence that children are malleable and that difficulties instigated by exposure to day care can be either reinforced or offset by other experiences.

Psychoanalytic Developmental Theory

The major contribution of the field of psychoanalysis has been to provide a refined view of the inner workings of the mind during development. Nuances of the child's relationship with others, in particular with the mother, have been delineated by Emde (1983), Emde and Harmon (1982), Sander and his colleagues (1978), and Stern (1985). Emde (1983) paid particular attention to the process through which the infant and the mother collaborate through interchanges fueled by a mutual capacity to monitor and respond to each other's affective state during the preverbal period. Emde explored the implication of this collaboration for the interpersonal process (e.g., "social referencing") later in childhood. Stern (1985) used Emde's data to construct a model of the infants' and toddlers' subjective experiences as they relate to the capacity to engage and interact with others, particularly the mother, and to progressively appreciate their separate existences and the meaning of their communications. Both researchers emphasized the equipment with which children and parents are prefitted to facilitate this mutual process and the interrelationship of events as they occur in the partners. Reflective of these perspectives are terms such as "affect monitoring" and "emotional referencing" (Emde 1983) and "affect attunement," "intersubjectivity," and "representations of interactions that have been generalized" (RIGs) (Stern 1985). The progressive elaboration of the child's internal world through age 2 or 3, and to a lesser degree to age 4 or 5, is traditionally thought to occur predominantly around the focus of the mother-child relationship. When this development goes smoothly, a child can explore and be progressively involved with others, at the same time crystallizing both an internal sense of certainty about his or her mother and a coherent sense of self. Somewhere between ages 2½ and 3, this initial progression is finalized and "libidinal object constancy," a stable internal image of a loving and available parent even when the parent is absent and when the child or the relationship is stressed, is clearly in evidence (Fraiberg 1969; Mahler et al. 1975). This development is complex and depends as much on the appearance of new cognitive capabilities as it does on the interpersonal and emotional events that precede its emergence (Greenspan 1979). Several authors (e.g., Jacobson 1964; Kernberg 1975; Kohut 1971; Tyson 1983) have provided models for deviations in the development of a sense of self and other that can result from problems in this progression.

The implications of these theoretical positions may be formulated as follows. The effect of excessive or poorly structured substitute care on the developmental process is a function of a child's age. Conceivably, the finely tuned interaction between mother and child that characterizes the early relationship can be diluted or distorted. This dilution may interfere with the child's developing abilities to identify and regulate affects and with the child's expectations of the responsiveness of others. The deviation may not be of pathological proportions but simply a departure from what would occur in the context of a more constant interchange with a competent parent.

From about 6 or 7 months, distinctions between key attachment figures and others are in the fore. If separation from parents and being placed in the care of a stranger exceed a child's tolerance, the child's sense of the reliability of others may be undermined. The result may be to create enough insecurity that the child feels a need either to cling or coerce in order to be assured of attention and love. Alternatively, as a result of the child's sense of vulnerability, he or she may prefer fantasized relationships or erect a defensive barrier against potentially hurtful involvements.

Between 15 to 18 months and 30 to 36 months, the child's focus shifts to the establishment of his or her prerogatives while still insisting on the continuous availability of a parent or another trusted adult. The absence of a regular and empathic adult relationship may lead to a chronic sense of deflation and ineffectiveness as well as exacerbate the already stormy feelings that separations and frustration tend to evoke during this developmental period. Relationships with key figures may then remain ambivalent, and an internal conviction that these relationships are secure may fail to materialize. The child's movement toward emotional independence—that is, libidinal object constancy—would then be impaired. These children may look like advanced versions of the Strange Situation anxious-resistant subjects, since their relationships are so ambivalent. Internal representations of others (object representations) may then be cast as untrustworthy or be suffused with aggression and be experienced as threatening (Kernberg 1975). Concomitantly, the child's sense of self or self-worth may be impaired (Kohut 1971; Tyson 1983). Finally, the capacity to use key figures effectively and then internal agencies (progressively) for the purpose of self-regulation may be compromised (Jacobson 1964) and result in deviations or deficiencies in impulse control or in the development of conscience.

Neubauer (1985) attempted to broaden the traditional psychoanalytic view that early relationships are essentially dyadic and took a position that is consonant with the observation that multiple bonds are available to children. He stated: "Under normal conditions of mother-child relationships, the simultaneous relationship to other adults and siblings during the first years of life does not dilute or divert the quality of the relationship to mother and father, but rather contributes to the shaping of primary objects" (p. 180). Regarding day care, Neubauer presented vignettes that emphasize that under usual circumstances the availability of multiple caregivers is tolerable for the child and may facilitate his or her development. The potential advantages of good-quality day care become especially clear in cases of stressed or otherwise inadequate mothering. Neubauer sounded a warning, however, for circumstances in which day care is used to "an inappropriate extent."

The earlier emphasis on the sanctity of the mother-child bond is reflected in a strong traditional psychoanalytic bias that the potential effect of day care is disruptive (Fraiberg 1977; Nagera 1975). This point of view emphasizes the potential for interference with the child's capacity to form meaningful and deep relationships. Neubauer's (1985) position, on the other hand, could point to a significant shift in that position.

Psychoanalysis offers a theoretical perspective for interpreting data on the impact of day care on development and possibly even for making predictions. It has produced thoughtful clinical studies and detailed case analyses. Until recently, however, research methodology has been deemphasized, resulting in a dearth of formal research on the disruption of the parenting relationship and, more specifically, on the effects of day care.

Nachman's (1986) paper entitled "A Study of Daytime Separation from Mother" illustrated both the advantages and limitations of the currently available research from a psychoanalytic perspective. (For a detailed look at this study, see Nachman, Chapter 8, this volume.) In brief, the study involved two groups of six children, one in the care of their mothers ("mother group") and one whose mothers worked full-time and who were cared for by a substitute caretaker at their home ("caregiver group"). Detailed observations were made beginning at 17 months of age. Compared with the mother group, accelerated functioning in many areas of development was reported for the caregiver group, including more symbolic play, an enhanced tendency to form groups and to interact with other children, and a greater inhibition of aggression facilitated by a greater strictness on the part of the caregivers. Also, there was a relative lack of emotionality in the children's relationships to their caregivers. Nachman's interpretation included the following: "Our impression is that [in the caregiver group] other children served as points of reference for each other to make up for the diminished contact (i.e., social referencing) with their adult partners" (p. 14). Nachman then suggested that imitation, intense doll play, and early onset of caring and helping behavior observed in the caregiver group are related to the child's identification with the absent mother.

If these observations can be replicated and tested over a variety of populations, a refined view of the effect of substitute care will begin to emerge. Currently, the data and conclusions must be regarded as tentative, since the population studied was small and specific. Further, the interpretation of the data remains inferential. In spite of these limitations, Nachman's detailed clinical perspective is potentially invaluable and not available from other types of research.

Provence (1974, pp. 13–14) was similarly focused on the child's inner world. She stated that

> infants and young toddlers have a difficult time maintaining the idea of the existence of a parent throughout the day. At home there are discontinuous but frequent encounters with mother. As the day lengthens, it must be difficult for the child to use evocative memory and call up the images of the familiar person. . . . If the child is in full-time day care from the earliest months of life, there will be some interference with and delay in forming close attachments . . .

We are again in the arena of inference, in spite of the enormous potential importance of these positions.

At this point, the greatest strength and potential contribution of psychoanalysis to the study of day care is also related to its greatest weakness. Psychoanalysis can provide detailed clinical observations and offers an extraordinarily refined view of the development and elaboration of the child's internal world. At the same time, it is currently weak in both its methods for research and its attempts at verification.

DISCUSSION

The available research suggests the following. Prior to the publication of some of the most recent studies, Rutter (1982) wrote: "It is clear . . . . that some of the more alarming stereotypes about day care can be rejected" (p. 21). Further, he acknowledged that "good quality day care does not disrupt children's emotional bonds without parents. Even day care for very young children does not usually result in serious emotional disturbances" (p. 22). Rutter claimed that day care may "influence social behavior" in ways that may be helpful or troublesome. He stated that a major question is whether it is essential or desirable for one parent to remain home during the early years. He answered by saying that since "day care research fails to show that day care commonly results in substantial emotional or social problems," it is obviously not essential (p. 23). Desirability, according to Rutter, is more complex. If economic conditions force the mother and father to work, the family will be stressed. If the mother likes working and is happier and a better mother when she works, then the maternal employment research indicates that she will do better. Rutter added: "The review of empirical research . . . concluded that strong assertions about what form of care would be best for young children would not be warranted in view of the lack of firm evidence" (p. 23). In making recommendations on child care, Rutter emphasized the quality of the center and the child's age, noting the special requirements of children under 3, since they make less use of interaction with peers and are more reliant on adults.

In a more recent publication, Gamble and Zigler (1986) were essentially in agreement with Rutter. They made note of the growing evidence that early entry into child care may be associated with disturbed parent-child attachments. Still, they acknowledged that even in the worst case (Vaughn et al. 1980) more than half the infants were securely attached at 1 year. Like Rutter, Gamble and Zigler emphasized the role of family stress and the accumulation of stressful experiences in influencing both near-term and presumably long-term outcome.

The malleability of the growing child is emphasized by research that demonstrates how readily attachment categories can shift in childhood (Egeland and Sroufe 1981; Vaughn et al. 1979), by the theories and research of child developmentalists such as Thomas and Chess (1980) and Kagan (1984), and by long-term studies of vulnerability such as those by Murphy (1987) and Felsman and Vaillant (1987). On the other hand, in concert with Werner and Smith (1982), there has been ample demonstration that unfortunate childhood experiences, including those that occur when a child has a psychiatrically disturbed parent (Brown et al. 1985; Siefer and Sameroff 1987), tend to predispose to the later development of psychopathology. Sometimes the effects are masked during long periods, or the character and locus of the problem shift over time. Wallerstein (1985) demonstrated such an effect in her 10-year follow-up of children whose parents had divorced. In that case, females, who previously seemed much less affected, came to manifest serious disabilities during and after adolescence. Males, who had early been most affected, seemed to do significantly better. The implication is that the assessment of the potential consequences of any day care situation necessarily involves knowledge of the individual child and his or her character, history, and family situation; the likelihood that the day care arrangement will be sustained; and the quality of the day care. Even with this knowledge, prediction is risky since the child's course will be influenced by intervening stresses and benefits.

IMPLICATIONS

My assessment of the available data, in spite of its ambiguity, adds reinforcement to the view that the child is capable of forming multiple bonds from a very young age. These bonds are apparently differentiated to the extent that attachment to parents is rarely if ever supplanted by attachment to caregivers. One possibility is that the child has multiple potentialities and can use these opportunities as they are made available to meet its needs. It remains to be seen whether children who are given an "optimal" dose of substitute care and exposure to peers differ in their outcome from those who are not. It is as conceivable that these experiences will facilitate the child's development as it is that they will be perceived by the child as a deprivation.

An additional possible explanation for the parents' retaining their centrality lies with the notion that children can interact with a high degree of selectivity. It is possible that children "save up" their more critical emotional needs and express these needs predominantly with parents. Others, even if they are present for long periods of time, may be dealt with in different and more restricted ways (see Nachman, Chapter 8, this volume). Finally, the advantage of day care for the family needs to be considered. The research suggests that if the mother and father can live a fuller and more satisfied life, or if stress can be decreased at home, then the effect of day care of at least adequate quality is likely to be salutary for the child.

My speculations then lead in the following directions. It seems likely that prolonged exposure to day care may result in a qualitative shift in the development of the child's personality. This shift may occur because of the shift in the focus of influence from parents to other caregivers, and because the child is subjected to a more fragmented and diffuse environment with many more influences during a large part of the day. Personality features that are based on modeling (imitation) and ultimately identification with parents may be altered. In addition, the internal regulatory capacities that a child develops through the vehicle of interacting with others may take on a different character. These internal agencies may be less rigorous and more vulnerable to disruption.

The following observations illustrate what I mean by subtle effects. They describe an impression I have formed from clinical observations of several children and adults who had spent more than two of their early childhood years in substitute care. These people showed a distinctly intensified need for contact and reassurance in a key relationship. The relationship tended to be with a parent, and in adolescence and later with a friend or in a romantic involvement. At times this need evolved into a desperate insistence. These people could easily feel abandoned, and the extent of their resulting loneliness was impressive. Alternately, when the relationship succeeded, there was frequently a sense of elation and even triumph. It was as if at some point in their earlier lives, perhaps in part as a result of a frustrating or excessive experience with day care, they felt deprived and potentially abandoned. Rather than fend off intimate relationships, they seemed to direct their later efforts toward greater valuing of these relationships. In contrast, these people were also somewhat compromised in their capacity to consummate the relationships they so much desired. Their sensitivity tended to be exquisite, and they would often recoil as a result of some perceived slight. Some defended themselves against these outcomes by developing a somewhat aloof and rejecting posture.

As a rough estimation, the characteristics described previously are at least consistent with the disturbance in attachment that has been identified by some studies for children who entered day care before age 1. The terms "anxious" and "avoidant" are apt. Further, these disturbances are thoroughly consistent with the kind of deviation in the child's sense of self and other that would be predicted by Mahler and her coworkers (1975) for children who experience a significant interference with the rapprochement phase of the separation-individuation process, during the period between 18 and 30 to 36 months of age.

Theoretically, disturbances in separation-individuation and anxious attachment are consistent with an early, troubled interaction between mother and child. Anxiety or confusion engendered by an anxious, emotionally unavailable, or ambivalent mother may be reinforced by subsequent experiences involving separation from the mother and substitute care. At this point these thoughts and observations are only speculative. They represent an attempt to think about possible relationships between research findings, clinical observations, and theory. In contrast, for example, to the ideas presented in the preceding paragraphs, it is possible that in some cases, substitute care provides a welcome respite for both the stressed child and mother and thus may have a reparative effect. Overall, we are looking for ways in which the day care experience may affect a child over time. If the effects that we are describing are both subtle and reside in the individual as potentialities, then they may not be manifest immediately (Wallerstein 1985). Indeed, to measure these effects one would have to use sensitive psychological instruments applied to individuals and, like Moore (1975), would have to follow these individuals over a long period of time.

Finally, the possible interactive influences between day care and the family need to be considered. These include the replacement of the extended family by day care and the movement of education about child rearing from family to agencies and possibly to society as a whole. Day care probably will need to be seen in the context of an evolving social form. In this framework, it may be viewed as an adaptive response to such factors as the mobility of families and the changing status of women as well as economic factors. One corollary is that upper middle-class families who use higher quality day care centers will receive more sophisticated guidance than parents of lower socioeconomic status, who become segregated into poorer quality day care centers.

TENTATIVE RECOMMENDATIONS

The position I have taken here is based on developmental criteria with an intrapsychic focus. It is a tentative and conservative position and is based on the knowledge that studies are emerging that demonstrate deviant attachment in some day care children, especially in those who enter day care at a young age (see Belsky, Chapter 3, this volume). In addition, studies such as Wallerstein's (1985) demonstrate unexpected long-term consequences for disruptive experiences in childhood and concern about the more subtle and qualitative effects that may go undetected. My position recognizes that the long-term effects of day care are unknown and that many factors (e.g., length of day in day care) have not been studied conclusively.

Children from birth to 18 and possibly 24 months appear to require the greatest degree of contact with their parents and, at the least, with a constant person in charge of no more than two other children in a stable environment (Kagan et al. 1978; Rutter 1982), preferably not a group center. Theoretically, movement into a position of greater independence would occur at the point at which a relatively resilient capacity for object permanence and the ability not just for locomotion and manipulation of physical objects but also for the translation of these capabilities into the manipulation of thought (Phase VI of Piaget's Sensory Motor Stage) are established. Accompanying and possibly reflecting this is the use of language, which begins to increase dramatically after about 18 months. Children up through this age seem to have limited tolerance, both cognitive and affective, for separation. In the absence of more conclusive data, it makes sense for parental absence throughout this period to be no greater than one-half of the child's day. Children from about 18 to 36 months are still highly dependent on adults for support and regulation. In addition, genuinely cooperative play remains unusual. These children lack the capacity to sustain relationships that are relatively immune to the effect of disruptive emotions. They lack libidinal object constancy; that is, anger and excessive frustration threaten the presence of the internal image of the love object. These children may be subject to a sense of deflation when excessively frustrated, and repeated experience of this sort might interfere with the substrate for a healthy sense of self-esteem. This notion suggests a need for the presence of one or a few stable adults who can be attentive and responsive. Family day care with a child-adult ratio of three or four to one seems adequate (Howes and Rubenstein 1985; Kagan et al. 1978; Rutter 1982). At about age 3, the rapid development of internal controls allows children to delay, deflect, and plan in such a way that they can consistently work to please adults. They are much more competent at managing the absence of their parents in a thoughtful and constructive manner. Nonetheless, these children remain predominantly dependent on adults, even though they may enjoy, and are much more competent at, relating with peers. Their ability to comprehend cause and effect is still limited and they are still relatively egocentric. Although a center-based day care experience may be manageable, it seems that the maximum child-adult ratio should be about seven to one (see Howes, Chapter 2, this volume), especially if the children are to attend day care on a full-day basis.

CONCLUSIONS

These recommendations represent an ideal that many parents cannot realize. The cost of day care is high, and the availability of high-quality care, whether on a family care basis or in centers, is limited. It is hoped, however, that these ideas can be used to help establish a direction in guiding selection and in the formulation of policy.

Finally, the rudimentary status of our knowledge needs to be underscored. Clearer, and perhaps more flexible, recommendations could be made if we had reasonably definitive longitudinal studies available to us. Beyond that, it would be reassuring if the potential subtle and qualitative shifts to which some day care–exposed children might be subject could be identified and measured. This lack of data represents a potent research challenge, one that has critical significance for influencing the future of our society.

REFERENCES

Ainsworth MDS, Blehar MC, Waters E, et al: Patterns of Attachment: A Psychological Study of the Strange Situation. Hillsdale, NJ, Erlbaum, 1978

Anthony E, Cohler B (eds): The Vulnerable Child. New York, Guilford Press, 1987

Belsky J, Steinberg LD: The effects of day care: a critical review. Child Dev 49:929–949, 1978

Bowlby J: Processes of mourning. lnt J Psychoanal 142:317–340, 1961

Bowlby J: Attachment and Loss, Vol 1: Attachment. New York, Basic Books, 1969

Bowlby J: Attachment and Loss, Vol 3: Loss, Sadness and Depression. New York, Basic Books, 1980

Bowlby J: Attachment and loss: retrospect and prospect. Am J Orthopsychiatry 52:664–678, 1982

Brown GW, Harris TO, Bifulco A: Long-term effects of early loss of parent, in Depression in Childhood: Developmental Perspectives. Edited by Rutter M, Izard C, Read P. New York, Guilford Press, 1985

Bryant B, Harris M, Newton D: Children and Minders. London, Grant McIntyre, 1980

Burlingham DT, Freud A: Infants Without Families: The Case For and Against Residential Nurseries. London, Allen and Unwin, 1944

Cochran M: A comparison of group day and family childrearing patterns in Sweden. Child Dev 48:702–707, 1977

Egeland B, Sroufe L: Attachment and early maltreatment. Child Dev 52:44–52, 1981

Emde RN: The prerepresentational self and its affective care. Psychoanal Study Child 38:165–192, 1983

Emde RN, Harmon RJ (eds): The Development of Attachment and Affiliative Systems. New York, Plenum, 1982

Felsman J, Vaillant G: Resilient children as adults: a 40-year study, in The Vulnerable Child. Edited by Anthony E, Cohler B. New York, Guilford Press, 1987, pp 289–314

Fraiberg S: Libidinal object constancy and mental representation. Psychoanal Study Child 24:9–47, 1969

Fraiberg S: Every Child's Birthright: In Defense of Mothering. New York, Basic Books, 1977

Gamble I, Zigler E: Effects of infant day care: another look at the evidence. Am J Orthopsychiatry 56:26–42, 1986

Greenspan S: Intelligence and Adaptation. Psychoanalytical Issues Monograph 47/48. New York, International Universities Press, 1979

Hock E: Working and non-working mothers and their infants: a comparative study of maternal caregiving characteristics and infant social behavior. Merrill-Palmer Quarterly 26:79–102, 1980

Hoffman LW: Maternal employment. Am Psychol 34:859–865, 1979

Howes C, Rubenstein I: Determinants of toddlers' experience in daycare: age of entry and quality of setting. Child Care Quarterly 14:140–157, 1985

Jacobson E: The Self and the Object World. New York, International Universities Press, 1964

Kadushin A: Adopting Older Children. New York, Columbia University Press, 1970

Kagan J: The Nature of the Child. New York, Basic Books, 1984

Kagan J, Kearsley R, Zelazo P: Infancy: Its Place in Human Development. Cambridge, MA, Harvard University Press, 1978

Kamerman S: Infant care usage in the United States. Report presented to the National Academy of Sciences Ad Hoc Committee on Policy Issues in Child Care for Infants and Toddlers, Washington, DC, 1986

Kernberg O: Borderline Conditions and Pathological Narcissism. New York, Jason Aronson, 1975

Kohut H: The Analysis of the Self. New York, International Universities Press, 1971

Lewis M, Feiring C, McGuffog C, et al: Predicting psychopathology in six-year-olds from early social relations. Child Dev 55:123–136, 1984

Mahler M, Pine F, Bergman A: The Psychological Birth of the Human Infant. New York, Basic Books, 1975

Moore T: Exclusive early mothering and its alternative: the outcome to adolescence. Scand J Psychol 16:255–272, 1975

Murphy L: Further reflections on resilience, in The Vulnerable Child. Edited by Anthony E, Cohler B. New York, Guilford Press, 1987, pp 84–105

Nachman PC: A study of daytime separation from mother. Paper presented at the Conference on Infant and Toddler Care, San Francisco, CA, June 1986

Nagera HC: Day care centers: red light, green light or amber light? Int J Psychoanal 2:121–137, 1975

Neubauer P: Preoedipal objects and object primacy. Psychoanal Study Child 40:163–182, 1985

Peters D: A Summary of the Pennsy Warrior Day Care Study. University Park, PA, Pennsylvania State University Press, 1973

Phillips D, McCartney D, Scarr S, et al: Selective review of infant day care research: a cause for concern. Zero to Three 7(3):18–21, 1987

Provence S: A program of group day care for young children, in Early Child Day Care. Edited by Neubauer P. New York, Jason Aronson, 1974, pp 11–17

Ramey C, Mills P: Social and intellectual consequences of day care for high risk infants, in Social Development in Childhood: Daycare Programs and Research. Edited by Webb R. Baltimore, MD, Johns Hopkins University Press, 1977, pp 79–110

Robertson J, Robertson J: Young children in brief separation: a fresh look. Psychoanal Study Child 26:264–315, 1971

Rutter M: Maternal Deprivation Reassessed, 2nd Edition. Harmondsworth, UK, Penguin, 1981

Rutter M: Epidemiological-longitudinal approaches to the study of development, in The Concept of Development. Edited by Collins WEA. Hillsdale, NJ, Erlbaum. Paper presented at the Minnesota Symposia on Child Psychology 15:105–144, 1982

Rutter M: Continuities and discontinuities in socioemotional development: empirical and conceptual perspectives, in Continuities and Discontinuities in Development. Edited by Emde R, Harmon R. New York, Plenum, 1984a, pp 41–68

Rutter M: Family and school influences: meanings, mechanisms and implications, in Longitudinal Studies in Child Psychology and Psychiatry: Practical Lessons from Research Experience. Edited by Nicol AR. Chichester, UK, John Wiley, 1984b, pp 114–137

Sander LW, Stechler G, Burns P, et al: Change in infant and caregiver variables over the first two months of life: integration of action in early development, in Origins of the Infant's Social Responsiveness. Edited by Thomas E. Hillsdale, NJ, Erlbaum, 1978, pp 66–79

Schaffer HR: Studies in Mother-Infant Interaction. New York, Academic, 1977

Schaffer HR, Emerson PE: The Development of Social Attachments in Infancy. Monographs of the Society for Research in Child Development, Vol 29 (ser no 94). Lafayette, IN, Child Development Publications of the Society for Research in Child Development, 1964, pp 1–77

Siefer R, Sameroff A: Multiple determinants of risk and invulnerability, in The Invulnerable Child. Edited by Anthony E, Cohler B. New York, Guilford, 1987, pp 51–69

Sroufe LA: The coherence of individual development: early care, attachment and subsequent developmental issues. 2:834–841, 1979

Sroufe LA, Fox ME, Pancake VR: Attachment and dependency in developmental perspective. Child Dev 54:1615–1627, 1983

Stern D: The Interpersonal World of the Infant. New York, Basic Books, 1985

Thomas A, Chess S: The Dynamics of Psychological Development. New York, Brunner/Mazel, 1980

Thompson RA, Lamb ME: Harmonizing discordant notes: a reply to Waters. Child Dev 54:521–524, 1983

Thompson RA, Lamb ME, Estes D: Stability of infant-mother attachment and its relationship in changing life circumstances in an unselected middle-class sample. Child Dev 53:144–148, 1982

Tizzard B, Hodges J: The effect of early institutional rearing on the development of eight-year-old children. J Child Psychol Psychiatry 19:99–118, 1978

Tyson R: Some narcissistic consequences of object loss: a developmental view. Psychoanal Q 52:205–224, 1983

Vaughn B, Egeland B, Sroufe LA, et al: Individual differences in infant-mother attachment at 12 and 18 months: stability and change in the family under stress. Child Dev 50:971–975, 1979

Vaughn B, Gove F, Egeland B: The relationship between out-of-home care and quality of infant-mother attachment in an economically disadvantaged sample. Child Dev 51:1203–1214, 1980

Wallerstein J: Children of divorce: preliminary report of a ten-year followup of older children and adolescents. J Am Acad Child Adolesc Psychiatry 24:545–553, 1985

Wallston B: The effects of maternal employment on children. J Child Psychol Psychiatry 14:81–90, 1973

Waters E: The stability of individual differences in infant-mother attachment: comments on the Thompson, Lamb and Estes contribution. Child Dev 54:512–520, 1983

Werner E, Smith R: Vulnerable but Invincible. New York, McGraw-Hill, 1982

Yarrow LJ, Klein RP: Environmental discontinuity associated with transition from foster to adoptive homes. International Journal of Behavior and Development 3:311–322, 1980

Part II

The Relationship Between Parents and Child Care Providers

Chapter 6

Balancing Working and Parenting

Shahla S. Chehrazi, M.D.

Although some attention has been paid to the experience of children in day care, little attention has been given to the experience of the parents. Yet we are aware that the relationship between parents and child is reciprocal, so that anything that affects one will affect the other.

Combining working and parenting, though desirable (Hock 1978), is difficult and stressful. In today's society, parents face the challenges of how to balance a career with child care and how to make child care arrangements that are best for both the parent and the child. In this chapter I will address the conflicts inherent in the situation and offer some guidelines for anticipating and confronting these challenges. In addition, I will report on a pilot study that interviews working mothers.

PARENTHOOD

Becoming a parent is associated with new tasks and new stresses, as well as with new sources of pleasure and satisfaction. Conceiving of parenthood as a developmental stage (Benedek 1959; Naylor 1970) is helpful in gaining perspective on the complexity of parenthood (see also Carter and McGoldrick 1980). Any developmental stage involves both new opportunities for growth and new potentials for vulnerabilities and regres-

103

sion. How well the particular task of each developmental stage is carried out depends in part on how well the conflicts of earlier phases have been resolved. Each developmental stage also presents a new opportunity for reworking earlier conflicts. Successful parenting provides the parent with an opportunity to work on the earlier unresolved problems, resulting in a new level of personality integration and maturity.

Learning to parent is a gradual process: new mothers and fathers do not become expert parents overnight. Developing a mutually gratifying relationship between infant and parent takes considerable time. But working parents are pressured for time and may feel torn between their work and wanting to spend more time with their child. Overall, working parents are often under considerable stress from multiple causes, including economic need and job pressures. Although the use of substitute care provides some relief from the demands on the parents' time, anxiety about the child care arrangement is in itself a source of stress. Most working parents interviewed in a pilot study felt that finding and supervising child care and adjusting to changes in caregivers are the most difficult and stressful parts of parenting.

A "good enough" parenting experience leads to the parent's development of confidence in his or her ability to parent, which is intimately related to the development of the child's confidence in the parent. The development of confidence or basic trust (Erikson 1964) in the caregiving environment is the main developmental task of the first year of life, and it is a prerequisite for later healthy emotional development. By the same token, the development of confidence as a parent is the most important achievement in the early stage of parenthood. This development is a mutually interwoven process that begins at the time of the birth of the infant and gradually evolves in the context of the parent-infant relationship. Between the infant's second and fourth months, there are usually observable signs of the parent's sense of confidence in his or her ability to comfort the baby. This confidence is also evident in the parent's response to the baby's smiling (Brazelton 1983); the parent demonstrates his or her awareness that the child is treating the parent differentially and is smiling specifically at him or her.

Parenting is a complex process, and at its core lies the parent's relationship with his or her own parents. Often parents find themselves repeating what was done to them, even when they consciously wish to do otherwise. Yet a common motivation for becoming a parent is the wish to be a better parent than one's own parents. Generally, this powerful wish helps parents to be more creative in their pattern of responses to their children and enhances growth in their parenting. Yet parents who have forgotten and repressed their own experiences of early childhood will repeat their parents' patterns. This situation often occurs without conscious awareness of the repetition, and such "forgetting" is common in child abuse.

As mentioned earlier, in the reciprocal interaction between the infant and the caregiver, a sense of trust gradually develops that later extends to the environment at large. The parent's confidence in his or her parenting ability is the first building block. Out-of-home work does not dampen the emotional intensity between the parent and child and should not compromise the development of confidence in the parent. The strength and constancy of the parents' emotional presence compared to that of other caregivers is an important reason for the child's attachment to them. Lieberman (1986, p. 3) suggests the following:

> Even more than the parent's daily presence, it is the parent's love for her child and the child's perception of and receptiveness to this love that enable the child to single the parent out from all other caregivers. A parent's passion for his or her child, with its many nuances of emotional intensity, ranging from delight to anger, is not dampened by a long working day. Even very young infants are smart enough to recognize this passion and to respond to it. Most likely this emotional claim is what mobilizes the integrative ego mechanisms that theorists postulate to explain why a baby recognizes his parents and prefers them in spite of other social input.

I would like to emphasize the importance and the primacy of the infant's attachment to his or her parents that is maintained in various caregiving environments. Because of feelings of anxiety and insecurity, parents tend to underestimate their primary importance to their infant. It is important for a parent to trust that the infant strongly distinguishes the parent's love and devotion in the midst of his or her experiences with other caregivers.

Although infants will make a more intense, specific attachment to one person, namely the primary caregiver, we have learned that when multiple caregivers participate in the caregiving environment, the infant is capable of attachment to all of them. For example, the father-infant relationship is separate from the mother-infant relationship and has its own distinct nature (Abelin 1971). Separate and distinct relationships are also established with siblings. Substitute care introduces yet another relationship. In the hierarchy of attachment (Bowlby 1969), siblings, grandparents, or extended family and caregivers follow the parents or the primary attachment figure. The infant's ability to relate to multiple caregivers seems to be related to his or her capacity to integrate the image of multiple caregivers with the image of the primary caregiver or the parents.

Our current theoretical understanding, drawn from observational research studies (Mahler et al. 1975; Stern 1985) and clinical work with young children (Fraiberg 1980; Greenspan 1981; Neubauer 1985), suggests that infants and toddlers gradually develop an inner or internal image of the parents, which is often an integrated image of all the caregivers but emphasizes the primary caregiver. Correspondingly, an internal image of the self develops in the interaction with the caregiver. The development of a basic trust and confidence in the external world is usually in progress when the child has a stable internal image of the parent and can mentally recall the parental image in the parent's absence. This stable parental image corresponds to a stable or cohesive image of the self, which gradually evolves into self and object constancy. It seems plausible that for the development of a stable internal image of the parent, the infant or toddler needs to be with the parent and have repeated interaction and visual and auditory input. These interactions reinforce the infant's memory and mental image of the parents. In other words, the repeated interaction between parent and child becomes internalized, leading to a cohesive sense of self and object.

In addition, we know that what is important is the continuity of relationships rather than the exclusive relationship with one person. For example, it has been demonstrated that parents almost always remain the primary attachment figures for the infants, which makes sense since parents are generally the only constant figures in the infant's life.

The foregoing theoretical considerations have implications for the number of caregivers and the length of time spent in day care. Changes in caregiver or stability of care are important determinants in the quality of care. Studies (see Howes, Chapter 2, this volume; Howes and Stewart 1987) showed that children who changed child care arrangements more often were less competent in their play with peers. The researchers concluded that the stability of child care arrangements was more important than the age at which the child began child care. An unstable caregiving environment or a setting that lacks continuity or predictability is detrimental to the infant's development (Farber and Egeland 1982).

The length of time in day care has only recently emerged as an important factor interacting with the quality of care. Early studies showed no differences in attachment to the parents when children were in part-time or full-time care. One study that examined the effect of the length of the time in day care (Schwartz 1983) showed that the infants who were in full-time care exhibited greater avoidance of their mothers. The infants in part-time care were no different in attachment to their mothers from infants not in child care.

The Yale Child Study Center findings (Provence et al. 1977) showed that children attending the day care center on a part-time basis did well, showing little evidence of delay in the development of attachment to their parents or in their cognitive and emotional development. This case was also true of the children whose parents stopped by during their lunch time.

The children who were at the center full-time seemed to have increasing difficulty toward the end of the day, expressing fatigue, lowered mood, clinginess, temper tantrums, and crying repeatedly and asking for their parents. In some cases, there was evidence of some delay in the development of attachment to the parents. Yet, the Provence study was a clinical one, and it was not designed with careful research methodology. Another limitation of the study is that the parents were all from the lower socio-economic class, which may represent an additional stress on the parent-child relationship.

Even though the current research findings on the implications of length of time in day care are limited and require replication, it seems likely that long hours of being away from the parents can often be stressful for the infant. In other words, the infant misses the parent. He or she is comforted if he or she can internally evoke the image of the absent parent. The missing of the parent and the associated internal evocation of the parent's image routinely and repeatedly occur when children are in substitute care. This process is related to the adaptive capacity of the infants and toddlers in coping with separation from the parents (see Nachman, Chapter 8, this volume). At this early age, however, the infant's or toddler's memory is somewhat limited, and fatigue and illness can seriously hamper his or her adaptive capacity for coping with separation.

Another source of concern is that when parents work full-time, they are away from the infant 9 to 10 hours a day. Being away from an infant or toddler for this long is not only a stressful situation for the child but is also stressful for the parents. The morning hours are very rushed, and the evening hours are burdened by fatigue and housework. Thus, the parent and child are left with only 1 to 2 hours a day to spend together.

It is important that these few hours be relaxed and enjoyable for both parent and child. Here, the parents' support of each other and sharing of child care responsibilities are essential. In a study of transition to parenthood, Cowan and his colleagues (1985) found that when men and women did not share parenting but instead drew apart into their respective stereotyped gender roles, there was greater dissatisfaction with the marriage following the birth of a child. When a parent is physically exhausted and emotionally drained, he or she may gradually react with emotional withdrawal and subsequently feel less connected to the child. This defensive withdrawal is also observed in some parents who are anticipating return to full-time work (Brazelton 1985).

A mistaken notion in parenting is the issue of quality time. Quality time is supposed to be the time that is in tune with the infant or toddler's needs. With the parents working full-time and the fatigue of the end of the day, scheduling a time that works out as quality time for both parent and infant is almost impossible. What is equally important is the quantity of time spent with the children, particularly with young children. Even though it is important for time spent with children to be enjoyable, one must not lose sight of the importance of simply being there. Clearly, some minimum amount of time must be spent by parents with their children if normal child-parent attachment is to develop with resulting optimal development in the children.

PILOT STUDY

Because of my interest in balancing career and parenting, I conducted a small, clinical pilot study to learn about the many different ways that working and parenting are currently combined. In this study I interviewed 20 mothers who had returned to work within 4 months of the birth of their infants. The mothers were a group of professional women who were in more or less successful marital relationships. Because of the difficulty of arranging interviews with the fathers, they were not included in the pilot study. According to the mothers, most of the fathers participated actively in the care of their child to varying degrees.

Like a number of other studies, this study found that, even though fathers attempted to be active participants in the child care, the burden was mainly left to the mothers. When parents chose to work part-time, it was usually the mother who, mostly due to financial reasons, cut back her work hours. The child care arrangements in this group varied among family day care, center care, and in-home individual care.

I interviewed the mothers in a semistructured interview setting for 1 hour. The clinical interview was designed to assess the parent's sense of confidence and satisfaction in her parenting. My findings were that maternal satisfaction was highest in the group who returned to work on a part-time basis. These mothers felt that they were lucky to be able to continue to work and also have enough time with their child to enjoy his or her growing up. This fact was independent of the type of care the parents had chosen.

In the group of mothers who returned to full-time work, mixed results were found, regardless of the type of care arrangements. One mother who had chosen in-home care felt competitive with her nanny and at times felt less confident in her mothering because she felt the child was very attached to the nanny. On the other hand, this mother was grateful that her nanny was so loving and emotionally responsive to her child. When frustrated by her conflicted feelings toward her nanny, she reminded herself that it was best for her child to feel comfortable loving them both. Another mother, whose job required frequent out-of-town trips, appeared defensive regarding the time away from her baby, denying any mixed feelings such as missing her baby, yet feeling that it was important for her career at this time to pursue her out-of-town commitments. During the interview, she repeatedly reassured herself and me that the baby was well taken care of and was receiving individual quality care at home.

In the group with out-of-home care arrangements, mixed results were observed. One full-time working mother whose child was in high-quality day care (staff-child ratio of 1 to 2) felt pleased about the care her child was receiving, seemed quite confident as a mother, and felt she was in tune with her child. Another mother who had returned to work full-time felt overwhelmed by the demands of parenting and her work. She had chosen a large family day care arrangement (10 children, with staff-child ratio of 1 to 5) mainly because of its location, since she needed to commute. This mother expressed feeling guilty that she hadn't been able to be as good a mother as she had wished to be. She felt somewhat depressed about having failed internally as a mother, that is, not living up to her own standards of mothering. This mother's description of her child and her interaction with her left me with the impression of a depressed mother-infant pair. What burdened this particular pair was the infant's recurrent infections and illnesses, possibly intensified by her attendance at family day care. The mother related in detail how her 3-month-old infant contracted one infection after another from the day she had entered the family day care. Even though she felt she was able to manage the illnesses and had only lost 1 day of work, the result was additional stress on the mother-infant relationship, with irritability and clinginess on the part of the infant. In this family, the father was working 4 days a week and was participating actively in the child care.

The findings of this small pilot study can only suggest criteria for a more systematic study; for example, a future study needs to include interviews with the fathers as well. Nevertheless, an interesting finding was the strong association between the mother's satisfaction with child care arrangements and a working relationship with the caregiver or child care provider. As a result of this study, I have become interested in the issue of full-time versus part-time work. It appears that two central questions require further exploration: 1) What is the impact of the length of time or number of hours on the experience of separation for both the parent and child? 2) Do long hours (9–10 hours a day) of being away from the parent delay the development of attachment in the infant? The answers to these questions require further research, since current research findings are ambiguous on this subject (Belsky 1986a, 1986b; Belsky and Steinberg 1978; Schwartz 1983).

THE ROLE OF THE FATHER IN DAY CARE

Research studies on fatherhood suffer from the absence of data on the role of the father in day care. The following discussion is derived from studies on the father's role in general. Several show that when mothers are employed, the degree of paternal involvement substantially increases (Lamb et al. 1985; Pleck 1983). It is plausible to assume that when both parents are employed, the use of substitute care is inevitable. Even though the focus of these studies is not on the use of substitute care or day care, we can nevertheless infer that with working parents who use substitute care, the amount of paternal involvement is substantially higher.

The studies of fathers who are responsible for at least 40% to 45% of the within-family child care are of interest. These studies show that the preschool-age children whose fathers share in or take primary responsibility for child care are characterized by increased cognitive competence, increased empathy, fewer sex-stereotyped beliefs, and a more internal locus of control (Pruett 1983; Radin 1982; Radin and Sagi 1982; Sagi 1982). Lamb's (1986, p. 17) discussion of these findings explains the following different variables:

> First, it is not surprising that the children have less sex-stereotyped attitudes themselves about male and female roles. Second, in the area of cognitive competence, these children may benefit from having two highly involved parents rather than just one; this assures them a diversity of stimulation that comes from interacting with different people who have different behavioral styles. A third important issue has to do with the family context with which these children are raised. In every study reported thus far, high paternal involvement made it possible for both parents to do what was subjectively important to them. It allowed fathers to satisfy a desire to become close to their children, and it allowed mothers to have adequately close relationships with their children while also being involved in pursuit of career goals that were important to them. In other words, increased paternal involvement in the families studied has made both parents feel much more fulfilled. Therefore, the positive outcomes obtained by children with highly involved fathers are largely attributable to the fact that the father's involvement created a family context in which parents felt good about their marriages and about the arrangements they had been able to work out.

In fact, in all the studies, the fathers were involved because both parents wanted this arrangement. The results might be quite different if the fathers were forced to become involved or were forced to stay home (e.g., if they were laid off or if they resented staying home and really wanted to work and support their families). This different constellation of factors may have an adverse effect on children. The central issue appears to be the reasons for the paternal involvement, rather than the extent of the involvement. Therefore, the positive effects of paternal involvement seem to have more to do with family context and the particular family dynamics. That is, high paternal involvement may have positive effects in some circumstances and negative effects in others. The recent changes in average levels of paternal involvement in the studies cited appear to be in the direction of the increasing number of families in which greater father involvement is associated with positive effects on children's development. In general, the characteristics of the father as a parent and the quality of the relationship with the child, rather than the characteristics of the father as a man, appear to influence child development. This situation is in contrast to earlier studies that emphasized masculine identification as the primary role of the father.

The key factors influencing paternal involvement are reported to be motivation, skill and self-confidence, institutional practices, and support from the spouse (Lamb 1986). Self-confidence and skill enhance the motivation factor. Parenting skills are mostly acquired on the job (see the "Parenthood" section in this chapter). In the context of the reciprocal parent-child relationship, the more time fathers or mothers spend with their children, the more confident and competent they'll feel about themselves as parents. In this vein, flexible time scheduling would be of great value to employed fathers as well as to mothers, enabling them to spend more time with their children. The absence of support on the part of the mother usually undermines and diminishes paternal involvement. However, my impression from the pilot study on mothers is that institutional practices are the most influential factors in determining the degree of parental involvement.

THE ROLE OF THE FATHER IN ATTACHMENT STUDIES

A serious limitation of studies on day care and attachment is the absence of the father in the study of attachment. It is likely that any inconsistent findings are related to overlooking this relationship to the father. It appears that attachment studies cannot be complete without evaluation and assessment of the attachment relationship to the fathers. More recent studies on attachment have paid attention to this omission and have applied the Strange Situation technique. Contrary to the assumption that if infants are securely attached to the mothers, the same type of attachment will be extended to the relationship with the fathers, Main and her colleagues (1985) found no relationship between security of attachment to the father and the mother in infancy. They found that an infant who is secure with the mother is almost equally likely to be secure or insecure with the father. This finding has been reported in two American studies (Lamb 1978; Main and Weston 1981) and one German study (Grossman et al. 1981).

Clearly, any conclusions about the role of the father in child care are preliminary and tentative. Future studies on the effects of day care need to include the child's relationship with the mother and the father, as well as the family context in which child care is chosen. In brief, the recent studies on increased paternal involvement in the families where both parents work show that the father's choice to participate more in child care is associated with positive developmental outcome in the children. Institutional practices are among the key factors that influence paternal involvement.

PARENTS AND DAY CARE

In a recent national study (U.S. Congress 1984), parents reported three main problems with child care: lack of information, unavailability, and expense. As a clinician, I consider the lack of information to be the major problem. For the most part, the available information is inaccurate, contradictory, or so ambiguous that it is of little assistance to parents. What is helpful to parents is clear and scientifically sound information. In fact, a parent need not be overwhelmed or confused. The three overriding issues confronting parents and about which they need to learn as much as possible are the following:

1. How to help the child with separation
2. How to assess and evaluate the quality of substitute care
3. How to develop a working relationship with the child care provider

How to Help the Child With Separation

Helping the child with separation is the central issue in substitute care. A parent must be sensitive to the child's experience of separation and at the same time be aware of his or her own feelings about separating from the child (see Kalmanson, Chapter 9, this volume). A parent may feel anxiety, guilt, doubt, uncertainty, and worry about the child's well-being. Experiencing the full emotional intensity of separation from the child, although burdensome, may reflect a parent's empathic understanding of the child's experience. In other words, by understanding the child's separation protests, a parent is less likely to react with irritation, anger, or rejection. Furthermore, the parent's empathic response prevents the formation of defensive reactions such as denial or avoidance of the separation experience. When this situation occurs, the parent reassures himself or herself that the child is well taken care of, ignoring the child's distress, and withdraws from an intense emotional relationship with the child.

It is important to understand that a parent's feelings of anxiety and guilt in response to daily separation is not only a normal reaction but one that needs to be cherished. Guilt and anxiety about separation from one's child are often signals of connectedness to the child and may reflect empathic understanding of the child's experience of separation. Of interest is the Stanford Day Care Study (Everson et al. 1984), which found that mothers who were reluctant to place their children in day care had children who did better in cooperation with an adult, were more compliant with the mother's prohibitions, and were more willing to share and help than children whose mothers were quite willing to place their infants in day care. This finding suggests that mothers who are sensitive to the emotional repercussions of early daily separations and group care can help their children cope with these stresses through empathic support. There is another interpretation as well: the group of mothers who wanted to place their children in day care included mothers who were more rejecting of their children. A more recent study (Barglow et al. 1987) found a high correlation between maternal separation reaction and secure attachment in infants.

There is a tendency in the recent literature, particularly as popularized in the media, to minimize the parents' guilt reaction and even to advocate the denial of any feelings of anxiety and guilt. Guilt, like any other human emotion such as love, joy, or anger, needs to be respected and understood. However, exaggerated guilt reactions that interfere with the parents' overall functioning or the attachment to the child require attention or intervention.

In the pilot study, most mothers reported missing their child, at times painfully, and felt conflicted and torn between their child and their work. Although the conflict is inherent in the situation, there are ways to minimize it. For example, the mothers who were able to arrange flexible work hours felt more in control and reported enjoyment in their working as well as parenting, in spite of the inevitable fatigue and exhaustion. In contrast, the mothers who had inflexible and rigid work hours felt overburdened and helpless in their situation.

Returning to the issue of separation, the parent's task is to help the child master the separation experience. This task is achieved by acknowledging the separation and helping the child participate in saying good-bye. The process of changing passive into active is an important step in the mastery of psychological tasks in children; consequently, it is important for the child to participate actively in separation rather than experience it passively. A common mistake is for the parent to suddenly disappear, a situation that is often encouraged by caregivers and teachers. The serious disadvantage of this approach is that it deprives the child of the opportunity to participate in, confront, and master the separation. It is important to remember that temper tantrums, crying, and separation protests can be healthy and normal reactions to separation. In other words, parents and caregiver need to be more worried about a child who does not respond to separation from the parent by crying or protesting than about the child who exhibits separation protest.

Needless to say, the separation protest needs to be understood within the context of reunion behavior. The child's behavior upon union with the parent has gained more significance in the recent research studies (Bretherton and Waters 1985). The gradual mastery of separation is accompanied by diminished anxiety at the time of parting. This decrease in anxiety is expressed in less crying and a gradual shortening of subsequent distress periods. Usually it takes 3 to 4 weeks for the child's visible stress to diminish and ultimately cease, and it accompanies the child's growing recognition that the parent will return. If there is no progress in separation distress within 3 to 4 weeks, a reevaluation of the situation is in order. For example, a different child care setting or delaying the placement of the child may be indicated. Often, a change to a smaller group setting (small family day care) and more sensitivity on the part of the parent and caregiver bring about marked improvement.

Exposing the child to continued overwhelming anxiety and distress (e.g., hours of unattended crying) undermines subsequent emotional development. In helping the child with separation, the parents and caregiver should follow the premise of "optimal frustration" for the child. Excessive frustration, which is frustration beyond the adaptive capacity of the child, provokes feelings of helplessness, despair, and exaggerated aggression (Lieberman, Chapter 4, this volume; Parens 1979). Optimal frustration refers to a level of frustration that matches the child's adaptive capacity and promotes the child's mastery of the situation. In other words, optimal frustration promotes development, whereas excessive or long-term frustration hinders development. Like other developmental tasks, separation needs to be mastered in gradual and increasing doses.

As a consultant to day care centers, I recommend a minimum 1-week transition period for parents and children. Initially, the parents are asked to stay with the child for about one-half hour and leave the child for about 1 to 2 hours. Gradually, as the child's need for the parents in the unfamiliar environment is decreased, the parents can reduce the time they spend at the center prior to the separation and the length of time the child spends at the center can be increased. Monitoring the transition is left entirely to the individual parent and child, and the staff remains supportive to both.

A transition period for the adjustment of parent and child to separation is, of course, impossible if the mother is returning to work at the same time. It is therefore necessary for the parent to plan the placement of the child at least 1 week prior to returning to work. My recommendation to mothers is to use this week as the "mental health" week, giving themselves and the child time to adjust to the separation. In addition, this week can help parents recover from exhaustion and fatigue so that they will be more prepared to return to full- or part-time work.

In discussions of separation at day care center staff meetings, the staff is trained to help the child with separation. For example, the use of transitional objects such as a blanket or a favorite toy from home is encouraged. Pictures of parents are also helpful to the child in recalling the image of the parent. In fact, at one center the staff designated one of the walls for pictures of the children and their parents. When a child is asking or crying for the absent parent, a staff member talks to the child about the parent and takes the child over to the pictures, reassuring the child that the parent will return soon. It must be noted that, even when separation is more or less mastered, during periods of stress such as illness the separation anxiety may reappear. The parent's or caregiver's sensitivity and understanding are helpful in supporting the child during these periods.

As stated earlier, a transition period seems to offer an opportunity for adjustment for both the child and the parent. In other words, the issue is not so much when to return to work but how to do it. The following case example illustrates the impact of an abrupt return to work.

Ms. G. returned to full-time work when her child was 7 months of age. She came to see me because her infant was showing some signs of depression. That is, the infant had lost her exuberance, joy, and curiosity about her environment and had become passive and withdrawn. In this case, both the age of the child and the abrupt way in which the mother returned to full-time work were factors. Ms. G. carefully selected an in-home caregiver for her daughter and was surprised with the child's strong reaction to her returning to work in view of the fact that she was receiving quality care at home. A highly sensitive and devoted mother, she observed the signs of depression in her daughter, and her awareness and empathy helped the resolution of the infant's depression over the subsequent 2 months. Retrospectively, it seems that this mother had focused all her energy on how long she could stay away from her job, disregarding the importance of a gradual transition back to work.

The transition period is a helpful guideline for babysitters as well. My advice in hiring new nannies or housekeepers is to begin their work on a weekend so that the child has the opportunity to be around the mother and the new person over a period of time. With new babysitters, it is helpful to have them visit the child on a couple of occasions and to start at least a few hours prior to the parent's leave-taking, so that the child has an opportunity to become familiar with the newcomer. Parents should also prepare their child for the separation and explain to him or her that they will be leaving shortly and will return at a particular time.

It is important for parents to be present when their child is being introduced to a new environment or person to develop trust in the strange situation. With younger infants who have not yet developed language, such introductions can easily be overlooked, and the parents may fail to prepare the infant when introducing a new person. Similarly, saying good-bye or preparing the child for separation may also be overlooked with infants and preverbal children. Recent infant observational studies on the origins of affective development are of interest in this regard (e.g., Emde 1983). They demonstrate the development of an affective, preverbal language between mother and child. In confronting a new situation or task, the preverbal infant looks to the mother for cues of safety or danger in order to proceed or withdraw. This study illustrates that the infant's point of reference for safety and trust in the environment is the parent. Put differently, the parent's confidence or trust in the new person or environment will be clearly communicated to the child at a preverbal stage.

To understand the child's experience in confronting new caregivers or caregiving environments, a helpful exercise for parents is to imagine how they would feel if every day at work they were confronted with a new boss, some of whom even changed the physical environment of the office. The child's feelings of shock and loss can be minimized if parents are prepared for the changes and can anticipate them.

Finally, where separation is concerned, another consideration in addition to the transition period is the length of time in substitute care, which is emerging as a significant determinant in the effect of child care. In the absence of any definitive research findings (Gamble and Zigler 1986; Phillips et al. 1987), a more cautious attitude about the length of time in child care is advisable. Parents need to consider seriously their return to full-time work during the infant's first year of life. They need to examine carefully any possible options. For example, one option is for each parent to work 4 days a week, which reduces the infant's or toddler's time in full-time care to 3 days a week or fewer. If the off days are spread through the week, a balance is created between the time spent with the child and the time spent away from the child (e.g., 2 days in child care, 1 day with one parent, 1 day in child care, the next day with the other parent, and the weekends with both parents). Five full days in child care and intense togetherness on weekends are often stressful for both parent and child.

How to Evaluate Quality of Substitute Care

Unambiguous information is available to parents about evaluating the quality of care. There is growing evidence that poor-quality care is detrimental to the child's development. Recent research studies on quality of care (Howes and Rubenstein 1985) have identified various guidelines for high-quality care. The experts are in general agreement regarding the following quality indicators:

1. Staff-child ratio—1 to 3 for infants, 1 to 5 for toddlers
2. Staff training—in particular, training in child development
3. Group size—smaller group size is preferred (5–6 children in a group)
4. Stability of care

In addition, other important quality indicators include family stress, the child's age at time of entry into care, and the length of time in care. (See Howes, Chapter 2, this volume, for discussion of staff-child ratio and staff training.)

Group size. Group size is an important consideration in evaluating the quality of care. Simply stated, the size of the group needs to be manageable for the caregiver. In most high-quality day care centers, groups of children are divided into smaller units of children and staff. Since this division requires more administrative work, some centers tend not to do it. Another consideration in group care is group mix. The group mix is an important factor (Kahn and Kamerman 1986) in addition to group size, particularly in family day care. Parents choosing family day care should inquire about the group mix: for example, how many children are under 2 years of age? Considering the ratio of 1 caregiver to 6 children, the number of infants and toddlers should probably not exceed 2. Reports on large family day care homes (2 caregivers to 10 or 12 children) are ambiguous. Some experts feel that mixing toddlers with older children is not advisable since they have different developmental needs (Rutter 1981).

Stability of care. The stability of care and the age of entry into child care appear to be interrelated. In other words, the sooner an infant is placed in child care, the higher the probability of change in the caregiver—simply because there is more time for changes to occur (Howes and Rubenstein 1985). Optimally, infants and toddlers experience no more than three to four changes in caregivers during the first 2 years of their lives. Even though research exploring the effect of these changes is lacking, it is likely that once the parent and the child establish a solid and secure attachment to each other, the child will more readily adapt to a reasonable number of changes in caregivers. This occurrence is illustrated in the following clinical vignette.

I saw Ms. B. in psychotherapy for job-related stress during her second pregnancy. She took advantage of her 6-month paid maternity leave and chose to stay home with her son and her 3-year-old daughter. When her son was 6 months old, she decided to return to school for further training. Periodically I saw Ms. B. with her son, when she brought him to the hour. When Ms. B. returned to school, she and her husband hired an in-home "babysitter" to care for their son, but the babysitter left within 8 months for a higher paying job. Subsequently, a younger relative, who lived with the family for 2 months, took care of the infant. When this relative left, the parents chose a family day care home with a ratio of 1 caregiver to 5 children. By the age of 18 months, Ms. B.'s son had experienced three different caregivers. I had observed the development of a secure attachment and a stable relationship between this mother and son from his early infancy. The caregiver changes were disruptive for both mother and son. However, Ms. B., who was her son's primary figure, was instrumental in helping her son's adaptation and mastery of these changes. More frequent changes in caregivers usually accompany family stress and appear to undermine infant development.

In reviewing the various kinds of quality substitute care, I was somewhat surprised by the frequency of changes in the caregiver in one-to-one in-home care. In most cases, the infant has three to four changes in caregiver during the first 2 years of life. The following vignette illustrates the frequency of the changes in caregivers.

M. returned to full-time work within 2 months of the birth of her baby. She hired an au pair, who took care of the infant for 6 months. After the au pair moved out of the area, she was replaced by a nanny, who lived with the family for 9 months. The nanny then decided that she wanted to pursue another career and was replaced by a housekeeper. Thus, by age 2, the child had had three changes in her special caregiver.

We are more familiar with changes in caregivers when it comes to center day care. The rate of turnover in the staff of day care centers (see Phillips and Whitebook, Chapter 7, this volume) approaches 50% to 60%. It is possible that high-quality center care offers fewer changes in caregivers compared to in-home care. We know little about the impact of these changes on the emotional development of infants and toddlers.

Based on the findings of the pilot study, it appears that the child care arrangement that offers the best continuity of care is small family day care—that is, family day care with a ratio of one adult to three to four children. Small family day care offers more continuity in care compared to in-home care or center care. A recent development in California, for example, is the large family day care, usually involving 10 to 12 children, with a ratio of 1 adult to 5 or 6 children. In my experience, the disadvantages of large family day care are the large size of the group, and since they are usually not as well equipped as center care, there is generally more exposure to various early childhood illnesses. This opinion, however requires further study.

One-to-one in-home care may give the illusion of being the best quality care because of the adult-child ratio and the familiar home environment. Yet what is important is not only the adult-child ratio but the relationship between the child and the caregiver. The crucial issue in child care is the quality of that relationship. The following case example illustrates the tendency for idealizing in-home care.

I was asked to see Danny, a 2½-year-old boy, in consultation for delayed speech development, lack of curiosity about his environment, and a withdrawn appearance. As part of the consultation, I routinely ask detailed questions about child care. In this case, I found out that Danny's first nanny had been with the family for 10 months. She was replaced by a housekeeper when Danny was 12 months old. I saw Danny and this housekeeper for one session as part of the consultation. A woman in her forties, she had left her country and her own family because of dire circumstances and appeared very depressed. She was not engaged in a relationship with Danny, and there was minimal interaction between them during the hour. The young parents, who were quite pressured by their concerns about advancement in their careers, felt that because they were providing one-to-one care for their child, they did not need to worry about the quality of care or the quality of the relationship between their child and the caregiver.

In our current sociopolitical climate, the burden of finding quality child care is laid squarely on the parents. Parents need to give themselves enough time to choose and locate affordable quality child care. They should plan for child care when they plan to have a baby. I know of parents who plan the pregnancy according to an expected opening on the waiting list of the local, high-quality child care setting.

In addition to the guidelines for quality care, parents need to follow their intuition and subjective experience. An open-door policy is a prerequisite for any high-quality care setting. Parents need to feel welcome to drop in to see the child—and should not feel like an intruder. Finally, I emphasize that parents need to choose the type of care that seems to fit their family needs best. It is important to find a match between parent child-rearing practices and the substitute care setting.

How to Develop a Working Relationship With Your Child Care Provider

A successful working relationship between parents and caregivers can provide a sense of continuity between home and day care, thus facilitating the mastery of separation for the child. It is therefore crucial for the parents to attempt to develop a working relationship with the caregiver—a relationship based on mutual respect and caring. This relationship needs to be developed in spite of the realistic pressures placed on both parties. Even though some attention has been paid to the importance of this relationship and how to promote the partnership between parents and providers, little progress has been made.

A study by Zigler and Turner (1982) found that parents spent an average of 7 minutes a day in their child's day care center and that 10% of the parents did not even enter the center. The failure of the relationship between parents and providers is alarming to most experts. This lack of relationship indicates that both parents and child care providers need to be educated about the importance of their partnership in child care, a partnership that is often forgotten in the hurry to get home after a long day. A failure in the relationship between the caregiver and the parents often results in the parents' avoidance of interaction with the caregiver, which often contributes to feelings of anger and isolation on the part of the parent or caregiver.

As noted earlier, the content analysis of the pilot study revealed a strong association between the mother's satisfaction with the child care arrangement and her relationship to the child care provider. Since the parent-provider relationship was not a focus of this study, the semistructured interview did not include any direct questions regarding the relationship with the child care provider. However, the issue came up during the interview when mothers volunteered information about their child care providers. One mother saw her child care provider as a model for herself. She had chosen a small family day care setting in which the provider was taking care of her own 2½-year-old daughter and another 18-month-old infant (adult-child ratio of 1 to 3). She perceived the provider as more maternal than herself and thus able to help her with her anxiety about her first child. Another mother perceived her day care provider as a grandmother to her child. She had chosen a woman in her fifties who was taking care of three children (one infant and two toddlers) in her home. The mother felt comfortable dropping by her family day care home and bringing food and cookies for the children. Another mother reported the same supportive relationship with her day care center; she had a particularly good relationship with one of the teachers and felt supported by the center in general. This mother had chosen a nonprofit, high-quality day care setting (staff-child ratio of 1 to 2) for her infant. The center had an open-door policy, encouraging parents to drop in and visit the child any time. This mother worked full-time, but since the day care center was close to her job, she was able to arrange to spend her lunch break with her infant three times a week.

Child care of any kind needs to be seen as a collaborative endeavor between parents and caregivers. There are three reciprocal, dyadic relationships in the caregiving environment: 1) the parents' relationship to the child, 2) the day care provider's relationship to the child, and 3) the parents' relationship to the day care provider. These relationships overlap and interact; they are not separate or independent. The working relationship with the day care provider is not only a source of support for the parents, but it is also important for the child's optimal development.

Understandably, the relationship between parents and the caregiver is burdened with intense feelings. To attribute a failure in the relationship between parents and caregiver merely to a lack of education or information is an oversimplification and an attempt to overlook the intense and complex emotional issues involved in the relationship. Powerful transferences to the caregiver either promote or interfere with the development of a working relationship between parents and the caregiver. In other words, the relationship is colored by feelings of anxiety, guilt, ambivalence, rivalry, envy, and competition. It is helpful for parents and caregivers to be aware of these feelings. When both parents and caregivers recognize that they are important to the child and that their partnership enhances the child's development, their relationship is strengthened by feelings of caring, mutuality, empathy, and joy.

Parents' intense feelings for the caregiver can be understood as positive, negative, and idealizing transferences. A parent may project his or her own feelings of guilt regarding the separation from the child onto the caregiver, perceiving him or her as critical and disapproving. This negative transference often leads to avoidance of contact and interaction with the caregiver and to the breakdown of the relationship. In an idealizing transference, the parents have a somewhat excessive admiration for the caregiver, associating him or her with an idealized parent image, and thus may be unaware of limitations and realistic shortcomings of the day care situation. A positive transference is, for the most part, helpful in establishing a feeling of trust in and a working partnership with the caregiver.

In a 1986 symposium entitled "Early Infant and Toddler Care," presented by the San Francisco Psychoanalytic Institute Extension Division, the most common feeling expressed by the providers was a feeling of being abused by both the system and the parents. The most common feeling expressed by the parents, on the other hand, was a sense of anxiety, discomfort, and avoidance of a relationship with the caregiver. The providers felt abused in general because of the long hours and low wages. However, in relation to the parent, they felt abused or mistreated specifically about late payments and parents' delays in picking up their child. In some cases, the feeling of being abused was extended to the child. Projecting their own feelings of mistreatment to the child, the providers felt that the child was also mistreated and neglected by the parents. If unrecognized, these feelings alienate parents and caregivers at the expense of the child. All too often, what each partner needs to hear is how he or she is appreciated by the other. Again, parents and caregivers need to recognize that their partnership is a key factor in enhancing the child's use of day care and in promoting his or her development.

During the early phase of parenting, because of anxiety and lack of experience, parents are insecure in their roles as parents and turn to others for advice, validation, and support. They may seek out their pediatrician, friends, and caregivers for support and reassurance. The substitute caregiver can play an important role in aiding the parents' sense of confidence and in enhancing their parenting skills. Often, caregivers underestimate their importance to the parents and the crucial role they can play in facilitating the parents' and child's optimal use of day care.

A helpful exercise for parents is a few minutes of reflection on their feelings regarding their caregiver. This reflection will help parents become aware of how the caregiver is perceived. Is he or she perceived generally as supportive and reassuring or as critical and rejecting? In examining and exploring their feelings, parents may be able to clarify some of the feelings that interfere with the development of a positive working relationship with the caregiver.

The caregiver is also in a vulnerable and difficult situation. He or she often feels overworked and underpaid, which undermines any capacity to empathize with the parents. Often the caregiver experiences the parents' visit or involvement in the program as intrusive. Training in child development usually helps the caregiver to be more aware of these issues and to be able to be sensitive and supportive toward parents. Most caregivers, however, feel that talking to the parents is an additional burden or another demand on their time; this feeling was expressed by most caregivers at the 1987 seminar of the San Francisco Psychoanalytic Institute Extension Division entitled "Mental Health Issues in Child Care." If parents are aware of these issues, they will not easily become discouraged by the lack of responsiveness on the part of teachers or caregivers. Parents need to accommodate to the caregiver's schedule and time limitations. The drop-in or pick-up time is not a good time for a relaxed conversation with the caregiver.

My suggestion to parents is to set up a special time (one-half hour) every week or two to talk comfortably with the caregiver, experience the day care environment, and interact with the children while helping the caregiver. In other words, unless asked to do otherwise, a parent should not behave as a neutral observer. Some caregivers may feel uncomfortable with an observer and prefer a parent who participates in the group setting. A parent needs to feel comfortable in the environment and imagine himself or herself as the caregiver's assistant. The most successful day care center I visited was a parent co-op. The parents took turns spending 1 day a week at the center. Other than their familiarity with the setting and the sense of continuity between home and day care, this setup increased the staff-child ratio without increasing the cost. In this center, all the parents worked full-time 4 days a week. This approach exemplifies day care as the extension of the nuclear family.

CONCLUSIONS

The following suggested guidelines are helpful in improving the child care experience for parents and children.

1. Network with other parents and request the help of your caregivers in developing an open-door policy at your child's day care setting.
2. Relate to your caregiver as an expert in the field of child care. Ask about his or her observations on your child. Express your concerns and ask advice. If you are a new parent, chances are that the caregiver knows much more than you do about child care. Find out if he or she belongs to the Association of Child Care Providers. Studies have shown this factor to be important in quality care, since it offers the provider a basis for support and education. If you are using a day care center, find out about its in-service training for the staff. Let the provider know you appreciate his or her advice and care.
3. Create bridges between your home and day care. It is important that you have an awareness of what goes on in your absence—the details of your child's daily schedule, nap time, meals, playtime, and so on. If you feel you do not know enough about your child's day, plan to spend some time at the center. This valuable experience provides you with a sense of continuity between home and day care. Your subjective experience of continuity and familiarity corresponds to your child's feelings and experience. Your child's transitional objects are helpful in creating a bridge between home and day care. Such special objects as blankets, soft toys, or your child's favorite toy have significant psychological meaning for your child. Pictures of you with your child posted on the wall are also helpful to your child.
4. Negotiate spending one-half hour a week or every other week at the center for a relaxed time during which you can observe and interact with all the children and the caregivers. Imagine yourself as a caregiver and participate in the environment. If you are working full-time, you can arrange to leave work earlier or start work later once a week or every other week. A long lunch break is another option.

The following suggested guidelines are helpful in promoting and enhancing parenting.

1. *Planning.* It is important to plan your child care when you plan to have a baby. Considering the scarcity of affordable quality child care, you need to give yourself enough time to locate and choose a high-quality child care setting.

2. *Conflict.* Feelings of being torn between time spent at work and time with your child are inherent in the situation. You need to compromise and realize that a sense of loss is unavoidable either way. By attempting to create a balance between your work and your parenting, you will be less conflicted and more able to enjoy both.

3. *Maternity leave.* The early months of an infant's life are the most important time for the development of attachment. Attachment theory has also shown that around 6 months or so, the attachment to a specific figure emerges. A minimum of 4 months' maternity leave is recommended by experts in the field (Brazelton 1985; Zigler and Muenchow 1984). Explore all your options at work and demand sufficient maternity leave with job security.

4. *Quality care.* Try to gain as much information as you can and take advantage of community resources. Review the literature available on selecting day care and become aware of the guidelines for evaluating quality care.

5. *Transition period in returning to work.* Plan a gradual transition to part- or full-time work. Trust your feelings and intuition as a parent, and be creative about your gradual return to work. This transitional period is not only for your infant but also for you. It is to help you and your child adjust to the gradual separation.

6. *Spouse.* Turn to your spouse for help and emotional support. A successful marital relationship is one of the strongest indicators of successful parenting (Cowan et al. 1985).

7. *Joy.* Plan relaxed time with your child when you are not struggling with fatigue or exhaustion and pressured by work or housework. Be determined to enjoy your experience of parenting and observe the joy in your child.

REFERENCES

Abelin EL: The role of the father in the separation-individuation process, in Separation-Individuation. Edited by McDevitt J, Settlage C. New York, International Universities Press, 1971, pp 229–252

Barglow P, Vaughn B, Molitor N: Effects of maternal absence due to employment on the quality of infant/mother attachment in a low-risk sample. Child Dev 58:945–954, 1987

Belsky J: Infant day care: cause for concern. Zero to Three 6(5):1–9, 1986a

Belsky J: Infant day care: cause for concern. Zero to Three 7(3):22–24, 1986b

Belsky J, Steinberg L: The effects of day care: a critical review. Child Dev 49:929–949, 1978

Benedek T: Parenthood as a developmental phase. J Am Psychoanal Assoc 7:389–409, 1959

Bowlby J: Attachment and Loss, Vol 1: Attachment. New York, Basic Books, 1969

Brazelton TB: Infants and Mothers. New York, Dell, 1983

Brazelton TB: Working and Caring. Reading, MA, Addison-Wesley, 1985

Bretherton I, Waters E (eds): Growing Points of Attachment Theory and Research. Monographs of the Society for Research in Child Development, Vol 50 (ser no 209), No 1–2, 1985

Carter EA, McGoldrick M: The family life cycle and family therapy: an overview, in The Family Life Cycle. Edited by Carter EA, McGoldrick M. New York, Gardner Press, 1980, pp 3–20

Cowan CP, Cowan PA, Heming G, et al: Transitions to parenthood. Journal of Family Issues 6:451–581, 1985

Emde RN: The prerepresentational self and its affective core. Psychoanal Study Child 38:165–192, 1983

Erikson E: Childhood and Society. New York, Basic Books, 1964

Everson, Sarnot, Abran: Day care and early socialization, in The Child and the Day Care Setting: Qualitative Variations and Development. Edited by Ricardo C, Ainslie LC. New York, Praeger, 1984, pp 63–97

Farber EA, Egeland B: Developmental consequences of out of home care for infants in a low income population, in Day Care: Scientific and Social Policy Issues. Edited by Zigler E, Gordon E. Dover, MA, Auburn House, 1982, pp 102–120

Fraiberg S: Clinical Studies in Infant Mental Health: The First Year of Life. New York, Basic Books, 1980

Gamble T, Zigler E: Effects of infant daycare: another look at the evidence. Am J Orthopsychiatry 56:26–42, 1986

Greenspan S: Psychopathology and Adaptation in Infancy and Early Childhood. New York, International Universities Press, 1981

Grossman KE, Grossman K, Huber F, et al: German children's behavior toward their mothers at 12 months and their fathers at 18 months in Ainsworth's Strange Situation. International Journal of Behavior and Development 4:157–181, 1981

Hock E: Working and non-working mothers with infants: perceptions of their careers, their infants' needs, and satisfaction with mothering. Developmental Psychology 14:37–43, 1978

Howes C, Rubenstein J: Determinants of toddlers' experience in day care: age of entry and quality of setting. Child Care Quarterly 14:140–151, 1985

Howes C, Stewart P: Child's play with adults, toys, and peers: an examination of family and child care influences. Developmental Psychology 23:423–430, 1987

Kahn A, Kamerman S: Child Care: Facing the Hard Choices. Dover, MA, Auburn House, 1986

Lamb ME: Qualitative aspects of mother infant and father infant attachments. Infant Behavior and Development 1:265–275, 1978

Lamb ME: The changing roles of fathers, in The Father's Role: Applied Perspectives. Edited by Lamb ME. New York, John Wiley, 1986, pp 3–28

Lamb ME, Pleck JH, Levine JA: The role of the father in child development: the effects of increased paternal involvement, in Advances in Clinical Child Psychology, Vol 8. Edited by Lahey BS, Kazdin AE. New York, Plenum, 1985

Lieberman A: Opening remarks presented at the Symposium on Early Infant and Toddler Care, San Francisco Psychoanalytic Institute Extension Division, San Francisco, CA, September 1986

Mahler M, Pine F, Bergman A: The Psychological Birth of the Human Infant. New York, Basic Books, 1975

Main M, Weston DR: The quality of the toddler's relationship to mother and to father: related to conflict behavior and the readiness to establish new relationships. Child Dev 52:932–940, 1981

Main M, Kaplan N, Cassidy J: Security in infancy, childhood and adulthood: a move to the level of representation, in Growing Points of Attachment Theory and Research. Edited by Bretherton I, Waters E. Monographs of the Society for Research in Child Development 50 (ser no 209):66–104, 1985

Naylor AK: Some determinants of parent-infant relationship, in What We Can Learn From Infants. Edited by Dittman L. Washington, DC, National Association for the Education of Young Children, 1970, pp 25–47

Neubauer P: Pre-oedipal objects and object primacy. Psychoanal Study Child 40:163–182, 1985

Parens H: The Development of Aggression in Early Childhood. New York, Jason Aronson, 1979

Phillips D, McCartney K, Scarr S, et al: Selective review of infant day care research: a cause for concern. Zero to Three 7(3):18–21, 1987

Pleck JH: Employment and fatherhood: issues and innovative policies, in The Father's Role: Applied Perspectives. Edited by Lamb ME. New York, John Wiley, 1986, pp 385–412

Provence S, Naylor A, Patterson J: The Challenge of Day Care. New Haven, CT, Yale University Press, 1977

Pruett KD: Two year followup of infants of primary nurturing fathers in intact families. Paper presented at the Second World Congress on Infant Psychiatry, Cannes, France, April 1983

Radin N: Primary caregiving and role sharing fathers, in Nontraditional Families: Parenting and Child Development. Edited by Lamb ME. Hillsdale, NJ, Erlbaum, 1982

Radin N, Sagi A: Childrearing fathers in intact families in Israel and the USA. Merrill-Palmer Quarterly 28:111–136, 1982

Rutter M: Social-emotional consequences of day care for pre-school children. Am J Orthopsychiatry 51:4–28, 1981

Sagi A: Antecedents and consequences of various degrees of paternal involvement in child rearing: the Israeli project, in Nontraditional Families: Parenting and Child Development. Edited by Lamb ME. Hillsdale, NJ, Erlbaum, 1982

Schwartz P: Length of day care attendance and attachment behavior in eighteen month old infants. Child Dev 54:1073–1078, 1983

Stern DN: The Interpersonal World of the Infant: A View From Psychoanalysis and Developmental Psychology. New York, Basic Books, 1985

U.S. Congress, House. Select Committee on Children, Youth, and Families: U.S. Children and Their Families: Current Conditions and Recent Trends. Washington, DC, U.S. Government Printing Office, 1984

Zigler E, Muenchow S: Infant day care and infant-care leaves: a policy vacuum, in Annual Progress in Child Psychiatry and Child Development, Vol 17. Edited by Chess S, Thomas A. New York, Brunner/Mazel, 1984

Zigler E, Turner P: Parents and day care workers: a failed partnership, in Day Care: Scientific and Social Policy Issues. Edited by Zigler E, Gordon E. Dover, MA, Auburn House, 1982, pp 174–179

Chapter 7

The Child Care Provider: Pivotal Player in the Child's World

Deborah Phillips, Ph.D., and Marcy Whitebook, M.A.

Medical and mental health professionals frequently rely on critical information provided by school teachers in diagnosing children. By enlisting the assistance of these educators, child psychiatrists, psychologists, and social workers develop and implement enhanced treatment plans for their young clients. With increasing numbers of preschool-age and school-age children now spending a substantial portion of their day in child care, it behooves professionals working with families to establish relationships with equally pivotal, but often overlooked, players in the child's world—the child care providers.

Unfortunately, this task is far more challenging than it may appear. Most elementary and secondary school teachers are readily accessible, work in familiar environments, and have received training that sensitizes them to the value of children's mental health. Not so for child care providers, whose workplace may be a private home, a large public or private institution, or a moderate-sized facility in a church or community center. Some are regulated by the state and are thus publicly visible; others operate underground. Some child care providers hold master's degrees in early childhood education; others have not completed high school. Effective collaborations between mental health practitioners and child care providers must begin, therefore, with an understanding of child care work and of those who make it their profession.

CHILD CARE TODAY

Contemporary social forces have led to the increasing amalgamation of the day nursery and the nursery school (Almy 1982; Scarr and Weinberg 1986). World War II provided the impetus to change. Child care centers staffed by nursery school teachers were established for women war workers, thus linking child care to mainstream, nonpoor families. Head Start and the emphasis on preschool education in the 1960s again challenged the autonomous traditions of the nursery school and day nursery. Although such programs are exclusively a service for disadvantaged children, emphasis is placed on education in the preschool tradition as well as on socialization. Child care remains a secondary function of these largely part-day intervention programs.

The relentless growth in the number of mothers of young children who work outside their homes has further contributed to the blurring of boundaries between day nurseries, nursery schools, kindergartens, and even some family day care homes. Many nursery schools now have extended-day programs to meet the needs of the middle-class working family. Similarly, many child care centers and family day care homes envision their roles as providing a preschool or kindergarten experience while providing care for children of working parents.

Perhaps nowhere does the controversy about services for young children emerge as clearly as in a discussion of what to call the child care practitioner. Is he or she a teacher or an educator? A babysitter or custodian? A professional? Some practitioners claim "day care" in their title and reject "teacher" in an effort to demonstrate the wide range of services they perform for children (Katz 1977). Others prefer "teacher," assuming this title includes caregiving functions but offers higher social status. Other "teachers" are insulted by being expected to perform tasks that are not strictly educational in nature.

The U.S. Department of Labor's *Dictionary of Occupational Titles* (U.S. Department of Labor 1977) reflects this confusion over titles and job descriptions for child care providers. Child care workers "read aloud," "organize activities of prekindergarten children," "teach children simple painting, drawing, and songs," "direct children in eating, resting, and toileting," "maintain discipline," and "help children to remove outer garments." Prekindergarten teachers "plan group activities to stimulate learning," "instruct children in activities designed to promote social, physical, and intellectual growth," and "prepare children for primary school." The dictionary notes that the use of the term "instruct" is restricted to preschool teachers, and descriptions of nonacademic responsibilities are reserved for child care workers (Phillips and Whitebook 1986).

This debate about nomenclature reflects strong differences of opinion related to philosophical and functional dimensions of the services provided by child care workers. Depending on how the service is envisioned, different ideas about preparing practitioners emerge. For some, the informal route of female socialization is thought to provide adequate training for the work. For those who view the work as skilled and who assume an educational component in the service, a more formal route involving specialized education is recommended. Bachelor degrees in early childhood education, child development, or home economics are frequently required for head teachers in public centers and many nursery schools. More recently, 2-year college certificates in early childhood-related fields have gained widespread acceptance as criteria for teaching jobs. Lying between the more formal educational route and the informal path is a third mode of occupational socialization, best embodied in the child development associate (CDA) credential. The CDA is an on-the-job training and certification program now available to family day care providers as well as center workers (see Zigler and Freedman, Chapter 1, this volume).

THE SIGNIFICANCE OF CHILD CARE WORK

Most seasoned child care consumers recognize that the quality of their children's child care hinges on the adults who provide the care. Too few adults for the number of children, too many changes in caregivers, and poorly trained or untrained staff are cause for concern. Parents often make such comments as "There didn't seem to be anything going on for the children," "I was worried that the provider couldn't handle an emergency," or "My child doesn't want to talk about her teacher."

Research lends support to parents' worries. Extensive empirical evidence has identified the skill, structure, and stability of staff in child care programs as primary ingredients of child care quality (Howes 1983; Howes and Olenick 1986; Phillips 1987; Phillips et al. 1987; Ruopp et al. 1979). Positive cognitive, social, and emotional development in child care are directly attributable to adult caregivers who are trained in early childhood education or child development, who establish consistent attachments with the children in their care, and who are responsible for a manageable number of children.

State regulations, the sole source of quality monitoring in governing child care, have largely ignored these research findings. Twenty-eight states require neither prior experience in child care nor training in child development for family day care providers. Twenty-seven states have no education or training requirements for child care teachers prior to employment. Some states mandate continuing education or in-service training, but others require as few as 3 hours annually. Neither preservice education nor ongoing training is required of center staff in seven states (Morgan 1986). Staff must only meet an age requirement (as low as 16 years in some states) and have no criminal record. Consequently, some providers are far better equipped than others to plan appropriate programs for children and facilitate the efforts of other professionals concerned about individual children.

A DESCRIPTION OF CHILD CARE WORK

Regardless of how child care practitioners label themselves, what the public calls them, or what their occupational socialization has been, all partake to some extent of the low status, poor compensation, and stressful working conditions endemic to jobs in the field of early childhood.

Those who have little direct experience with young children consider child care work unskilled. Because young children spend much of their time playing, it is assumed that the adults in their midst function in a similar carefree manner. And because the work of caring for children has long been performed by women without pay, it is regarded as something natural and unlearned, an outgrowth of female nurturing, rather than skilled work that requires training and deserves adequate compensation.

A wide range of skills is required to perform the diverse functions involved in caring for young children. The image of a jack-of-all-trades replaces that of the unskilled babysitter. An examination of typical responsibilities included in job descriptions for center personnel sheds more light on the actual tasks child care providers perform: curriculum planning and implementation, parent contacts (meetings and conferences), meal preparation, janitorial services, clerical tasks, administrative duties (budgeting, fund-raising, and staff supervision), indoor-outdoor supervision of children, and staff meetings (Whitebook et al. 1982). Listing responsibilities, however, gives only a partial picture of what caregivers actually do.

Consider curriculum planning and implementation. In order to perform these tasks, good caregivers must begin by assessing the children and the program environment. They must be keen observers of behavior and must be able to recognize appropriate and inappropriate responses in children of different ages. They must also have an understanding of the range of needs within the population of children under their care. Which activities are appropriate for facilitating the particular skills one is seeking to build? Of those activities, which will be most engaging for this particular group of children? Are there sufficient materials and staff to implement the planned activities? In addition, caregivers must have alternate activities prepared in case of a weather change or another unpredictable occurrence. The time actually spent implementing curriculum constitutes only a small portion of the work; preparatory tasks consume a large part of the caregiver's day (Almy 1975).

Of course a caregiver's activities are not restricted to creating a rich environment for learning and development. Attending to the physical needs of children over the course of a long day also consumes a great deal of energy, and the younger the children, the more physically demanding the caregiving (Katz 1977).

Keeping the program financially afloat is a task that would tax the most experienced corporate executive. Although the burden of activity in this arena falls most heavily on the director or administrative staff, teachers and family day care providers may find themselves embroiled in budgeting, fund-raising, purchasing insurance, seeking legal advice, or scrounging for goods and services in the local community.

Staff relations and management may pose the most serious challenges caregivers face. Some skill in training or supervising other adults is essential to effective communication with coworkers. Staff must also manage relationships with parents, which often involve intense feelings (Kontos and Wells 1986; Powell 1980).

Negotiating these myriad responsibilities requires flexibility and careful organization. The work of caring for children, like other household chores, is never done. One cannot prepare for a snack, help a child to sleep, comfort a distraught parent or coworker, or change wet clothes and assume that these chores can be permanently crossed off this week's "to do" list. Not only are these demands likely to be repeated frequently, but they are likely to compete with equally compelling pleas, perhaps in the midst of a carefully planned, not easily interrupted project—such as cooking corn bread with seven impatient 4-year-olds. Although there are moments of calm during the day, they too are unpredictable.

Differences in caregiver experiences emerge, of course, depending on the setting, the ages of the children served, job responsibilities, and funding options. For example, the pace of a day with infants is quite different from one with older children. With babies, workers typically experience several slow times in a day, but seldom do all children rest simultaneously. Preschoolers, on the other hand, maintain high energy throughout the morning with little opportunity for breaks before the afternoon nap.

For the center worker, the role as aide, teacher, director, or support staff (cook, nurse, social worker, etc.) further shapes the caregiving experience. A San Francisco study found that aides, teachers, and teacher-directors all performed the same range of duties (Whitebook et al. 1982). Job title reflected no differences in paid or unpaid time spent in curriculum planning and implementation, maintenance, and meal or snack preparation, but it did suggest differences in time spent communicating with parents and performing clerical or administrative chores. Similar results were obtained by Kontos and Stremmel (1988) based on interviews with 40 center-based staff persons in northeastern Pennsylvania. Regardless of job title, indoor-outdoor supervision of children and curriculum implementation were the most time-consuming tasks for all staff. Directors and assistant directors were almost exclusively responsible for clerical, budget, and administrative duties. Daily parent communication was shared equally among all staff.

Job titles also indicate differences in power and control over major policy decisions and day-to-day decision making. In the Kontos and Stremmel (1988) study, for example, decision-making was almost exclusively reserved for directors and assistant directors.

THE CHILD CARE WORK FORCE TODAY

Overall, it is estimated that the number of child care workers providing direct service to children lies between 2.8 and 3.4 million (National Association for the Education of Young Children 1986a). The number of child care workers grew by 13% between 1983 and 1985 alone. The most dramatic growth is among child care workers who work outside private home settings, increasing by 90% since 1972 and 43% since 1982. This child care work force remains predominantly female, with women comprising 95% to 99% of employees, compared to 44% in the total labor force (U.S. Department of Labor 1985). The available evidence on child care providers consists of three relatively independent literatures. One relies on survey methods to examine the demographic characteristics of child care workers, including their age and sex composition, their salaries, their preparation, and job turnover. The second, more empirical literature (reviewed by Howes, Chapter 2, this volume) examines the relationship of staff training and stability to child care quality. The third, which examines job satisfaction among child care workers, is among the newest areas of child care research.

Demographic Characteristics of Child Care Providers

According to the National Day Care Study (Coelen et al. 1978), the 200,000 center-based child care workers in the United States in the mid-1970s were primarily female and under 40 years of age. About one-third were ethnic minorities. In 1984, the Department of Labor (U.S. Department of Labor 1985) reported 677,000 child care workers (excluding those who worked in private households) and an additional 330,000 workers who defined their employment as prekindergarten or kindergarten teacher. Assuming these numbers are comparable, they indicate that the number of nonhousehold child care workers has tripled in the past decade.

The National Day Care Home Study (Fosburg 1980) described the family day care provider population 10 years ago as predominantly female and 25 to 55 years of age. About 60% were ethnic minorities. Interesting patterns emerged when the age, race, and site of the family day care providers were examined together. White women providing informal care outside the regulatory system were substantially younger (median age: 30.4 years) than any other group of providers (median age for total sample: 41.6 years). Most of these mothers chose to provide family day care during the early years of their own children's lives, and they tended to come from households with relatively high incomes. Black and Hispanic caregivers, by contrast, were older and were typically not living in high income households. The modal annual income category for the total sample was $6,000. No comparable current data exist for family day care providers, but it is known that since 1977 there has been a 46% increase in the number of registered or licensed family day care homes (National Association for the Education of Young Children 1986b). In light of consistent growth in the demand for child care over the past decade (Hofferth and Phillips 1987), it is likely that a similar growth pattern has occurred in unregulated family day care and other forms of home-based care such as baby-sitting, thus further expanding the less visible child care work force.

A recent study by the National Committee on Pay Equity ranked child care teachers and providers as the second most underpaid workers in the nation (only the clergy earned less) (National Committee on Pay Equity 1987). The earnings of child care workers fall below those of animal caretakers, bartenders, parking lot attendants, and amusement park workers (see Figure 7-1).

In 1984, 58% of nonhousehold child care workers earned poverty level wages, with median annual incomes of $9,204. The poverty level in 1984 for a four-person household was $10,610 a year (National Association for the Education of Young Children 1986b). By 1986, the median annual income of child care workers remained under $10,000, whereas the poverty level had risen to $11,200 (Child Care Employee News 1987). For workers who care for children in private homes, the median annual income was $4,732 in 1986.

Although many believe these low wages typically supplement the higher earnings of spouses, this belief is far from the truth. In 1977, 30% of center-based child care providers were the sole income earners for their families, and 70% provided more than half their families' income (Coelen et al. 1978).

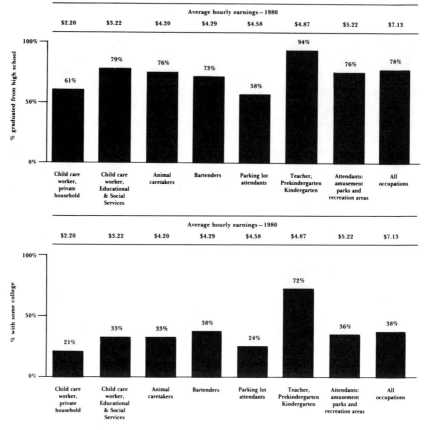

Figure 7-1. Earnings and education of child care workers compared with other occupations. From U.S. Bureau of the Census 1984.

These striking salary data are not solely attributable to lack of education or training among the child care work force. In 1977, family day care providers had, on the average, 11.3 years of education; the majority (57%) had completed high school, and about 30 percent had received some postsecondary education. In 1977 center-based providers had, on the average, 14 to 15 years of formal education. Close to 30% had 16 or more years of education—twice the percentage among all employed females in the United States at that time (Coelen et al. 1978). Anecdotal evidence, however, suggests that there was a general decline in both the level and appropriateness of the training among child care workers in the 1980s.

Moreover, the low wages of child care workers are compounded by the unpaid overtime work that this profession entails. A majority of the workers in the San Francisco study reported several unpaid hours spent each week in curriculum planning and preparation, staff meetings, parent contacts, and general center maintenance. Almost half received no compensation for working these extra hours. Kontos and Stremmel (1988) found that center-based staff reported an average of 59.73 hours spent on center responsibilities per week, compared to their paid work weeks of 37 hours. Only 7 of the 40 staff members were compensated for overtime. Annual wages, therefore, fail to reflect the true hourly wage of child care workers.

Low salaries are not offset by excellent benefits. Kontos and Stremmel (1988) report that 42.5% of the 40% of the center-based staff in their study had no medical insurance and 70% had no dental insurance. Unpaid maternity leave was available to 45% of the sample. The majority of the staff (75%) received some paid vacation days, averaging 9 days per year. Other state and local data from isolated staff surveys (National Association for the Education of Young Children 1986a, 1986b) reveal that the 42.5% estimate for no health care coverage is typical (Child Care Employee News 1987; National Association for the Education of Young Children 1986a, 1986b), and further, that at most, 20% of child care workers report participating in a retirement plan. Staff working in publicly funded centers are usually the highest paid child care workers in any community and those most likely to receive benefits.

With respect to job turnover, child care workers have among the highest turnover rates of any occupation tracked by the Department of Labor. The department estimated that 42% of all nonhousehold child care workers and 59% of private household workers would need to be replaced each year between 1980 and 1990 just to maintain the current supply of child care providers. These rates, which may underestimate actual turnover rates according to studies done in several local communities reporting 60% turnover rates, were more than double the average replacement rate of 19.4% for all occupations (Child Care Employee News 1987; "New Occupational Separation Data" 1984). Low pay, lack of benefits, and stressful working conditions are the major reasons why child care workers leave their jobs in such great numbers (Kontos and Stremmel 1988; Whitebook et al. 1982).

Staff turnover is an important source of inconsistent child care. Initial research suggests that caregiver stability is related to children's adjustment in child care (Cummings 1980). In a similar vein, Berk (1985) found that career-committed caregivers interacted with young children in more age-appropriate and stimulating ways than did caregivers who approached their work as a temporary job.

This brief demographic profile of child care workers reveals remarkable growth in a work force that is predominantly female, that receives very low wages and few benefits (despite levels of education that match national averages), and that exhibits extremely high turnover rates. The data on which this profile is based, however, are seriously flawed and outdated. The federal data bases on child care workers are based on outmoded definitions of the child care work force, rely heavily on self-reported information, and fail to tabulate data to permit, for example, an examination of wages for workers with different levels of education or varying levels of experience (Phillips and Whitebook 1986). The National Day Care Study and the National Day Care Home Study, the only other sources of national data on child care workers, were conducted 10 years ago when the supply of child care was about half what it is today. Despite the significance of this profession, we have at best only sketchy information about the adults who provide child care in this country.

EMPIRICAL STUDIES OF RELATIONS AMONG TRAINING, JOB SATISFACTION, AND CHILD CARE QUALITY

After an initial wave of child care research that compared children reared at home with those who attended child care centers, growing recognition of the wide diversity of child care environments prompted a new emphasis on studies of variation in child care quality and its effects on child development (Belsky 1984; Clarke-Stewart and Fein 1983; McCartney and Phillips 1988; Phillips 1987). This second wave of child care research identified several staff-related factors as central ingredients of high quality child care: training, ratios, stability, and staff-child interaction (see Howes, Chapter 2, this volume, for a discussion of quality indicators).

In a study conducted by Pettygrove and colleagues (1987), variations in costs related to staffing requirements were analyzed for 25 state-funded infant-toddler programs in California. Programs with a larger share of their budget devoted to staff reported lower turnover rates and shorter delays in finding substitute and replacement staff. In 1986, Olenick analyzed quality reviews for 16 state-funded preschool programs in California and found that quality positively related to budget allocations for teacher salaries and benefits and negatively related to costs for supervisory personnel (Olenick 1986). These California studies found that the percentage of total budget spent on personnel—not the total cost of care—was related to quality and to staff turnover qualifications (Child Care Employee News 1987).

In sum, characteristics of child care staff (particularly their child-related training), workload as assessed by staff-child ratios, stability and job commitment, and competence to engage in stimulating verbal interaction with children have been linked directly to the quality of care received by children and to children's healthy development in child care. The next question concerns factors that predict and promote these staff characteristics. It is surprising that this issue is largely unexplored despite its apparent significance.

JOB SATISFACTION AMONG CHILD CARE WORKERS

Although job satisfaction is among the most widely researched topics in psychology (Moos 1979), child care workers are only beginning to be studied in this context (Berk 1985; Jorde-Bloom 1986a, 1986b, 1986c). Yet the job turnover statistics for child care workers, combined with evidence that the training and commitment of this work force have major implications for the children in child care, have highlighted the need for research on factors that enhance job satisfaction in child care.

Anecdotal evidence suggests that low morale, stress, and job burnout are not uncommon among child care workers (Hyson 1982; Jorde 1982; Kontos and Stremmel, in press; Whitebook et al. 1982). The same literature, however, suggests that these workers find the day-to-day challenges of their work highly satisfying. For example, the 40 center-based staff persons studied by Kontos and Stremmel (1988) reported contact with children and coworker relations as the most satisfying aspects of the jobs. The study also reported that wages and benefits were the most dissatisfying aspect. When asked to make recommendations for improving their jobs, about one-third of the staff persons interviewed cited reducing the child-staff ratios and one-fifth mentioned better pay and better administration. It is clear that job satisfaction in child care is a complex, multifaceted issue requiring multidimensional measurement.

Preliminary work in this area suggests that caregiver job satisfaction is related positively and significantly to such caregiver behaviors as encouragement, development of verbal skills, and age-appropriate instruction (Berk 1985). On the other hand, low levels of satisfaction are related to greater limit setting and disparagement of children on the part of the caregivers. Berk's study also differentiated intrinsic sources of job satisfaction (e.g., feelings of accomplishment) and extrinsic sources (e.g., pay, employee policies) and found generally stronger links between extrinsic satisfaction and caregiver behavior. Finally, caregivers with higher levels of career commitment were found to be more educated and more satisfied with their work, to show fewer restrictive encounters with children, and to place more emphasis than less committed caregivers on the development of children's verbal skills (Berk 1985).

A second empirical study of job satisfaction among child care workers (Jorde-Bloom 1987) yielded results that contradict those of Berk. Specifically, caregivers with higher levels of education were found to be less satisfied with their salaries and promotion opportunities. Length of time on the job also showed a negative relation to satisfaction with pay and promotion opportunities.

Kontos and Stremmel (1988) reported a nonsignificant correlation between staff job satisfaction and center quality assessed with the Early

Childhood Environment Rating Scale (Harms and Clifford 1980), although significant relations were found for two more refined measures. High-quality centers had staff persons who reported receiving compensation for overtime work and who spent more time with curriculum planning than did low-quality centers. The lack of a relation between overall job satisfaction and quality may be attributable to the minimal variation in satisfaction yielded in this study. Most staff persons were satisfied with their jobs.

Although implying a link between job satisfaction, caregiver background, working conditions, and quality of care, this area of research is in its infancy. These initial results require replication and extension to other settings and to a more diverse sampling of providers. Studies of child care as an adult work environment need to develop more differentiated conceptions of job satisfaction and to relate worker perceptions to characteristics of the child care programs, to staff stress and career commitment, and to the development of children in child care. Staff-parent relations examined in the context of employment issues constitute additional unexplored territory (Kontos and Wells 1986; Powell 1980).

GAPS IN THE RESEARCH LITERATURE ON CHILD CARE STAFF

In addition to the problems of timeliness and reliability, the available data on child care staff are limited by three additional unaddressed issues. First, the three focuses of information on child care staff reviewed here have remained largely independent paths of inquiry. Yet several of the most pressing issues concerning child care staff require that these literatures be interwoven into a single study. For example, how do the family structure and income of child care staff interact with job satisfaction and commitment to child care work? How do caregiver characteristics interact with characteristics of program clientele? Do indicators of caregiver satisfaction vary reliably with other indicators of program quality such as ratios, group size, and quality of the physical environment?

Second, with the single exception of the National Day Care Study, the literature that includes caregiver measures in studies of child care quality have been restricted to single-site investigations, which fail to reflect national diversity in the child care market. This diversity becomes particularly significant in light of the large differences in state child care regulations pertaining to staff qualifications. Similarly, regional variation in economic conditions is also expected to affect the basic parameters of child care work, such as pay schedules, alternative job opportunities, and the financial means of the families who use child care.

Third, other than the flawed Department of Labor data, no research addresses trends in the child care work force. Have the basic characteristics of this work force changed over the last decade? Have wages kept up with inflation? Have changes in the nature of the children in care, such as the growing number of infants, prompted higher salaries or greater demands for trained staff? The National Child Care Staffing Study returned to the cities examined in the National Day Care Study so that several of these important issues could be addressed (Whitebook et al. 1990).

POLICY IMPLICATIONS

Almost every news story about child care begins with statistics describing the rapidly expanding percentage of mothers in the work force. These figures conjure up a variety of images of women on the job—some with briefcase in hand, others wielding heavy equipment, and of course, clerical and factory workers, nurses, schoolteachers, and waitresses. Seldom imagined, however, are the child care providers who enable millions of women and men to balance, however precariously, the dual roles of worker and parent.

At this time of increasing demand for child care services coupled with growing recognition of the developmental value of preschool education, the field of early childhood education faces a severe shortage of qualified, trained providers. Child care centers throughout the country report difficulty in recruiting and retaining adequately prepared staff. In many communities, extensive efforts to recruit family day care providers are under way (Lawrence 1987). Without adequate numbers of providers, expansion of the child care supply is severely hampered. Either programs simply cannot be developed, or those that emerge are forced to hire inadequately trained or uncommitted personnel—both of which alternatives severely compromise the caliber of services. Recruitment and retention of multiple cohorts of untrained staff drain program budgets. Yet increases in salaries and benefits needed to attract and retain qualified staff generally require increased fees for families, many of whom already find child care costs unmanageable.

Several factors have converged to constrain the rapid growth of a qualified, stable work force of child care staff. First, the rising demand for teachers in the elementary grades and recent efforts to enhance the salaries of public school teachers have created competitive pressures that place those seeking to recruit and retain child care staff at a distinct disadvantage. Given that starting salaries for a 9-month school position exceed 12-month earnings for most child care teachers after years on the job (Whitebook 1986), it is not surprising that early childhood teachers with bachelor's degrees and/or credentials find public schools a relatively more attractive option.

Second, decreasing interest in educational careers among college students and the declining size of the young adult population further aggravate the problem. And third, growing interest among young women in fields traditionally closed to females further limits the pool of potential applicants. The low pay in child care offers little economic incentive for people to pursue, let alone make a long-term commitment to, a child care career. Sadly, however, the better trained staff are precisely those who are meeting the rising need for public school teachers.

Keeping child care an attractive option entails substantially higher salaries and benefits, and thus higher costs to parents. Increasing salaries also decreases the number of spaces supported by government dollars at current funding levels. Thus, efforts to rectify the child care staffing crisis are in direct conflict with the equally pressing need for affordable services for families.

The convergence of rising demand for child care and trends that appear to be eroding the child care work force has implications for each of the three primary issues identified with child care: supply, quality, and costs. As child care services continue to play a major role in the lives of growing numbers of American children, the question of who will care for them becomes increasingly important. As Young and Zigler (1977, p. 53) pointed out: "When a family chooses day care, it is not buying a service that permits both parents to work, but rather it is purchasing an environment that influences the development of its child." As the research evidence accumulates that caregivers with child-related training are indeed the backbone of quality environments for young children, it becomes imperative that mechanisms be developed to attract and retain qualified staff despite the economic implications.

With the cost of child care in some areas now as high as $4,000 to $6,000 a year for just one child, it is easy for us to see why high-quality child care is beyond the financial capabilities of most American families. Unfortunately, there are those who will argue that the way to keep child care affordable and to respond to the shortage of child care teachers is to lower regulations and standards—standards that in some states are already frighteningly inadequate (Phillips and Zigler 1987; Zigler and Freedman, Chapter 1, this volume). The argument put forth is that with lower qualifications and higher adult-child ratios, child care programs will be able to hire fewer providers and pay them less to care for the same number of children. Thus the cost of child care can be held relatively steady.

But can we afford to use low standards as a means of containing costs? In raising the question of affordability we must not only ask what parents can afford to pay but also what will be the consequences for children if we continue to rely on teachers and providers to subsidize the cost of child care. What will be the short- and long-term effects on the education and development of children if they are cared for in programs with insufficient numbers of adults and in which the adults are not trained in early childhood development? Ultimately, what is the cost if children experience a constantly changing group of adult caregivers during their early years?

Others are looking for ways to balance parents' needs for affordable care with those of providers for fair and decent employment without compromising quality. Massachusetts allocated close to $10 million between 1985 and 1987 to raise day care salaries in publicly funded programs. When advocates realized that wage-upgrading efforts led to higher fees in centers for families who had not simultaneously received state-supported services, they fought for and won funds for an affordability project to expand the economic range of families receiving subsidies.

In Toronto, Canada, government grants to centers for the sole purpose of raising salaries have been awarded annually for the past 4 years. These grants are explicitly intended to help programs attract and retain qualified workers without raising parent fees at a higher rate than the cost of living. The success of this program is evidenced by a recent decision by the provincial government to assume responsibility for the grants program and to extend it to other communities. Day care workers holding an associate of arts degree in nonprofit centers in Toronto now average $17,200 a year, a several-thousand-dollar increase since the program began.

Sen. Christopher Dodd (Democrat-CT) recently sponsored legislation to provide scholarships to employed providers pursuing the CDA credential, a national on-the-job training program. Although this project does not increase salaries per se, it minimizes the drain of training costs from child care providers' meager incomes. Expanding eligibility to child care workers for college loan deferments (now available through both state and federal sources to students who pursue teaching careers in kindergarten through 12th grade) would also constitute a potential incentive for young adults to enter the child care profession. Congressman George Miller (see Chapter 15, this volume) describes the various legislative efforts that are evolving and clarifies the role of government in child care.

CONCLUSIONS

Because most families cannot afford to pay the real cost of child care, staffs are expected to subsidize parent fees and accept salaries that are far below the value of the job they perform. Sadly, we are beginning to understand the consequences of this form of subsidy. By relying on early childhood professionals to keep the cost of child care affordable, we are running the risk of exhausting a valuable national resource—a resource that is critical to the future education and development of our young children. However, if we recognize the importance of giving our children the highest quality care and education in their earliest years, then we must value the individuals who are providing that care and thus compensate them accordingly.

As medical and mental health professionals establish working relationships with child care workers, the disparity between the actual value of this profession and its economic and social position will become readily evident. Perhaps some will join other advocates who are seeking reforms to enable child care to become an economically viable and socially respected career.

REFERENCES

Almy M: The Early Childhood Educator at Work. New York, McGraw-Hill, 1975

Almy M: Day care and early childhood education, in Day Care: Scientific and Social Policy Issues. Edited by Zigler E, Gordon E. Dover, MA, Auburn House, 1982, pp 476–496

Belsky J: Two waves of day care research: developmental effects and conditions of quality, in The Child and the Day Care Setting: Qualitative Variations and Development. Edited by Ainslie RC. New York, Praeger, 1984, pp 1–34

Berk L: Relationships of educational attainments, child oriented attitudes, job satisfaction, and career commitment to caregiver behavior toward children. Child Care Quarterly 14:103–129, 1985

Child Care Employee News, Vols 1–3, 1987

Clarke-Stewart A, Fein GG: Early childhood programs, in Handbook of Child Psychology, Vol 2: Infancy and Developmental Psychobiology. Edited by Haith M, Campos J. New York, Wiley, 1983, pp 917–1000

Coelen C, Glantz F, Calore F: Day Care Centers in the United States: A National Profile, 1976–1977. Cambridge, MA, ABT Associates, 1978

Cummings E: Caregiver stability and day care. Developmental Psychology 16:31–37, 1980

Fosburg S: Family Day Care in the United States: Summary of Findings. Final Report of the National Day Care Home Study, Vol 1. Washington, DC, Department of Health and Human Services, 1980

Harms T, Clifford RM: Early Childhood Environment Rating Scale. New York, Teacher's College Press, Columbia University, 1980

Hofferth SL, Phillips DA: Childcare in the United States, 1970 to 1995. Marriage and the Family 49:559–571, 1987

Howes C: Caregiver behavior in center and family day care. Applied Developmental Psychology 4:99–107, 1983

Howes C, Olenick M: Family and child care influences on toddlers' compliance. Child Dev 57:202–216, 1986

Hyson M: Playing with kids all day: job stress in early childhood education. Young Children 37(2):25–31, 1982

Jorde P: Avoiding Burnout in Early Childhood Education. Washington, DC, Acropol, 1982

Jorde-Bloom P: Early Childhood Work Attitudes Survey. Evanston, IL, National College of Education, 1986a

Jorde-Bloom P: The Early Childhood Work Environment Survey. Evanston, IL, National College of Education, 1986b

Jorde-Bloom P: Teacher job satisfaction: a framework for analysis. Early Childhood Research Quarterly 1:167–183, 1986c

Jorde-Bloom P: Factors influencing overall job commitment and facet satisfaction in early childhood work environments. Paper presented at the annual meeting of the American Educational Research Association, Washington, DC, April 1987

Katz L: Teacher's developmental stages, in Talks With Teachers: Reflections on Early Childhood Education. Edited by Katz L. Washington, DC, National Association for the Education of Young Children, 1977

Kontos S, Stremmel AJ: Caregivers perceptions of working conditions in a childcare environment. Early Childhood Research Quarterly 3:77–90, 1988

Kontos S, Wells W: Attitudes of caregivers and the daycare experiences of families. Early Childhood Research Quarterly 1:47–67, 1986

Lawrence M: California Child Care Initiative, Year End Report. San Francisco, CA Resource and Referral Network, 1987

McCartney K, Phillips D: Motherhood and child care, in Different Faces of Motherhood. Edited by Birns B, Itay D. New York, Plenum, 1988, pp 157–183

New occupational separation data improve estimates of job replacement needs. Monthly Labor Review 107(3):3–10, 1984

Moos R: Evaluating Educational Environments. San Francisco, CA, Jossey-Bass, 1979

Morgan G: The National State of Child Care Regulations, 1986. Washington, DC, National Association for the Education of Young Children, 1986

National Association for the Education of Young Children: In whose hands: a demographic fact sheet. Washington, DC, NAEYC, 1986a

National Association for the Education of Young Children: The Child Care Boom: Growth in Licensed Child Care From 1977 to 1985. Washington, DC, NAEYC, 1986b

National Committee on Pay Equity: Pay Equity: An Issue of Race, Ethnicity and Sex. Washington, DC, NCPE, 1987

Olenick M: The relationship between quality and cost in United Care programs. Unpublished doctoral dissertation, University of California, Los Angeles, 1986

Pettygrove W, Howes C, Whitebook M: Cost and Quality of Child Care: Reality and Myth. Child Care Information Exchange 11:40–42, 1987

Phillips D: Quality in Child Care: What Does Research Tell Us? Research Monographs of the National Association for the Education of Young Children, Vol 1. Washington, DC, NAEYC, 1987

Phillips D, Whitebook M: Who are the child care workers? The search for answers. Young Children 41:14–20, 1986

Phillips D, Zigler E: The checkered history of federal child care regulation, in Review of Research in Education, Vol 14. Edited by Rothkoph E. Washington, DC, American Educational Research Association, 1987, pp 3–41

Phillips D, Scarr S, McCartney K: Child care quality and children's social development. Developmental Psychology 23:537–543, 1987

Powell D: Toward a sociological perspective of relations between parents and child care programs, in Advances in Early Education and Day Care, Vol 1. Edited by Kilmer S. Greenwich, CT, JAI Press, 1980, pp 203–206

Ruopp R, Travers J, Glantz F, et al: Children at the Center: Final Results of the National Day Care Study. Cambridge, MA, ABT Associates, 1979

Scarr S, Weinberg, RA: The early childhood enterprise: care and education of the young. Am Psychol 41:1140–1146, 1986

U.S. Bureau of the Census: 1980 Census of the Population, Vol 2: Subject Reports: Earnings by Occupation and Education. PC-80-2-8B. Washington, DC, U.S. Bureau of the Census, May 1984

U.S. Department of Labor: Dictionary of Occupational Titles, 4th Edition. Washington, DC, U.S. Government Printing Office, 1977

U.S. Department of Labor, Bureau of Labor Statistics: Annual Report for 1984. Washington, DC, U.S. Government Printing Office, 1985

Whitebook M: The teacher shortage: professional precipice. Young Children 41:10–11, 1986

Whitebook M, Howes C, Darrah R, et al: Caring for caregivers: burn-out in child care, in Current Topics in Early Childhood Education, Vol 4. Edited by Katz L. New York, Ablex, 1982, pp 211–235

Whitebook M, Howes C, Phillips D: Who Cares? Child Care Teachers and the Quality of Care in America. Final Report of The National Child Care Staffing Study. Oakland, CA, Child Care Employee Project, 1990

Young KT, Zigler E: Infant and toddler day care regulations and policy implications. Am J Orthopsychiatry 56:43–55, 1977

Chapter 8

A Comparison Study of Toddlers Cared for by Mothers or Substitute Caregivers

Patricia A. Nachman, Ph.D.

Historically the mother-child relationship has been the prime focus of concern to those interested in the influence of early experience upon emotional development. The prevailing view in the psychoanalytic literature has been that the preoedipal years are primarily dyadic and that any arrangement that deprives the child of a continuous and caring relationship impairs the development of maternal attachment and thereby adversely affects the child's emotional security.

The rapid change in our society during the past decade in the number of children who are being cared for by multiple caregivers has alerted us to the need to reexamine our conceptualization of primary objects during the early years. An increasing number of children under the age of 3 will have caregivers other than their parents who will play a significant role in their lives.

Ainsworth's (Ainsworth and Wittig 1969) Strange Situation paradigm has frequently been used to assess the "security" of children in varying caregiving arrangements (for a review, see Belsky and Steinberg 1978;

147

Belsky, Chapter 3, this volume). At the Margaret S. Mahler Observational Research Nursery, our approach was systematically to observe children at play in a naturalistic nursery setting. The conceptual framework used in this study for understanding children's behavior stems from the work of Mahler et al. (1975) on the separation-individuation process. The concept of the separation-individuation phase of personality development refers to the development of object relations. There is a complex circular interaction, however, among progressive psychosexual development, the maturing ego, and the separation-individuation process, the outcome of which is the differentiation of self and object representations and the beginning attainment of self and object constancy.

Separation-individuation involves two interdependent and complementary kinds of development. "Separation" concerns an intrapsychic process that leads to self-object differentiation and "objectivation" (Hartmann 1956), a process in which the other comes to be perceived as separate from the self. "Individuation" centers around the child's developing self-concept, brought about by the evolution and expansion of the autonomous ego functions. The separation-individuation process normally takes place within the setting of the child's developmental readiness for and pleasure in independent separate functioning, together with the physical and emotional availability of the mother, who also, under optimal conditions, encourages the child's growing autonomy.

Mahler's observational research led to descriptions of four characteristic subphases of separation-individuation, beginning at the peak of a symbiosis-like mother-child unity in the third quarter of the first year and evolving into the subphases of differentiation (from about 5–6 months through 10–11 months), practicing (10 months through 15–16 months), and rapprochement (from about 15–24 months), and culminates in the object constancy subphase at the end of the third year. These subphases overlap and the various ages are an approximation. Progressively, these sequences describe the stages leading to the acquisition of the sense of self and to the development of a separate identity from that of the mother.

Our aim in this study was not to evaluate the effects of different caregiving arrangements on the children. Rather, it was to learn through observation about the daily transactions, adaptations, and ego modifications of the children who were cared for by employed caregivers during the day.

For this purpose a comparison was made between two groups of children, with six children in each group. The first group (the mother group) was brought to the Margaret Mahler Nursery by their mothers and remained in their care throughout the nursery session. The second group (the caregiver group) were children of full-time employed mothers. These children were cared for in the nursery by the substitute caregivers, who were in charge of them while their mothers were at work. The mothers and caregivers were told that they had the major responsibility for their children throughout the nursery session. The groups were never in the nursery together. Each group attended the nursery two mornings a week on different mornings. The two groups of children were within 3 weeks of age of one another. The children and their adult partners were observed from the time the children were 17 months old until they were 36 months old. In terms of Mahler's subphases, we observed the children from the beginning of the rapprochement subphase through what Mahler called the on-the-way-to-object-constancy subphase. All of the children were first born except two, and there were three boys and three girls in each group.

The children were from intact, upper middle-class families. The parents had at least 4 years of college. The substitute caregivers were from lower socioeconomic circumstances, and all had children of their own. Only one of the six caregivers had completed high school. The children in the caregiver group had been with the same caregiver since they were a few months old, with the exception of two children who had had a change of caregivers during their second year.

A substantial portion of the following comments were derived from running narrative samples. Two observers made simultaneous but independent records of the children for 120 observation sessions. Video recordings of the children and their adult partners were also collected monthly in the nursery and in a laboratory situation. This report is based on preliminary findings from these data.

The comments that follow focus primarily on group differences. It should not be inferred from our highlighting the overall comparisons between the groups that there were not significant individual differences and wide variation within each group. The individual story of each adult-child relationship is of ultimate importance. However, with the advantage of two distinct groups that were matched for age and many other variables, our focus was on an overall comparison between the groups.

Observations of Interactions

One of the most consistent observations made throughout the year was that the affective interchanges between the children and their caregivers were remarkably more subdued than those observed in the mother group. In general, we did not observe the same intensity and range of emotions that we observed in the mother group, with the exception of one toddler who had an exceptionally close relationship with her caregiver. Direct scoring of our video and nursery data revealed significantly more expressions of laughter, excitement, and enjoyment as well as more crying, distress, and upsets in the mother group.

There were also significantly more incidents of hostile aggression in the mother group, particularly of anger outbursts directed specifically at the mother. Early on we noted that the substitute caregivers were quick to curb any signs of hostile aggression in the children. Hitting, pushing, biting, banging, throwing, and grabbing toys were quickly stopped by the caregivers. In general, the children were obedient when they were with the caregivers, and at an early age they inhibited the fussing, tantrums, and minor skirmishes with other children that were observed in the mother group. The caregivers were clear and straightforward about their prohibitions. A "no nonsense" attitude seemed to prevail, and we often remarked how much calmer practically all the transactions were between the caregivers and the children.

When the children in the caregiver group were seen with their own mothers at home, a different picture emerged. The children were more cranky and irritable at home. Almost all the mothers reported that after the age of 2 the children actively protested their mother's leaving for work in the morning. This situation continued with some modifications until the study was completed. With one exception, separation protests subsided in the mother group during the same time period.

In addition, general dissatisfaction, disgruntlement, and temper tantrums with anger directed specifically toward the mother, which Mahler (Mahler et al. 1975) described as characteristic of the height of the rapprochement subphase (at about 19 months), were delayed, occurring months later for some of the children of employed mothers. The mothers were clearly the objects of these disputes, whereas the children's relationship with the caregivers continued to remain calm and relatively free of aggression. In two children, rapprochement reactions to their mothers were subdued but prolonged. In the other four, reactions were intense, or what Mahler described as more than average reaction.

Nonverbal signals and communicative exchanges between the caregivers and the children were also subdued. Our analysis of the appeals (i.e., the child's signals for help, approval, and attention from the mother), of social referencing (i.e., of visually checking the mother's facial expressions to regulate affect or activity), and of nonverbal signals of communication (e.g., pointing, reaching, and indicating) confirmed that the children who were with their mothers gestured, made visual and physical contact, and appealed to them for help and approval significantly more frequently than the children in the caregiver group.

An important behavioral sign of the beginning of the rapprochement subphase is the continual bringing of things to the mother, filling her lap with objects found in the child's expanding world. Only the one child who had an exceptionally close relationship with her caregiver participated in this kind of sharing.

Although the children and the caregivers did not seem to participate in the routine exchanges that we observed in the mother group, particularly those having to do with sharing, it is of importance that the children became noticeably upset when the caregivers were out of the room for a long period of time. For example, one little boy kept on saying his caregiver's name over and over and seemed dispirited one morning when his caregiver was one-half hour late arriving at the nursery. When she did arrive, he glanced at her, accepted her greeting, and then barely attended (at least noticeably) to her again for the rest of the session, except that we noticed he had recovered his usual playfulness and was able to go about his business freely in the nursery. Most of the children seemed to need and want the caregivers "there," even though they did not appear to be actively engaged with them. The fact of their presence seemed to override all communications.

Observations of the Children

During the first months of our study, when the children in the caregiver group were 17 to 19 months old, we noted that they seemed to have developed an intense interest in each other. In some circumstances the behavior toward one another was similar to the behavior we observed between the children who were in the nursery with their mothers. They visually checked with each other in moments of uncertainty; they imitated each other frequently; they offered toys and bottles to each other; and they waited for each other to assemble before starting an activity. It is interesting that the children in the caregiver group also knew each other's names at least 2 months before the children in the mother group.

The use the caregiver children made of each other and the group deserves further discussion. Many observers of young children (e.g., Mahler et al. 1975; Neubauer 1985; Sander 1980) have commented on the impressive adaptive capacities of children that enable them to extract emotional satisfaction from the surroundings. For the caregiver children, the peer group became quite significant psychologically. Feelings of solidarity and group identity were readily formed.

The strength of the children's adaptive capacities to form peer attachments is supported by research in other contexts. The functional significance of early peer relationships, particularly during periods of separation from the mother, has received extensive documentation in the primate literature (e.g., Suomi and Harlow 1979), in the work on kibbutz children (e.g., Rabin and Beit-Hallahmi 1982), and in numerous reports from day care centers (e.g.. Clarke-Stewart 1973; Rubinstein and Howes 1979).

Probably the most vivid portrayal of this same phenomenon was written by Freud and Dann (1951) about the group upbringing of six war orphans. The children were described as having centered their positive feelings exclusively on their own group; they cared for each other, wished always to be together, and showed many examples of sharing, considerateness, and helpfulness to each other. Freud and Dann concluded that in the absence of a parent relationship the children were able to attach their libido to their companions and the group—much the way identical twins often identify with each other's needs (Burlingham 1949). Although our nursery situation was clearly not as extreme or severe as that described by Freud and Dann, it is likely that we were observing a modified version of this same adaptation.

The play between the children and the caregivers was also of interest. Despite the reticence (because of cultural factors) of the caregivers to participate in pretend and imaginative play and the unavailability of the children's mothers to facilitate their interest in the external world, we observed an earlier onset of symbolic functioning in the caregiver group of children. In general, the caregiver children's use of symbolic representational play was at a higher level than it was for the children in the mother group.

An interesting example is that we saw more doll play and more elaborate doll play in the caregiver group. Also, when the research assistants initiated pretend activities such as cooking, going to the supermarket, or building a house with blocks, the caregiver children responded eagerly and caught on to the "pretend" aspect at an earlier age than the children who were with their mothers. Moreover, when they were older, the caregiver group were able to participate in shared fantasy play such as playing house or going to the store together, activities we still had not observed in the mother group by the end of the study. Thus, as social partners, the caregiver children took a more initiating role in interaction, and they did so earlier than the children with their mothers. They also expressed considerable knowledge in extended play sequences, which reflected the realities of their everyday life, and, communicatively, they made reference to nonpresent people and events earlier than their counterparts.

Almost all new developments that had to do with language and cognition emerged earlier in the caregiver group. Observers frequently commented that the caregiver children acted older and seemed more alert to what was going on around them than did the children in the mother group.

Several comments need to be made about this apparent advance in development. First, the children who were with their mothers were actively involved in the interpersonal give and take and struggles of the separation-individuation process, which may have temporarily deterred their interest in the world around them. The children in the caregiver group, as previously noted, were relatively free during the day of interpersonal struggles and conflicts over aggression with their caregivers. Therefore, during this period, the caregiver group may have been able to attend more readily to the external world.

Second, the apparent advance in functioning we observed may have been precipitated by premature activation of certain aspects of the ego. With one exception, all the children in the caregiver group had an adequate relationship with their parents and their caregivers. For these children, we can assume that the daily deprivations were not so extreme as to impede their adaptive capacities; in fact, they may have hastened them. According to Werner and Kaplan (1963), the child's motive for symbolic development is the maintenance of a shared reference with an "other" with whom he or she initially enjoyed a close affective relationship. It is possible that as the caregiver children became more acutely aware of the separateness of their own from the maternal point of view, the early onset and eagerness for pretend and symbolic play served to bridge the affective distance they were experiencing.

We have evidence to suggest that the children who were separated from their mothers during the day made what seemed to us extensive efforts to sustain the memory or representation of their absent mothers and fathers. Our scoring of doll play sequences revealed significantly more frequent doll play in the caregiver group. Not only were the dolls more frequently selected as playthings, but the caregiver children played with them for significantly longer periods of time. This play usually involved caregiving activities such as giving the dolls a bath. feeding them, or putting them to bed.

A related phenomenon was observed in two of the little girls in the caregiver group. These little girls took on characteristics that made them seem like "little mothers" in a manner that made them appear quite precocious for their age. These children also showed concern and empathy for the other children at an earlier age than has been reported in the developmental literature (Dunn and Kendrick 1979; Mahler et al. 1975; Zahn-Waxler et al. 1979). We also observed some of the children in the caregiver group frequently performing caregiving-type activities on each other, such as feeding another child or patting or offering a toy to another child when the child was crying. One little girl brought bottles when they were empty to the caregivers of the children to whom they belonged. We observed this same little girl bringing a child from across the room when he was missing from the table at snack time, and on several occasions we heard a child call another child's name when that child was about to embark on a prohibited activity. There was an aspect of "the adult" in all these instances that was startling in the way it made the children seem quite grown-up for their age.

The frequent use of the words "mommy" and "daddy" when the children were 17 to 18 months old was also of interest, particularly for reasons having to do with evocative memory of the absent parents. Although it is common to hear children of this age call other adults "mommy" or "daddy," what was unique to the caregiver group of children was the spontaneous use of the word "mommy" when no adult was nearby. This occurrence was especially noticeable during moments of high intensity or excitement such as when a child went down a slide alone or did something for the first time, For example, one little boy built a high tower of blocks and squealed "mommy, mommy" to no one in particular. Another little girl repeated "mommy" several times as she picked up a large peg board from the floor and placed it on a nearby table. A third little girl said "mommy" when she climbed up on the rocking horse by herself.

These examples were interspersed with many instances when the children were obviously reminded of "mommy" and said her name, such as when playing with the toy telephone or when looking down the long corridor outside the nursery. Altogether it seemed to us that the absent mothers and fathers were very much on the children's minds and that a variety of processes were at work to enable the children to bridge the separation.

On an observable level, it seemed to us that the frequent use of imitation and intense doll play, and the early onset of the caring and helping behavior (i.e., the "little mother" aspect of the caregiver children), were related to the children's identification with their absent mothers and fathers. It is important to keep in mind that from the time of Freud's earliest formulations of identification, the idea that identification is related to object loss has continued to influence psychoanalytic thinking.

The children's experience of loss of their parents during the day may have intensified the identification process for them and also may account for the mild precocity we observed in their development. As the children grew older, at around 32 to 36 months of age, we noted that differences in gender identity formation were remarkably pronounced in the caregiver group of children in the form of exaggerated masculinity in all of the boys and exaggerated femininity in one of the girls. The subdued aggression that we observed in the nursery at an earlier age in the caregiver group gave way to group aggressivity. Phallic strivings and male identifications were particularly strong among the boys, who began to exclude the girls, sometimes rather harshly, from their play activities. By the end of the study, when the children were 36 months of age, the intensity of such behaviors had never been observed in the mother group.

Before concluding, it should be emphasized that as competent and as caring as many of the substitute caregivers were, in most instances they did not respond as mothers do to their own children. In all likelihood the caregivers were "mothers" to their own children and were competent and responsible caregivers to the children for whom they were in charge. It seemed apparent that the employed mothers, despite the limited time they spent with their children, remained the primary objects around whom the children's wishes, identifications, separation-individuation conflicts, and libidinal and aggressive attachments centered.

Neubauer (1985) raised the question of how the inner unification toward primary objects occurs. He proposed that the ego may have at its disposal an autonomous function, a kind of integration mechanism in which the importance of the mother is maintained despite her absences and the presence of multiple caregivers. Two decades ago Mahler (1961, p. 334) commented on this same issue:

> The primitive ego seems to possess an amazing ability to absorb and synthesize complex object images without adverse effect, and on occasion even with benefit. Thus, the Gestalt of the nurse who may be relegated to the function of providing immediate need satisfaction, is synthesized with the Gestalt of the mother, who may be available only as an additional or transient external ego. However, it is truly impressive that although the mother may be less involved in the actual care of the infant, her image seems to attract so much cathexis that it often, though not always, becomes the cardinal object representation.

The nature of the construction of an inner representational world, particularly of primary objects, is central to understanding more about the experience of infants and young children in the care of multiple caregivers. Recent work in developmental psychology has demonstrated that infants have some ability to represent averaged or generalized information preverbally (Fagan 1976, 1977; Rose et al. 1983; Strauss 1979). Other experimental studies with children (Rosch 1978) and infants (Strauss 1979) have demonstrated the infant's ability to aggregate experiences and distill or abstract out an averaged prototype. The notion that prototypes arise within flexible structures of generalized episodes of memory has important implications for the nature of the earliest internal representations of the mother. The confluence of memories that make up the prototype "mother" may not be restricted exclusively to past occurrences with the maternal object. For the very young child, mother may be, in part, a composite of an assembly of past relationships that are affectively organized around a variance of pleasurable and unpleasurable experiences.

CONCLUSIONS

It is no surprise that in this study we concluded that the children's relationship to their parents was the primary factor in their adjustment to the long absences from them during the day. However, had the caregivers not been steady, reliable, and reasonably caring, it seems unlikely that the children would have been able to sustain either the ego adaptations we observed or a favorable balance of libidinal and aggressive forces directed toward themselves and their parents.

We leave unsettled the question of the mild precocities and strong rapprochement reactions of some of the children and the intensity of their identifications. Even short-term predictions appear to be rather precarious.

Whether the ego is compromised because of the urgency of the defensive and the adaptive functions, such as those we observed regarding socialization, symbolization, and identification, awaits further developments and follow-up observation of the vicissitudes of the children's libidinal and aggressive drives.

REFERENCES

Ainsworth M, Wittig B: Attachment and exploratory behavior in one-year-olds in a strange situation, in Determinants of Infant Behavior. Edited by Foss BM. New York, John Wiley, 1969, pp 111–136

Belsky J, Steinberg LD: The effects of day care: a critical review. Child Dev 49:929–949, 1978

Burlingham D: The relationship of twins to each other. Psychoanal Study Child 3/4:57–65, 1949

Clarke-Stewart KA: Interactions between mothers and their young children: characteristics and consequences. Monographs of the Society for Research in Child Development 38(ser no 153):1–109, 1973

Dunn J, Kendrick C: Interaction between young siblings in the context of family relationships, in The Child and Its Family: The Genesis of Behavior, Vol 2. Edited by Lewis M, Rosenbaum L. New York, Plenum, 1979, pp 143–168

Fagan JF: Infants' recognition of invariant features of faces. Child Dev 47:627–638, 1976

Fagan JF: Infants' recognition of invariant features of faces. Child Dev 48:68–78, 1977

Freud A, Dann S: An experiment in group upbringing. Psychoanal Study Child 6:127–165, 1951

Hartmann H: On the reality principle. Psychoanal Study Child 11:31–53, 1956

Mahler M: On sadness and grief in infancy and childhood: loss of the symbiotic love object. Psychoanal Study Child 16:332–351, 1961

Mahler MS, Pine F, Bergman A: The Psychological Birth of the Human Infant. New York, Basic Books, 1975

Neubauer P: Preoedipal objects and object primacy. Psychoanal Study Child 40:163–181, 1985

Rabin AL, Beit-Hallahmi B: Twenty Years Later: Kibbutz Children Grow Up. New York, Springer, 1982

Rosch E: Principles of categorization, in Cognition and Categorization. Edited by Rosch E, Floyd BB. Hillsdale, NJ, Erlbaum, 1978, pp 27–40

Rose SA, Gottfried AW, Bridger WH: Infants' cross-modal transfer from solid objects to their graphic representations. Child Dev 54:686–694, 1983

Rubinstein J, Howes C: Caregiving and infant behavior in day care and in homes. Developmental Psychology 15:1–24, 1979

Sander L: Investigation of the infant and its caregiving environment as a biological system, in The Course of Life. Edited by Greenspan S, Pollock G. Washington, DC, U.S. Department of Health, Education, and Welfare, 1980, pp 177–202

Strauss MS: Abstraction of prototypical information by adults and ten-month-old infants. J Exp Psychol 5:618–632, 1979

Suomi SJ, Harlow HF: The role and reason of peer friendships in rhesus monkeys, in The Child and Its Family: The Genesis of Behavior, Vol 2. Edited by Lewis M, Rosenbaum AL. New York, Plenum, 1979, pp 219–244

Werner H, Kaplan B: Symbol Formation: An Organismic-Developmental Approach to Language and Expression of Thought. New York, John Wiley, 1963

Zahn-Waxler C, Radke-Yarrow M, King R: Child rearing and children's prosocial initiations towards victims of distress. Child Dev 50:319–330, 1979

Chapter 9

Understanding Children's Responses to Separation

Barbara Kalmanson, Ph.D.

How do we assess a child's response to a daily separation from his or her parents? How does the child demonstrate his or her feelings? How can the adults involved assess which behaviors are worrisome responses to the separation and which are healthy and expectable protests? The following vignettes illustrate common experiences related to separation in day care and indicate the complexity of the issue to be addressed.

Vignette 1

A mother enters the home of her neighbor where she leaves her 11-month-old daughter for family day care while she is at work. She is exhausted from the day's work and the long commute home. As she approaches her baby, the infant scowls and begins to scream, crying in loud, hard sobs. As this mother lifts her baby to her shoulder, the neighbor says, "I just don't know—she's happy all day 'til she sees you!"

Is this child's crying a separation response? What can it mean to the mother and her neighbor?

Vignette 2

A father rushes into the day care center with a briefcase in one hand and the hand of his toddler son in the other. Out of breath, he speaks rapidly to a child care worker who greets the pair. He tries to pass his child's hand into the caregiver's hand, but his young son clings to his pants leg instead. The caregiver lures the boy into the room to play with a new toy. Once the child is engaged, she motions to the father to slip out unnoticed. Within the hour the boy becomes very active. He dumps containers of toys and searches in closets and drawers. Later in the day, he refuses to stay in his cot during nap time. He spends the late afternoon staring out the window while running a toy bus up and down the window pane.

The child care worker had a simple solution to the father's need to rush off to work: distract the child and let the father slip out unnoticed. What was the effect on this toddler? What was his response to the disappearance of his father? Does such a separation make the day easier or more difficult for a young child?

The preceding vignettes highlight the complexities of understanding adults' and children's responses to separation. Children can exhibit behaviors that are perplexing to observers but can be understood in the context of the effect separation has on the expression of anxiety and defenses. The child care provider's behavior is motivated by a desire to be seen as competent, as someone who makes the child happy and helps the parent get to work on time and home again with a minimum of stress. Parents are often harried in the morning and pressured by the demands of work. They may be anxious about leaving their child in someone else's care and worried about the effects on the parent-child relationship because the child spends so many hours with another caregiver.

A child's response to separation from the parents has been an important area of exploration for better understanding the nature of the child's tie to the parents. Early psychoanalytic theory linked the child's distress at separation to the infant's dependence on the parent for fulfillment of bodily needs (Freud 1926/1959). There is increasing evidence, however, that the absence of the psychological relationship to the parent is the source of the distress, not the availability of someone to meet the infant's physical needs (Bowlby 1973).

The daily separation creates a situation of stress for both the child and the parents. This stress needs to be openly addressed so that parents and caregivers can work together to alleviate the stress as much as possible. How well a child copes with separation depends on a complex network of factors. These factors include the developmental status of the child; the quality of the relationship between the child and parents; the quality of the relationship among the child, the parents, and the day care providers; and the competence of the day care providers in attending to the emotional needs of the child and the parents (Provence et al. 1977). It is extremely rare for parents to be untroubled about leaving their child in the care of others for long hours on a daily basis. Parents who have positive feelings about their work or careers express concern about losing so much time with their child. Quality day care, then, is not a program in which parents can have so much confidence that they can leave their child easily but a situation in which the feelings about the separation can be recognized and addressed.

RESEARCH ON SEPARATION IN DAY CARE

In one way or another, most research on the effects of day care on children is an attempt to measure and understand the effects of separation. Most studies look at the effects of day care on groups of children, the statistical averages of which may not be central to parents' decision making about their own child's day care needs. Studies repeatedly find that the quality of care is a consistent variable affecting the outcome measures (Howes 1987; Phillips et al. 1987). Many of the quality dimensions considered in the research only address the issue of separation indirectly. Variables such as child-staff ratios, characteristics of the physical plant, available curriculum materials, and staff training are all related to how well prepared a day care setting will be to attend to a small child's needs. But ratings along these dimensions cannot tell parents how well prepared a particular day care provider is to notice a particular child's method of coping with the stress of separation, nor how he or she may alleviate the distress of the moment.

Researchers commonly employ the Strange Situation methodology to assess a child's response to a separation experience (Ainsworth 1982; Ainsworth and Wittig 1969; Ainsworth et al. 1971; Belsky, Chapter 3, this volume). Yet such an experience in a research setting is not equivalent to the nature of the separation imposed by day care. The meaning of being left with a relative stranger is very different to the child from being left with a familiar caregiver in a familiar environment. The limitations of group research thus leave many unanswered questions for the couple considering day care options for their young child.

Because of these limitations, in this chapter I rely on clinical experience to assist parents in assessing an individual child's response to a separation during day care. Discussion focuses on how to interpret a child's behavior and how parents and caregivers can work together to mediate the separation experience for the child.

EXPECTABLE AND PROBLEMATIC
RESPONSES TO SEPARATION

All children are expected to protest the departure of a parent (Bowlby 1973; Field 1984). If left to choose, a baby would want to be cared for by the most loved and familiar person, the person who usually mediates the events of the baby's life, who smells right, feels right, and sounds right. It makes sense that infants and young children do not like to be left without their most significant attachment figure. Parents often wonder why their child becomes upset, yet the child's capacity to understand that the parent will return depends largely on age and stage of development. For example, a 5-year-old girl may become upset when her mother leaves her at the kindergarten door, but, depending on her prior separation experiences, she is probably well aware that her mother is not going to disappear. This child's cognitive capacity to retain a memory of a person out of sight and her understanding of a plan related to the passage of time should be stable by this age. In contrast, a 10-month-old boy may be just beginning to realize that his mother has not disappeared forever, yet he may also be actively working on his capacity to call her back with a cry or protest.

The Role of Memory in Separation Responses

As the infant develops, there is an important interplay between the emergence of cognitive and emotional aspects of memory. The development of memory plays a key role in how the child interprets the separation experience. For example, a child who knows that her father will pick her up at five o'clock and that five o'clock is right after story time, feels far less threatened by the separation than the infant who has only some idea that his parents still exist when out of sight.

The cognitive aspects are most frequently referred to as recognitory and evocative memory and the achievement of object permanence (Piaget 1952). Recognitory memory relies on familiar cues to elicit remembering and is thought to emerge very early in infancy, perhaps in the womb (DeCasper and Fifer 1980). As early as 3 months of age, infants appear to recall cues that elicit events they have experienced previously and perform motor acts such as kicking or sucking to demonstrate recall (Rovee-Collier and Fagan 1981). Experimental research suggests that by 6 or 7 months the specific conditions that elicit particular affective experiences can be remembered (Nachman 1981; Stern 1985). Clinical data, however, suggest that recall of affective experiences develops as early as the first days of life (Gunther 1961).

Evocative memory is the symbolic capacity to remember an image with relative autonomy from a stimulus. This type of memory does not appear until about 18 months and may be an important cognitive development on the way to consolidating a sense of a sustained emotional presence of a parent despite his or her absence (Fraiberg 1969). The emotional aspects of memory are referred to as object constancy or libidinal object constancy (Hartmann 1965; Mahler et al. 1975). These aspects refer to the child's capacity to maintain stable memories and the emotional tie to loved ones. It is assumed that the child's ability to feel the parents' nurturing qualities enables him or her to function well even in the parents' absence. This capacity is thought to develop between 24 to 36 months (Mahler et al. 1975).

The increasingly autonomous capacities for memory directly affect how an infant perceives the absence of a parent and what kinds of supports are needed to assist the infant in coping with a separation. A young infant's fear of the loss of the actual person becomes complicated with age, for the child—no longer afraid of the actual loss—is now able to imagine and fear the loss of a parent's love and approval. Although memory becomes more sophisticated, one must keep in mind that fantasy is also elaborated, just at an age when a child is learning to cope with emerging aggressive feelings. Thus, the child who has achieved object permanence and object constancy presents a new constellation of emotional needs related to both imagined and real fears. For example, a 30-month-old boy in the midst of toilet training may worry during the day about his early morning refusal to use the toilet. In his mother's absence he may feel anger toward her for her insistence, concern over his angry feelings, and sadness about her withdrawal of approval. These feelings can affect his entire day in substitute care because he needs his mother's warmth and reassurance to alter the fantasy that he could make her disappear.

The Issue of Control Over People and Events

Separation protest is a healthy and normal reaction in young children, because these children lack a sense of control or ability to have an effect on their environment; despite the child's protest, the parent can leave anyway. The child's expectation that his or her signals will be met with a contingent response from a parent is violated by the parent's leave-taking. Yet a child is more likely to protest a separation when the environment and caregiver are unfamiliar. Therefore, it is important for parents to accustom their child to a new surrounding or a new day care provider before any leave-taking.

If a young child has a familiar and attentive caregiver and has not experienced prolonged or uncertain separations in the past, a clear, vociferously expressed protest is a healthy sign of a positive attachment to the parents. In general, if parents acknowledge the child's dissatisfaction with their leave-taking, the child will readily adjust when the parents are gone. Once parents understand that active protest can be a positive sign of their child's feelings about them, it is easier for the parents to announce their departure, commiserate with their child, and leave for work.

EVALUATING DIMENSIONS OF DISTRESS

Given the expectability of a strong protest, how can a parent determine when or whether protest behavior signifies a separation problem? Three dimensions of the child's response can be helpful in evaluating the meaning of the behavior: the nature of the distress, the pattern of the distress, and the magnitude of the distress.

The Nature of the Distress

Young children can show a variety of distress responses, some more obvious than others. The clearest is vociferous protest at the time of departure. It is easy for both parents and caregivers to identify the precipitant and respond to the child in a manner that connects his or her distress to the parents' leave-taking. Indirect or delayed responses are more difficult to interpret and are harder for parents or caregivers to connect to separation distress. For example, a young child may stay rooted to one corner of a room, appearing disinterested in the available play opportunities. Although this behavior may reflect feelings of insecurity about exploration and play in the absence of the parent, the child may also show no obvious departure protest when the parent leaves for work.

In evaluating the nature of a child's separation distress, then, it is important to keep in mind that distress in some form is expected during the early weeks of the separation. Therefore, caregivers should be alert for any indirect expressions of distress. This understanding makes the child's behavior more meaningful and provides an avenue for helping the child with his or her feelings. Similarly, parents may notice differences in the child's behavior at home, such as increased crying when the child is put in the crib or expressions of distress when the child is put down after being carried. Slightly older children may protest going to bed or prolong bedtime rituals. They may become clingy or whine. Conversely, some children respond defensively by feigning disinterest in the reunion with the parent. They may seem strikingly independent and unconcerned with the separation, making their parents wait for them at the end of the day or neglecting to greet them when they arrive because they are "too busy."

The Pattern of the Distress

Over time, a natural decrease in separation distress should occur. If a child has not experienced previous traumatic separations and has been prepared for day care, the expression of distress should gradually lessen over the course of a couple of months as the day care provider becomes increasingly familiar and accepted into the child's hierarchy of significant people. The constancy of the setting, the familiarity with the separation, and most important, the reunion with the parent at the end of the day, should all function to decrease the child's sense of stress. A pattern of distress that increases over time needs to be carefully evaluated. Sometimes an early indirect expression of distress, such as withdrawing behavior, will not be observed or will seem disconnected from feelings about the separation. These feelings can escalate and eventually be transformed into more overt expressions of distress. In this case, failure to recognize early signs of distress can exacerbate the problem. If a child's separation distress increases over time, various aspects of how the separation is handled and the quality of the day care environment need to be assessed.

How do the parents feel about the separation? Ambivalence may be inadvertently communicated to the child, causing the child to feel that the day care environment is less nurturing or stable than the child needs. The parent or child may also feel that the parent-child relationship is endangered if the child allows the parent to leave easily. The day care setting can be investigated to learn whether there is an adequate number of personnel to provide individual attention to a child in distress, whether each child has a consistent special person with whom to negotiate the separation each day, and whether the child is forming relationships with adults and peers. Information about a child's prior experiences with separations can provide crucial data for assessing the current difficulty. How the child's behavior is being dealt with by parents and day care providers can often give clues to whether the source of the distress is being fully recognized, understood, and translated into empathic means for helping the child adapt.

The Magnitude of the Distress

Some distress from a separation is expectable and healthy, but sustained, high-intensity distress indicates separation problems. For example, in preschool-age children, intense distress does not seem to indicate problems with separation during the first week or two, but its continuation into the seventh or eighth week signals an emerging problem with adjustment to the separation (Bloom-Feshbach 1987). Thus, an intense early protest can be understood as a natural response to a painful event, but intense prolonged protest indicates some disturbance in the adjustment.

One must then look at the particular situation for clues to the source of the problem. Does the parent's behavior toward the child at the time of departure inadvertently encourage an intense response? Is the child forming a trusting relationship with a substitute caregiver? Is this caregiver regularly available to the child at the moment of the parent's departure? What are the child's previous experiences with separations? Do the caregiver and the parents discuss the departure and coordinate a plan that helps the child experience the departure as a less threatening event?

In summary, the nature, pattern, and magnitude of distress can assist parents and caregivers in determining whether there is a cause for concern about the child's response to the separation. Children who actively protest, cry, cling, or seek attention from day care providers during an initial period of adjustment tend to function well in day care within a few months. In contrast, children whose withdrawn or difficult behavior persists or escalates over time tend to have more separation problems.

DETERMINANTS AFFECTING THE CHILD'S CAPACITY TO MANAGE THE SEPARATION EXPERIENCE

Developmental theory assumes that a certain degree of stress can evoke adaptive responses that promote positive development. Because the needs of young children are so multifaceted, there is always a risk that a particular situation will overtax a specific child's capacity to form such adaptive responses. Among the factors to be considered in assessing any child's potential to adapt positively to the stress of the separation imposed by day care are the developmental status of the child, the quality of the child's relationship with the parents, the child's previous experiences with separations, and the characteristics of the day care setting.

Developmental Status of the Child

What are the constitutional capacities of the child? Is he or she easy to care for or fussy, vulnerable to overstimulation or resilient? Does his or her physical health present any special considerations? What is the child's developmental ability to sustain mental images of his or her parents in their absence? How well can he or she use the social and play experiences offered by day care? Such questions pertaining to the age, stage of development, and constitutional factors for a particular child can be useful in assessing a child's readiness for day care and in anticipating an individual child's special needs in making the adjustment.

In general, the younger the child, the greater the vulnerability to stress, because the young child has fewer internal resources with which to master stressful situations. Paradoxically, it is usually thought to be easier to begin substitute care with young infants because it is believed they are less aware of the specific qualities of the people caring for them. In fact, the effects of the separation on an infant may only be more difficult to identify as such, making the separation more tolerable for the adults involved. An infant who is not yet mobile has few resources for expressing distress except to cry, and if the cries go unheard or are responded to unpredictably, the child may stop crying, losing even this one expression of his or her feelings.

In a day care setting, where there are many demands on the provider's time, it is often too easy to leave infants in a crib or playpen, to overlook responding to their first vocalizations, or to let them go wet or hungry beyond the infant's perception of a tolerable length of time. The infant's response may be subtle: for example, changes in visual alertness, body tension, or smiling and vocalizing. A decrease in crying and withdrawal into prolonged sleep may be misunderstood as signs of adjustment to the day care environment, whereas they may actually reflect the onset of apathy and depression. Physical symptoms such as rashes, diarrhea, or vomiting will arouse concern. Although these symptoms may not initially stimulate questions about the emotional quality of the care provided, when they do occur, the emotional atmosphere should be investigated.

The toddler's improved mental representation, mobility, and verbal ability give him or her an expanded repertoire of internal resources for adapting to day care. But at the same time, toddlerhood presents caregivers and parents with a host of new challenges. The toddler's increasing sense of autonomy, emerging capabilities to manage aggressive feelings, alternation of assertiveness and dependence, emotional lability, and toilet training can create struggles with adults that make it difficult to provide substitute care, especially in a group setting. Keeping groups to no more than four children can protect the caregiver from the level of exhaustion that caring for toddlers expressing healthy development can produce.

A 3- or 4-year-old usually has more resources for coping with a daily separation than a 2-year-old, but such an older child may still have some of the needs of the toddler. A preschooler may have habits not ordinarily thought of as age appropriate, such as using a pacifier, blanket, or bottle. Toilet training may not yet be accomplished. These habits may be responses to normal stress for the child, or they may have grown into problems of some magnitude, depending on the child's history and his or her response to previous efforts to influence his or her behavior on such matters.

The Quality of Family Relationships

The nature of the affectionate tie between child and parents can affect a child's ability to form a relationship with a substitute caregiver as well as influence how a particular child responds to the separation during day care.

A child's sense of trust in his or her parents and the accumulation of positive experiences with the parents interact with the child's developmental status to help promote adaptive responses to day care. A child who has not established secure attachment relationships with his or her parents may show little apparent response to separation from them but may be upset by a strange environment. Depending on the child's history and the reasons for failure to develop a strong bond, such a child may form a significant attachment to a nurturant caregiver or be unable to form a new relationship. If the attachment relationship is healthy, the child is apt to protest vigorously initially and then adjust to the separation. This reaction, without denial of the feelings of loss, enables the child to make good use of the playful social environment and nurturant substitute care.

Previous Experiences With Separation

A child who has experienced few prior lengthy separations and is well prepared for even temporary losses is better able to adjust to the separation imposed by day care than a child who has experienced unpredictable or lengthy separations. It is unlikely that a child will come to day care never having experienced prior separations. Even the parent who has not left the child with a substitute caregiver will have established patterns for leaving the child's sight, a brief but recurrent separation experience that is likely to have occurred several times daily. The parent who, as he or she moves out of the baby's visual field, announces where he or she is going and that he or she will be right back sets up a model for coping with separations. The infant simultaneously learns to anticipate the separation and to be reassured of the parent's return. Parents who slip out when the baby is not attending to them, sneak out of the house leaving the child with an unfamiliar baby-sitter, or leave while the child is asleep only to have him or her wake up to the care of a stranger are engendering in their child a different model for anticipating, managing, and mastering separations than the child who is well prepared for leave-taking. A child exposed to such separations is likely either to be anxious for some time about the parent's leave-taking or to show little reaction to the parents' departure but be apathetic or anxiety-ridden throughout the day. In general, the more traumatic the departure, the greater in number and length, and the less empathetically responded to in the past, the greater the child's difficulty is likely to be in adapting to a new separation.

Characteristics of the Day Care Setting

The most important characteristic of the day care setting in predicting the child's adjustment is the nurturant qualities of the substitute caregiver. How well this person understands a particular child's needs and can attune himself or herself with the rhythms and personality of the child and the emotional tone of the family most significantly affect the child's experience of the separation. The caregiver needs to be as sensitive to the parents as to the child on this issue. Many parents find it difficult to directly discuss their feelings about leaving their child, and it is up to the caregiver to find ways to address the issue without being perceived as intrusive.

It is generally easier for an infant or toddler to adjust to a substitute caregiver who comes to the child's home than to adjust to an unfamiliar person and place. In contrast, a preschool-age child may welcome the adventure of leaving home for a day care or nursery experience. Younger children can more readily adjust to care by a friend or relative who has spent a great deal of time with the child in the context of the family prior to the initiation of a day care arrangement. In general, familiarity increases the ease of adjustment. Such familiarity can occur naturally, as in at-home care with a grandparent, or it can be engineered by having parent and child spend adequate time together with a new provider or in a new environment until a feeling of familiarity has been established.

The length of the separation is a major factor affecting a child's capacity to cope adaptively with the separation. The longer the day, the more taxing on the child's internal resources for sustaining an internalized sense of parental nurturance. Even for preschoolers, the predictable end-of-the-day fatigue can overburden the child who otherwise manages the separation.

If a child is in group care, the ratio of staff to children is a crucial factor in determining the quality of the setting (Ruopp and Travess 1982). The recommended ratio for infant care is one to three; for older children it is one to five. Every child should have access to a special person whom he or she can identify as specifically available to substitute for his or her parent. Thus, if all the children are hungry, there must be enough staff so that everyone can be fed. In addition, at the close of a long day, an adequate number of staff allows all the cranky children to be soothed with a lap or a story.

A day care setting should have a curriculum flexible enough to follow an individual child's lead and developmental needs. Most children in day care are not yet ready to spend their time in a structured instructional program in which they are expected to take direction from staff all day long. A certain amount of structure in daily events will assist children in developing a sense of familiarity and mastery in the day care setting, as it would with parental care. But a scaled-down version of first grade tends to overstress the child's capacity to organize himself or herself around the demands of a caregiver.

Whatever the day care arrangement, coordination between the family and the day care provider can create strong links between family life and substitute care. The caregiver is thus in a position to help the child integrate the day care experience into his or her conception of extended family life. This capacity requires that the caregiver know considerably more about the family than simply the child's eating or sleeping patterns. Coordination of child-rearing practices such as toilet training or methods of dealing with unacceptable behavior is also important. A caregiver should be able to talk to a child about his or her family with familiarity. The sense of separation from home and parents is eased when current events in the child's life can be referred to during the day. In practice, therefore, the parent and caregiver must have opportunities to talk to each other at the beginning and end of every day, a sometimes difficult task when everyone is in a hurry or several parents wish or need to talk to the caregiver simultaneously.

HELPING CHILDREN AND PARENTS ADAPT TO THE SEPARATION

A Primary Caregiver

Children of any age find the adaptation to day care least painful if they are able to form a relationship with one provider who becomes their primary parental substitute. Children in center-based care need a primary provider with whom they are secure in looking to for help and solace throughout the day, especially at those times when feelings about the separation are apt to surface, such as just after being left, just before being picked up, when food is served, and at nap times. The primary provider can further alleviate stress for the child by talking about the child's home life throughout the day.

Complications that can arise from cultivating a close relationship between a child and caregiver require careful monitoring and open discussion. Some parents worry that their child will spend so much time with the caregiver that he or she will come to love the caregiver more. A child can become caught in a web of competition between a parent and a caregiver that can make the daily separation feel dangerous and cause the child to display more severe separation reactions. Feelings of competition can also cause a parent to change child care arrangements frequently, which creates instability for the child.

For example, in Vignette 1 (see above), the caregiver communicated to the parent that the baby never cries until the parent arrives. Such a revelation can make a parent feel that he or she makes the baby unhappy and that the child may prefer the caregiver to the parent. Unwittingly, in an effort to reassure the parent that the baby is content in her care, the caregiver inflamed the parent's feelings of loss and guilt about leaving the baby. In such a situation, it is important for the caregiver to understand that it is the strength of the attachment to the parent that enables the baby to cry. It does not reflect poorly on his or her care during the parent's absence, nor does it indicate the child's preference for the caregiver. Knowledge of child development, outside consultation, and a warm, mutually supportive relationship between the parents and the caregiver can guard against potential pitfalls when a child is provided with one primary substitute caregiver. From the child's point of view, the benefits of having one special person almost always outweigh the potential for complications.

Easing the Transition to Day Care

There are several ways parents and providers can help young children ease into day care arrangements and lessen both normal and extreme separation distress during the initial weeks of day care. If the parent remains with the child and the provider until the child is comfortable with the new setting and the new person, the child will not feel an abrupt loss of the parent or the anxiety produced by unfamiliarity. Further, the time spent together allows the caregiver to experience directly the quality of the parent's relating to the child and to take on some of the attributes of the parent. If the parent has arranged to be available for some time, small separations of 15 minutes increasing to several hours can be engineered to introduce the separation to the child gradually. Such a plan means that parents should begin day care several weeks before they actually plan to return to work, sometimes a difficult prospect for a parent who hates the thought of leaving the child and whose parental work leave is all too short. These benefits need to be carefully explained to a caregiver who may worry that the parents want to hang around to "spy." They also need to be explained to the center that advertises the convenience of easy curbside drop-off, never expecting the parents to want to come inside.

Even a child who is well acclimated to day care is likely to have days when the separation feels threatening. For example, a mother may think nothing of an early morning fight with a toddler who insists on eating cereal from a particular bowl. But the toddler may worry about having angered the mother or about his or her own angry feelings toward her. These factors may influence the separation response when the mother leaves the child with the day care provider. When parents can stay with the child and help him or her engage in some familiar and pleasurable activity with the provider, a difficult day or the onset of a new pattern of distress can be avoided. Of course, caregiver understanding of the causes of a particularly upsetting separation can prevent further disturbance, although the reassurance of the parent's presence can relieve the immediate distress.

The length of the separation can be an important factor in the child's experience of the loss of the parent. Keeping the parent-child relationship alive during the day with representations of the parent can assist the child in managing the length of the parent's absence. Children can be encouraged to bring significant objects from home: a photograph book with pictures of the child with the parents; an audio tape of the parent reading a favorite book for a toddler or preschooler, or just talking for an infant; a transitional object like a blanket or teddy bear; or an object that belongs to the parent. To serve their purpose as on-call parent substitutes, these objects need to be available to the child throughout the day. They are not intended to be kept in a cubby for an emergency or looked at only during "sharing time," as is often the approach in day care centers. Providers can easily manage the hassles of sorting through toys for personal possessions or maintaining a child's sense of ownership when the benefits of ready availability of these significant objects can be seen in positive changes in the child's mood and flexibility.

Feelings of loss or loneliness from a long separation can also be relieved by encouraging parents to phone or visit during the day. Calls and visits break the length of the separation for the child and reassure him or her of the parent's presence as object constancy develops. Many day care providers object to midday calls or visits because the child is likely to become upset when the parent hangs up or leaves. It is a false saving to spare the child from becoming upset by a midday contact with the parent. The brief, active protest following midday contact can prevent ongoing distress that may be expressed more passively. Empathizing with the child's distress and experience of loss can help him or her to express feelings directly and prevent other, more serious, disturbances.

Curriculum for Mastering Separations

Many play experiences can specifically enhance a child's capacity to cope with separation. For infants, variations of peek-a-boo provide a sense of control over appearance and disappearance. Toddlers enjoy games of hiding and finding. Games that enact themes of coming and going, and role playing departures and reunions, provide toddlers and preschoolers with opportunities to control others' comings and goings and to master feelings of loss or anger through play.

Clear Reunions and Departures

Parents may need assistance in making their departures and reunions explicit. In Vignette 2 (see above), the boy searched for his father all day (dumping containers, looking in drawers, waiting at the window) because his father had slipped out unnoticed, without saying good-bye. Children who are uncertain about their parents' departures often become needlessly anxious, expecting to lose their parents at any time. Infants can become hypervigilant and fussy, and toddlers can become distracted and agitated. Although sneak departures are often favored because they avoid upsetting the child at the moment, they create unfavorable reactions later in the day and obstruct the natural development of object permanence and healthy departure protest.

CONCLUSIONS

How a child manages daily separations imposed by day care depends on multiple factors related to the child's developmental status, the family's relationships, the child's prior experiences with separations, and the nurturant qualities of the day care provider. Parents and providers can assess a child's response along the dimensions of the nature, pattern, and magnitude of the distress. Whereas initial vigorous protest can be seen as integral to healthy adaptation, withdrawal or prolonged intense protests can be seen as signs of disturbance.

Day care providers can assist children in adjusting to substitute care by helping parents provide a gradual transition to day care and by offering the child many opportunities to master the experience of separation through play and through the relationship with the primary caregiver. Parents, providers, and day care consultants cope best with separation responses by keeping in mind that separation is not a single event. Separation is a natural, recurring phenomenon that requires continuous emotional work throughout life.

REFERENCES

Ainsworth M: Attachment: retrospect and prospect, in The Place of Attachment in Human Behavior. Edited by Parkes CM, Stevenson-Hinde J. New York, Basic Books, 1982, pp 25–37

Ainsworth M, Wittig B: Attachment and exploratory behavior in one-year-olds in a Strange Situation, in Determinants of Infant Behavior, Vol 4. Edited by Foss BM. New York, Wiley, 1969, pp 111–136

Ainsworth M, Bell S, Stayton D: Individual differences in Strange-Situation behavior of one-year-olds, in The Origins of Human Social Relations. Edited by Schaffer HR. New York, Academic, 1971, pp 17–57

Bloom-Feshbach S: Variations in adjustment to nursery school, in The Psychology of Separation and Loss. Edited by Bloom-Feshbach J, Bloom-Feshbach S. San Francisco, CA, Jossey-Bass, 1987, pp 207–231

Bowlby J: Attachment and Loss, Vol 2: Separation. New York, Basic Books, 1973

DeCasper A, Fifer W: Of human bonding: newborns prefer their mothers' voices. Science 208:1174–1176, 1980

Field T: Leavetakings and reunions of infants, toddlers, and preschoolers, and their parents. Child Dev 55:628–635, 1984

Fraiberg S: Libidinal object constancy and mental representation. Psychoanalytic Study Child 24:9–47, 1969

Freud S: Inhibitions, symptoms and anxiety (1926), in The Standard Edition of The Complete Psychological Works of Sigmund Freud, Vol 20. Translated and edited by Strachey J. London, Hogarth Press, 1959, pp 87–175

Gunther M: Infant behavior at the breast, in Determinants of Infant Behavior, Vol 1. Edited by Foss B. London, Methuen, 1961, pp 37–44

Hartmann H: Essays on Ego Psychology: Selected Problems in Psychoanalytic Theory. New York, International Universities Press, 1965

Howes C: Quality indicators in infant and toddler child care, in Quality Indicators for Child Care. Edited by Phillips D. Washington, DC, National Association for the Education of Young Children, 1987

Mahler M, Pine F, Bergman A: The Psychological Birth of the Human Infant: Symbiosis and Individuation. New York, Basic Books, 1975

Nachman P: Memory for positive emotional events in 7 month old infants. Paper presented at the National Center for Clinical Infant Programs Fellows' Conference, Yale University, New Haven, CT, 1981

Phillips D, McCartney K, Scarr S, et al: Selective review of infant day care research: a cause for concern. Zero to Three 7(3):18–21, 1987

Piaget J: The Origins of Intelligence in Children. New York, International Universities Press, 1952

Provence S, Naylor A, Patterson J: The Challenge of Daycare. New Haven, CT, Yale University Press, 1977

Rovee-Collier C, Fagan J: The retrieval memory in early infancy, in Advances in Infancy Research, Vol 1. Edited by Lipsitt LP. Norwood, NJ, Ablex, 1981, pp 226–252

Ruopp R, Travess J: James faces day care: perspectives on quality and cost, in Day Care: Scientific and Social Policy Issues. Edited by Zigler EF, Gordon EW. Dover, MA, Auburn House, 1982, pp 72–101

Stern D: The Interpersonal World of the Infant. New York, Basic Books, 1985

Part III

Pediatric Issues in Day Care

Chapter 10

Health and Safety in Child Care

Susan S. Aronson, M.D., F.A.A.P.

Data on the health status of children in child care are scarce. Unfortunately, there is no national surveillance system for child care. The nation's five injury prevention demonstration projects have only begun to look at this issue. One, the Statewide Comprehensive Injury Prevention Program of the Massachusetts Department of Public Health, collects age-specific injury data on childhood injury. However, data on the sites of injury are not currently available. A few studies conducted in the United States and Scandinavia on the incidence of injury in child care suggest that the types of injuries that occur in the child care setting are not different from those experienced by children generally (Chang et al. 1989; Elardo et al. 1987; Jacobsson and Schelp 1987; Landman and Landman 1987).

The United States also lacks a surveillance system for infectious diseases in day care. Outbreaks of infection in child care settings are sensationalized by the lay and medical literature. These reports create the illusion of child care as a setting where outbreaks are common. Although outbreaks give us the opportunity to study how to control the spread of infectious diseases in child care, they do not give us the needed information on the incidence of disease in this setting. Because common infectious diseases occur so frequently among young children in any child care arrangement, the question research must answer is how much, if any, increased risk do children experience by receiving care in groups? In addition, how child care can promote health by meeting the needs of the families who use child care must be addressed.

One of the first priorities for health professionals should be to establish adequate surveillance systems to monitor health and safety problems in the child care setting. Such monitoring systems are likely to improve the quality of care by themselves, since monitoring results in heightened awareness of the risks being measured.

Injury control and prevention, management of infectious diseases, and health promotion are top priorities for all children and especially for those in child care. We can profit by a look at each of these areas.

INJURY CONTROL

Incidence Data

Without widespread surveillance, we do not know whether children are safer or at increased risk of injury in child care. A preliminary assessment of the types of injuries that occur in child care was conducted on insurance claims received by Forrest T. Jones & Company, Inc., during 1981–82 (Aronson 1983). During this period, 422 claims were filed under accident insurance policies covering 14,502 children in child care programs across the United States. Some of the insured child care programs included many sites in several states; others were individual child care centers. Family day care homes were included as well, although all the claims came from centers. This finding may not represent a lesser injury rate in family day care, however, since center users may be more likely to file claims. Although the data are neither complete nor a statistically valid representation of child care as a whole, they are the first available compilation of the types of injuries in a large child care population.

In the insurance study, the products most frequently associated with the severest injuries were, in descending rank, climbers, slides, hand toys and blocks, other playground equipment, doors, indoor floor surfaces, motor vehicles, swings, pebbles or rocks, and pencils. By far, climbers accounted for the greatest number of the most severe injuries. For those injuries in which the location of the accident was specified, nearly two-thirds occurred on the playground. Subsequently published studies have confirmed the incidence data from the analysis of insurance claims (Rivara et al. 1989; Sacks et al. 1989).

Corrective Action

Six implications for corrective action emerge from these injury data:

1. Climbers, slides, and swings used in day care should be modified to reduce injury. The risk is so high with climbers that if the program cannot afford to modify the apparatus, it should be removed. In an extensive study, the U.S. Consumer Product Safety Commission (1978a, 1978b, 1978c, 1981) found climbers, slides, and swings to be associated with a high frequency of severe injury in the general child population. The commission recommended a number of measures to reduce the hazardous use of these play structures:

   - Limiting the maximum climbing height by making the top of the structures closer to the ground.
   - Mounting the structures over at least an 8-inch depth of loose fill materials such as loose sand or pine bark to help absorb impact.
   - Spacing the structures far enough away from other structures and child traffic patterns to prevent collisions.
   - Covering sharp edges and exposed bolts.
   - Limiting the number of children using the structures at one time.
   - Teaching children how to "play happy, play safely," as suggested by a preschool curriculum of the same name developed by the U.S. Consumer Product Safety Commission to help parents and teachers foster safe play habits in children (U.S. Consumer Product Safety Commission 1978b, 1978c).

2. Activities associated with more frequent and more severe injuries, such as climbing and block building, require closer supervision than activities that are less commonly associated with injuries. Because the playground accounts for such a large share of the injuries, staff persons must avoid the understandable tendency to relax their vigilance during large-muscle playtime. This part of the curriculum not only provides opportunities for children to let off steam and build gross motor skills but should also teach children the safety rules that will help them avoid injury.

3. Certain architectural features of child care facilities need modification to reduce the risk of injury, for example, slowing door-closing devices, interrupting open floor space in areas where running is hazardous, and eliminating floor surfaces where children might trip.

4. The majority of motor vehicle injuries are preventable through use of age-appropriate seat restraints, and close attention to driver training and drop-off and pick-up routines.

5. A systematic study of injury in child care programs should be undertaken as a well-planned, prospective, epidemiological effort. Individual child care programs must begin to collect and routinely review reports of injuries occurring in their own programs. These data

should also be aggregated to identify high-risk areas so that preventive strategies can be developed.
6. The staffs of child care programs need training and resources to change hazardous conditions. Training for child care personnel on injury prevention should be focused on the known causes of injury in the age group served. This training should include transportation safety as well as hazard control in the child care facility.

PREVENTION AND MANAGEMENT OF INFECTIOUS DISEASES IN CHILD CARE

Opportunities for Health Promotion

Young children who are brought together in groups for care are exposed to infectious disease agents in a manner analogous to that of a large family. But these children can also benefit from opportunities for health promotion made possible by frequent interaction among parents and caregivers. Child care programs that implement appropriate health and safety policies promote prevention of infectious diseases by requiring that children receive needed immunizations and routine health care. Many child care providers also promote health by giving young and inexperienced parents day-to-day instruction about hygiene, appropriate nutrition, and management of minor illnesses. The success of child care providers as advocates for immunization has been documented; nationally, a greater proportion of children in day care meet American Academy of Pediatrics and United States Public Health Services immunization standards than children not using day care services (Hinman 1986).

Child care personnel must understand immunization schedules well enough to check an individual child's record and identify deficiencies. Child care staff can help allay parental concerns about the use of diphtheria-tetanus-pertussis vaccine evoked by adverse and often inappropriately sensationalized publicity about the risks associated with the vaccine. To serve in this role, child care staff must become familiar with the issues involved and learn how to identify children who need immunization. Children should be directed to health resources for catch-up doses.

Incidence of Infectious Diseases in Child Care

As increasing numbers of younger children become involved in group care settings, health professionals have become more aware of the opportunities for transmission of infection in these environments (The Child Day Care Infectious Disease Study Group 1984; Goodman et al. 1984). A few studies have evaluated the specific characteristics or practices of child care settings that promote or inhibit transmission of infectious disease. With such data, the risk of infection from child care attendance can be reduced.

Outbreaks of gastroenteritis, bacterial meningitis, hepatitis A, and vaccine-preventable diseases have been documented in child care programs. For example, recent reports of higher incidence of shedding of cytomegalovirus (CMV) among child care staff and children have raised concern. Such reports must be kept in perspective. CMV is a cause of birth defects in some fetuses of women who become infected for the first time during pregnancy. However, the virus is widespread in the community; immunity-producing infection during childhood is common and usually occurs without any evidence of illness. Until more data are available on the risk to pregnant workers in child care, the Centers for Disease Control (CDC) advise that no special precautions are needed other than routine handwashing after contact with urine or with respiratory or other body secretions (CDC 1985).

Another area of concern for child care personnel and parents is the correlation between entry into child care and frequency of illness. In one study in which this issue was examined, the overall burden of respiratory infection was not greater for children in a stable child care program, but there was a shift of illness to younger ages (Denny et al. 1986). In this study, conducted at the Frank Porter Graham Child Development Center in North Carolina, infants under 1 year of age had 9.5 respiratory illnesses per child per year. This rate can be compared with 6.7 for children cared for at home, as reported in the Cleveland Family Study (Dingle et al. 1964). However, unlike the Cleveland Family Study, the North Carolina group found that the frequency of respiratory infections in child care children steadily diminished as the children grew older, to less than that for children at home by age 2. By age 5, the North Carolina study found that child care children had only 3.8 respiratory illnesses per child per year, compared with 7.6 for children in the Cleveland Family Study who were receiving care only at home. The significance of the shift of age incidence for common respiratory disease is unknown.

More recent studies by the CDC used telephone surveys and self-reporting by families to determine how the incidence of common respiratory infection is affected by child care attendance, smoking in the home, and crowding (Fleming 1987). The CDC data suggested that all three factors contribute to the reported incidence of respiratory infection, both individually and in aggregate fashion.

Young children have a high frequency of illness under any circumstances. In a large study based on the 1981 National Health Interview Survey, prevalence of reported medicated respiratory illness was highest among children under 3 years of age in child care centers, lower in family day care homes, and lowest when only own-home care was used. After 3 years of age, the difference between child care centers and family day care homes disappeared (Presser 1988). The prevalence of reported illness for children who received care only in their own homes was almost 30%. Children in child care are ill more frequently, but consideration of the magnitude of this increase must include the fact that so many children are reported to be ill in a given 2-week period in any setting.

The data from retrospective surveys may be flawed by parent perception. Parents who use child care may have a heightened awareness of their children's illnesses. They may take them to physicians more readily to avoid work loss due to child illness. Survey data may be biased by these factors and should be viewed with some caution. Based on a growing number of studies of respiratory disease, however, it seems that children under 2 years of age attending child care have an increased number of respiratory tract illnesses and an increased risk of developing otitis media than age-matched control children cared for only in their own homes (Frenck and Glezen 1990).

Recent reports have confirmed the suspected increased risk of primary disease caused by *Haemophilus influenzae* type b among day care users (Band et al. 1984; Redmond and Pichichero 1984). The magnitude of risk varies by geographic area, age of child, and type of child care program. The risk of subsequent cases of *H. influenzae* type b infection after a single case occurs in child care and the use of Rifampin for chemoprophylaxis remain controversial (Osterholm 1990). *H. influenzae* type b is a bacteria that causes brain-damaging meningitis and other serious, deep-tissue infections.

A vaccine against *H. influenzae* type b has been developed and is widely administered to protect children who are 15 months of age or older. However, the largest risk for disease is for children under the age when the current vaccine is effective. A new vaccine is being readied for licensure that will protect most (but not all) recipients over 2 months of age. The American Academy of Pediatrics recommends universal immunization of children aged 15 to 60 months with the currently available conjugate vaccines, and it especially encourages immunization of children who are at increased risk, e.g., children in child care. When effective vaccines for younger children become available, health professionals and child care providers should encourage parents to have one of them administered to their children.

The CDC recommend that Rifampin be given to all children and staff who were exposed to a child who developed *H. influenzae* type B disease in a family or center setting. The American Academy of Pediatrics also recommends that consideration be given to use of postexposure Rifampin prophylaxis but notes that the issue of whether secondary cases occur in child care is still unsettled. The problem with Rifampin prophylaxis in child care is that, to be effective, the drug must be given within 7 days of contact with the infected patient, must be given to at least 75% of the members of the group, and must be given in repeated doses for a prescribed course. Compliance with this type of regimen is best achieved by providing the medication in the child care setting and notifying the personal physicians of those involved. If each individual must seek the drug from a personal physician, compliance is nearly impossible to achieve.

An effective measure for control of gastrointestinal infections in child care has been suggested by studies that compare the incidence of vomiting and diarrhea in child care programs in which conscientious handwashing is practiced with the incidence in child care programs in which no special handwashing program is followed. Without conscientious handwashing practices, children in child care experience two to four episodes of gastroenteritis per child per year, twice as many as do children receiving care at home (Black et al. 1981; Dingle et al. 1964; Pickering and Woodward 1982). With handwashing, the incidence of gastrointestinal disease among child care children drops to near the levels found among children cared for in their own homes.

Measures to Reduce Infectious Diseases in Child Care

The challenge is to reduce the transmission of infectious disease agents in the child care setting without loss of developmentally desirable features of child care. Measures to consider include the following:

1. Assign soft, cuddly toys to individual children where possible.
2. Sanitize frequently mouthed objects and surfaces contaminated by body fluids by washing them with dishwashing detergent and water, followed by a rinse in a dilute bleach solution. A 200-ppm solution can be made by mixing ¼ cup bleach diluted with 1 gallon of water (or 1 tablespoon per quart). To maintain the minimum required strength, the solution must be made fresh daily.
3. Establish routines for handwashing for staff and children.
4. Establish routines for handling fecally contaminated materials and surfaces.
5. Require immunization for child care participation. If immunizations are delayed for any reason, systems must be in place to follow up where needed.
6. Establish reasonable, scientifically supportable policies for excluding children with transmissible infection. Considering the lack of evidence that exclusion for respiratory infection makes any difference, the decision about permitting a child to remain in child care with respiratory illness should depend on the availability of the parent to

provide sick-child care and the ability of the caregivers to provide the extra attention that an ill child requires. On the other hand, it is prudent to exclude children with infectious diarrhea from child care because they pose a significant risk for transmission of the disease if they remain in the program.

7. Establish criteria for parents and child care professionals to differentiate suspected cases of infectious diarrhea from other causes of loose stools. Because of the potential public health consequences of infectious diarrhea among children in child care, health providers may need to be reminded to use laboratory testing more freely to identify causative agents of gastrointestinal disease among children in child care.

Many states lack specific regulations requiring sanitation inspections of child care facilities by personnel trained to conduct such inspections. Few communities have public health officials willing and able to provide consultation to local child care programs. Many areas need improved standards and public health inspections of day care programs at the local level. Where these safeguards are lacking, the responsibility for prevention and management of infectious disease problems in child care programs falls to child care staff and individual child health professionals whose patients are using child care.

HEALTH NEEDS OF INDIVIDUAL CHILDREN

Injury control and prevention and management of infectious diseases in child care are areas in which the need for action is apparent. A more subtle health implication of child care program use is the need to assure that the unique requirements of individual children are met during the many hours children spend in this setting. In this area, pediatricians and other health professionals should work closely with parents and the child care staff.

The health professional's role in meeting the needs of individual children whose families plan to use child care begins with helping families evaluate their plans. Some parents are highly conflicted about arranging for child care outside their immediate family. Some may not be aware of alternatives such as using flex time, deferring employment, or sharing parenting within their own families.

Once the decision to seek care outside the family is made, the health professional can use knowledge of the family, of the child, and of available community child care resources to help families find appropriate child care settings for their children. Health professionals can guide parents in the search for alternative child care by referring them to child care resource and referral centers in communities where such services exist. Where there are no such centers, health professionals can give parents the telephone number of the child care licensing agency to call for a list of licensed programs convenient to them. At the very least, health professionals can share the information gathered from other parents about community programs used by patients in their practices.

To carry out these roles, health professionals must be as well informed about child care in their community as possible. Some child care programs help educate local health professionals by contacting them about child care children who are their patients, by sending them child care newsletters and program brochures, and by inviting them to open houses at the child care facility. A late morning visit to a child care program (during peak activity time) extended through lunch and the beginning of nap time can provide valuable understanding of a particular child care program.

Child health providers should use periodic health assessments to collect information from caregivers about early signs of correctable problems and to provide health-promoting advice and services. Child care program regulations often require that children have periodic health assessments, usually documented by having the health provider complete a form. This chore accomplishes more than one purpose. The presentation of the form by the parent alerts the health provider that the child is a child care user and opens the door for discussion of the child care experience.

For some families, the requirement to deliver a completed form for the child to attend the program may be the incentive for making an appointment for a preventive health care visit. Despite pediatric advocacy, many children do not receive preventive care as frequently as is appropriate to their age and developmental status. Data from the 1975–76 National Health Interview Survey indicated that 14% of children and youth did not meet the guidelines of the American Academy of Pediatrics for routine care (U.S. Department of Health and Human Services 1981a, 1981b). Among children from large families and among black children, about one-fifth did not see a physician frequently enough to receive adequate preventive care. Child care professionals usually collect information about community resources for child health care to help families with special health or social problems find services.

By sharing their observations, caregivers help health providers shape recommendations to promote more effectively the healthy development of individual children. Communication among parents, health professionals, and day care personnel is essential to mobilize all persons involved with the child on the child's behalf. The child whose behavior or development is of concern may be recognized sooner by an experienced caregiver who observes the child in a peer group than by a parent who lacks opportunities for comparison.

To be effective, there must be two-way communication between health providers and day care staff. The physician has important information about unique features of the child's health to share with the child care personnel. The child care staff have information about the child's behavior on a day-to-day basis to share with the physician. Admittedly, effective communication between the child's physician and regular caregivers is sometimes difficult to achieve. Usually, parents convey information about the child between the doctor and caregiver; but, with prior approval from a parent, telephone calls or notes between the child care staff and doctor may be more efficient and effective.

Appropriate topics for routine communication between a child's physician and child care provider include 1) the child's current state of health and nutrition, including any special needs for management of the child in health and illness; 2) growth and development of the child in relation to adaptations that might be required of the child care facility or program; 3) social and behavioral skills of the child; and 4) family strengths and weaknesses that affect the use of child care and health care services. It is especially important for the child's doctor to engage in interactive communication with the child care staff about children with behavior problems, developmental difficulties, or chronic disease. Parental consent for such communication is often easily obtained.

Parents whose children use child care need to be reminded to find and maintain appropriate emergency contact arrangements. Many parents are unaware that they must always be available to give at least telephone consent for medical treatment. Except in a life-threatening situation, medical-legal considerations preclude providing treatment to a child without informed consent from the parent. Consent forms for medical care signed by the parent in advance, without knowledge of the treatment required, are not considered informed consent. Many child care programs collect signatures authorizing any necessary emergency treatment when the only valid consent that can be obtained in advance is for transport of the child to a facility for emergency care.

Parents and caregivers usually appreciate a doctor who takes the time to share information about child care and who communicate with child care staff. Physicians who foster communication among all those involved with the child are often mentioned by child care professionals when parents ask for suggestions about where to go for good health care for their children.

THE NEED FOR A HEALTH CONSULTANT FOR CHILD CARE

Child care program administrators are becoming increasingly aware of the need to identify a specific health professional to serve as an overall program health consultant. The role of the health consultant includes providing and interpreting the advice of national, standard-setting bodies to develop site-specific policies for the child care program, and serving as a point of access to technical information when health issues arise. Advice might be needed about what should be done when an outbreak of disease occurs in a child care program or how to handle a child whose biting behaviors are disrupting the program. For infectious disease issues, health professionals can stay informed by subscribing to *Morbidity and Mortality Weekly,* the report of new information disseminated by the CDC. Other good sources are the publications of the American Academy of Pediatrics. Child health providers can also stay abreast of the most current recommendations for handling specific infectious disease problems by contacting local departments of public health.

When advice is sought about how to handle other health or behavior problems, health professionals would do well to use the same problem-oriented approach they would use in the office setting: gather all the subjective data by talking with those who are involved in any way with the problem, collect whatever objective information is available, formulate an assessment (and check for concurrence with those who are involved), and formulate a plan that includes all parties. The plan may involve collection of additional objective data, a strategy to use in the interim, and education of all those involved about the plan and the rationale for it. Additional health and mental health consultation is often valuable.

One of the most helpful roles a health consultant can play is to participate in the development of program-specific health policies. The policies serve as guidelines for day-to-day operations, which necessarily go on with little health professional input. As a minimum, child care program policies should address topics related to health, safety, and sanitation in the child care program (see Table 10-1).

Yet another role for health professionals is child care staff training. Few workers in child care programs have had any health education beyond that provided to most of the public. Because aspects of child care have health implications, there is a need for preservice orientation and ongoing training on health promotion for child care staff. The essential elements of the health component should be covered in such training and should be recorded for regular reference in the day care program health policies.

CHILD CARE FOR ILL CHILDREN

The care of ill children who use child care deserves special attention (see Oremland, Chapter 11, this volume). Studies have shown that young children can be expected to have six to eight upper respiratory infections

Table 10-1. Checklist of health policies for child care

Inclusion or exclusion of children with health problems at enrollment and on an ongoing day-to-day basis

Daily admission and ongoing surveillance for infection and illness

Care of ill children

Management of injuries, emergency preparedness, and first aid

Safety surveillance in the facility, on the playground, and on trips

Transportation safety for routine pick-up, drop-off, and pedestrian or motor vehicle travel

Medication administration

Routine health assessments for children, including information exchange among providers of health care, child care staff, and parents

Nutrition, food, and formula handling

Sanitation routines, including handling of contaminated clothing and furnishings, as well as routine cleaning

Dental hygiene practices

Provision for bathing or swimming if appropriate

Health promotion and health education activities

A mechanism for routine annual review of health policies by child care staff, parents, and health consultants

---

and one or two gastrointestinal infections per year, whether cared for at home or in child care (Black et al. 1981; Dingle et al. 1964; Loda et al. 1972).

All parents and child care providers need to plan how children will be managed when they are ill. Although home care by parents may be the ideal approach, this alternative is not practical and probably not truly necessary for every illness. Employers need to modify sick leave policies so more parents can use their benefits to care for their children during significant illnesses.

If sick children are to remain in child care, provision must be made to attend to their needs for extra nurturance without depriving the other children in the group of the attention they require. Many illnesses are most contagious when the children have no symptoms; for these, exclusion should be required only when the child's need for extra attention exceeds the child care staff's resources to provide the care. Whenever possible, child care programs should provide supplemental staffing to groups in which children are ill but not contagious. In this way, ill children can remain with familiar caregivers in familiar settings while they recover.

New options for sick-child care are being explored, including sick-child centers and in-home caregivers available to care for children who are ill and whose parents can afford the high costs of home health workers. As alternative options are developed, child care and health care professionals must advocate for children, to be certain that while arrangements are made so parents do not miss time from work, children are not punished for being ill by being sent to unfamiliar caregivers in strange environments.

CHILD CARE HEALTH AT THE COMMUNITY LEVEL

At the community level, there is much to be done. It is unrealistic to expect parents to provide adequate monitoring of child care quality on an ongoing basis. Parents of young children often lack the experience required to recognize hazardous conditions and may accept risks because of their need for child care. Maintenance of adequate regulations and competent monitoring of compliance are essential to protect young children who are in child care. Many state child care regulations lack specific statements about health, safety, and sanitation requirements. Inspections are not uniformly conducted, and they often omit observations for significant health risks (Schrag 1984; U.S. Department of Health and Human Services 1981a, 1981b).

Like caregivers, regulators assigned to inspect child care programs often lack any health training. Even if they are trained in a health discipline, they may lack any pediatric expertise to guide their observations. Health professionals can help provide training for licensing staff and improve the guidelines used by public agencies for the protection of children. Rational application of realistic guidelines will help protect the staff and children from significant health and safety risks in the child care environment.

CONCLUSIONS

In health as in other aspects of child care, when an interdisciplinary approach is used, children will benefit. Integrating health with other concerns in child care is essential to achieving quality in child day care. Child care professionals, health professionals, and parents must work together to make this aspect of child care work well.

REFERENCES

Aronson S: Injuries in child care. Young Children 38:19–20, 1983

Band J, Fraser D, Ajello G: *Haemophilus influenzae*. Diseases study group: prevention of *Haemophilus influenzae* type b disease by Rifampin prophylaxis. JAMA 251:2381, 1984

Black RE, Dykes AC, Anderson KE: Handwashing to prevent diarrhea in day-care centers. Am J Epidemiol 113:445–451, 1981

Centers for Disease Control: Prevalence of cytomegalovirus excretion from children in five day-care centers in Alabama. MMWR 34:49–51, 1985

Chang A, Lugg M, Nebedum A: Injuries among preschool children enrolled in day-care centers. Pediatrics 83:272–277, 1989

The Child Day Care Infectious Disease Study Group: Public health considerations of infectious diseases in child day care centers. J Pediatrics 105:683–701, 1984

Denny F, Collier A, Henderson F: Acute respiratory infections in day care. RID 8:527–532, 1986

Dingle H, Badger F, Jordan S: Illness in the Home. Cleveland, OH, Western Reserve University Press, 1964

Elardo, R, Solomons HC, Snider BC: An analysis of accidents at a day care center. Am J Orthopsychiatry 14:60–65, 1987

Fleming DW, Cochi SL, Hightower AW, et al: Childhood upper respiratory tract infections. Pediatrics 79:55–60, 1987

Frenck R, Glezen W: Respiratory tract infections in children in day care. Seminars in Pediatric Infectious Diseases 1:234–244, 1990

Goodman A, Osterholm MT, Granoft DM, et al: Infectious diseases and child day care. Pediatrics 74:134–139, 1984

Hinman A: Vaccine-preventable diseases and child day care. Reviews of Infectious Diseases 8:573–583, 1986

Jacobsson B, Schelp L: Home accidents among children and teenagers in a Swedish rural municipality. Scand J Soc Med 15:31–35, 1987

Landman PF, Landman GB: Accidental injuries in children in day care centers. Am J Dis Child 141:292–293, 1987

Loda FA, Glezen WP, Clyde WA: Respiratory disease in group day care. Pediatrics 49:428–437, 1972

Osterholm M: Invasive bacterial diseases and child day care. Seminars in Pediatric Infectious Diseases 1:222–233, 1990

Pickering LK, Woodward WE: Diarrhea in day care centers. Pediatr Infect Dis J 1:47–52, 1982

Presser H: Place of child care and medicated respiratory illness among young American children. Journal of Marriage and the Family 50:995–1005, 1988

Redmond SR, Pichichero E: Hemophilus influenzae type b disease. JAMA 251:2581–2584, 1984

Rivara F, DiGuiseppi C, Thompson R, et al: Risk of injury to children less than 5 years of age in day care versus home care settings. Pediatrics 84:1011–1016, 1989

Sacks J, Smith J, Kaplan K, et al: The epidemiology of injuries in Atlanta day-care centers. JAMA 262:1641–1645, 1989

Schrag E: Infant and toddler care in the states: a comparative licensing study and beyond. Zero to Three 4(3):8–11, 1984

U.S. Consumer Product Safety Commission, Division of Human Factors: Human Factors Analyses of Injuries Associated With Public Playground Equipment. Washington, DC, U.S. Government Printing Office, 1978a

U.S. Consumer Product Safety Commission: Play Happy, Play Safely: A Child-Centered Playground Safety Curriculum Approach. Washington, DC, U.S. Government Printing Office, 1978b

U.S. Consumer Product Safety Commission: Play Happy, Play Safely: A Look at the Playground Education Materials. Washington, DC, U.S. Government Printing Office, 1978c

U.S. Consumer Product Safety Commission: A Handbook for Public Playground Safety, Vol 1: General Guidelines for New and Existing Playgrounds. Vol 2: Technical Guidelines for Equipment and Surfacing. Washington, DC, U.S. Government Printing Office, 1981

U.S. Department of Health and Human Services: Better Health for Our Children: A National Strategy. Washington, DC, U.S. Government Printing Office, 1981a

U.S. Department of Health and Human Services: Summary Report of the Assessment of Current State Practices in Title XX Funded Day Care Programs: Report to Congress, Washington, DC, DHHS, 1981b

Chapter 11

Childhood Illness and Day Care

Evelyn K. Oremland, Ph.D.

Parents become aware rather early that sustained perfect health for their young children, no matter the degree of effort toward that ideal, is not possible. Although reports of statistical frequencies vary somewhat as to the extent of ill health in normally well young children, there is complete agreement that the minor illnesses of childhood occur and recur frequently throughout the early years. For example, Work/Family Directions (1985) cited the following: young children typically get 8 to 10 viral infections per year (Skold 1985), each lasting from 3 to 7 days (Pantell et al. 1982), and more than 46% of preschool children studied were ill 10 or more days during the year (Chang et al. 1978).

CURRENT ISSUES AND PRACTICES IN SICK CHILD CARE

In the United States, more than half the mothers of young children are now employed. It is no surprise, then, that child care becomes particularly complicated during times of illness. Accepted practice used to reflect the guidelines of the 1930 White House Conference: Sick children should be excluded from school. Similarly, sick children were excluded from day care or isolated until taken home by their parents. Currently, taking care of one's sick child at home is a "luxury" that many cannot afford. No longer is the child's state of health the only consideration in planning for care during his or her illness. Workplace demands on parents and the difficulty of finding care for sick children have affected standard practice.

Pressures are such that today's experts recommend what may have seemed routine before: serious illness calls for parent care at home. Brazelton (1987, p. 184), for example, suggested: "Working parents should save up their sick leave so they can take a day at home with a sick child." Similarly, Fredricks and her colleagues (1985, p. 5) wrote: "When children become ill . . . parents usually take time off from work. At these times the right solution is for the parent or a close member of the family to be with the child. Parents need to be free to choose to stay home with their children without fear of reprisals by [work] supervisors."

Although some surveys indicate that mothers generally do stay home with sick children (Clinton 1985), there are reports of pressures to stay on the job from employers and parent concerns regarding job maintenance, continuing income, and career advancement that interfere with the stay-at-home practice. Kahn and Kamerman (1987, p. 190) noted: "Many parents, even when they manage to find an affordable, reliable, and satisfactory child care arrangement, still speak with something akin to horror when they describe their fears about a child getting sick on a work day." For parents, the dilemma is in deciding when it is necessary to stay home with a sick child and for how long. The current direction, as indicated in the literature on sick-child care models and by pediatric and day care professionals, is toward some form of continuing day care during the onset of illness and in extended recuperative phases.

Appeals have been made for greater flexibility at parents' workplaces, including allowances for leave when children are ill and establishment of employer-sponsored day care/sick-child care. The latter could benefit employers by creating a situation in which parents could stay on the job, knowing their children were being well cared for. But economic rewards for employers must be soundly demonstrated before an employer will risk the practice. In situations in which employers are financially unable to make the desirable changes, the implementation of governmental contributions is essential. These contributions can include grants for sick-child leave for parents, or advantaged tax considerations for employers who support appropriate sick care arrangements.

Sick-Child Day Care Regulations

Fredricks and her colleagues (1985) noted that the challenge in sick-child care is to require exclusion when it is necessary while recognizing when it is unnecessary or counterproductive. Regulations should specify when it is safe for mildly ill children to be in group care as well as provide guidelines for quality care for such children.

Most states specifically require isolation of a child who becomes ill during the day. Variations among states reflect a range of perspectives and degrees of regulatory standards. Often, vague legislative directives leave many of the decisions to the child care providers themselves (see Miller, Chapter 15, this volume).

State regulations are in a transitional phase. California, for example, established a Sick Child Care Task Force to develop "regulations regarding the care of children with non-life-endangering illnesses" (California Department of Social Services 1987). California currently maintains interim licensure of day care centers that care for ill children, pending adoption of the regulations. The interim procedures require that waivers be implemented, providing exceptions to the requirements still in effect that completely exclude sick children.

The California plan calls for the creation of a segregated area of the center, one not to be used by the well children. During the day in which the sick child enters the sick-child area, he or she is not permitted to use the rest of the center. The regulation guidelines offer extensive detailing of physical environment and personnel practices. In addition, they offer criteria for exclusion of sick children with the following symptoms or illnesses: rapid or difficult breathing, stiff neck, undiagnosed rash, persistent vomiting, persistent diarrhea, yellowing of the eyes or skin, fever of 100.5°F (oral) associated with any one or more of the foregoing, chicken pox, mumps, or measles. Yet children with any of these conditions may be accepted for day care when a health professional determines that the child is not seriously ill or in a contagious stage of the illness (California Department of Social Services 1987).

Formats for Sick-Child Care

Although a variety of day care arrangements attempt to meet the needs of sick children and working parents, their availability is still limited. A growing series of publications covering sick-child care issues lists models, giving specific examples and localities of each (e.g., Fredricks et al. 1985; Mohlabane 1983).

Parent care at home. Parental care in the child's own home is the simplest to arrange if the parent is not regularly employed outside the home or if the two parents can arrange a system of turns, given part-time or flexibly scheduled employment. Familiarity of relationship and environment is maintained, allowing the child the potential for use of his or her primary relationship in responding to the situation.

Given the propensity and employer allowances to do so, care at home by a parent is common, particularly during acute phases of the illnesses. Parents and employers are quick to report the difficulties inherent in such arrangements, including the inability to anticipate the onset of the illness, the effects of the disruptions on work, and, with repeated illness episodes, the risk to productivity and job stability.

Substitute care at home.   Calling a special sitter for daytime care during illness is another alternative, albeit an expensive one. Reduced hourly fees are available through special sick-child care programs in some communities. Parents hasten to note, however, not only that such programs are insufficiently available, but also that they introduce a stranger to the child at a time of increased vulnerability. In addition, parent confidence in an unknown child care worker at such times may be less than firm.

The sick-child center.   Operating under such names as Wheezles and Sneezles (Fasciano 1985), special centers for the care of sick children have evolved in a number of communities. These centers frequently use a nurse to screen entering children. Children with infections may be rejected, with instructions to the parent to consult a physician. Such centers are often used during the recuperative phase. In commenting on a sick-child care center, one mother recognized that the quieter nature of the center more closely fit the capacities of her child during recuperation than did the more challenging activities of the regular day care center. Family day care homes may also become sites for sick-child care. "Day hospitals," in which mildly ill children are cared for in underutilized areas of hospitals, have also emerged recently.

Sick-child care in a regular center.   Most models for this kind of care are relatively recently established and are frequently referred to as "pioneer" projects. There is little memory of the Kaiser Center, established in Oregon during World War II, which had an infirmary in each of its two units (Hymes and Eliot 1978). The infirmary children were those who were not well enough to be with their regular groups, yet not sick enough to be home. Generally, these children's conditions were not contagious: many had minor colds; others were in recuperative phases following illnesses. Children could be assigned to the infirmary as needed, either at the beginning or during the course of a day.

Each infirmary was staffed by a registered nurse, with overall supervision from a physician who consulted daily with the nurse. The number of teachers from the child care center assigned to the infirmary depended on the number of sick children on a particular day and on the developmental or other specific needs of those children. A maximum of 10 to 12 children could be cared for in each of the infirmary units (J. L. Hymes, personal communication, April 1987).

Where state regulations permit, some day care centers have developed areas in their facilities for sick children. Assignment of special staff in this use of a "sick bay" repeats the Kaiser design. Parents may deliver sick children directly to these areas, and a child who becomes ill during the day can easily move to the sick bay area.

Combination models. A more recent innovation has been the development of a specialized family day care home, which is set up as an adjunct to a particular day care center. The family day caregiver is an assistant in the regular center and is thus familiar to the children. If a child becomes ill during the day, this caregiver will take the child to the family day care home, or a parent may bring a sick child there directly if appropriate notice is given.

Day Care and Infectious Illness

The occurrence of illness because of day care is also an issue in current discussions. Some take the position that day care represents a danger to children's health. Schuman (1983, p. 76), for example, wrote that "studies . . . of infections contracted at day care centers support a growing suspicion that these infections are an important problem." Brazelton (1987, p. 131), too, suggested that children in day care are liable to contract more disease: "As new children move into an area crowded with other children, they are bound to be sick over and over until they get immune to all the new germs." He went on to note, however, that after this initial period, "they'll be well for years to come—their immunity will be high."

A 1985 report from the Centers for Disease Control concluded:

> Child care settings should be recognized as special epidemiologic environments, just as schools are. . . . Parents need to accept that placing a child in a DCC [day care center] adds new parental considerations and responsibilities, including the possibilities of disease transmission within DCCs. (Child Day Care Infectious Diseases Study Group 1985, p. 134)

The preceding positions are challenged by others who believe that children contract the same number of illnesses regardless of whether they are in day care or at home (see Aronson, Chapter 10, this volume, for a discussion of this issue). In a recent review, however, higher incidence of illness and complications within the younger group of children in day care is reported (Wald et al. 1988).

This issue remains unresolved. Regardless of whether children contract as many or more illnesses at day care than at home, and regardless of whether they are cared for at home or elsewhere, ill children require special care. Finding ways to address the specific needs of ill children is the issue addressed here.

VULNERABILITIES AND BEHAVIORS OF CHILDREN DURING ILLNESS

Studies indicate that children are particularly vulnerable during illness (Freud 1952; Oremland and Oremland 1973). Illness in early childhood heightens their sense of vulnerability and may thus intensify the needs of children for their parents. This situation may be expressed in increased clinging and irritable behavior. Such regression occurs in sick children whether they are cared for by day care providers with whom they have strong attachments or whether they remain under the care of their mothers at home, although the quality of this response may differ from one circumstance to the other.

Regressive behavior during illness includes mood swings, loss of self-confidence, and temper tantrums. Symptoms such as bed wetting, soiling, feeding and sleeping troubles, and anxiety about separation that had existed and had been overcome earlier in life may reappear. At times, children who are considered brilliant in their intellectual performance before illness appear dull and apathetic afterward. "Others surprise their parents and teachers by emerging from the same experience curiously ripened and matured." (Freud 1952, p. 70)

In regressions secondary to illness, newly acquired developmental achievements are frequently lost (Oremland and Oremland 1973). Emerging capabilities are particularly threatened when an overwhelming experience occurs, for such experiences have not yet become consolidated.

The degree or severity of disease may have less meaning to children than does the experience of illness itself. Infants and young children may perceive the symptoms of minor, major, or chronic illness in terms of pain, separation, or immobilization rather than in terms of particular diagnoses. The sick child's self-concept or his or her sense of security with relationships may be imperiled, regardless of the seriousness of the disease.

Mattson and Weisberg (1970) conducted a particularly informative study of the reactions to illness of nonhospitalized children cared for by their mothers at home. The researchers followed 35 children, aged approximately 2 to 4, from one pediatric practice. Over a 3-year period, 76 illnesses were reported, covering acute, febrile infectious illnesses (usually viral upper respiratory infections but also otitis media and chicken pox). The average duration of illness was 5 days. Some of the children were reported to show irritability and fatigue before any specific physical symptoms were evident. Most verbalized pain or discomfort as these symptoms developed. Several of the mothers of the youngest children reported clinging and crying at illness onset.

During the acute phase of illness, all children showed behavioral changes. They became less active, slept longer, and had diminished appetites. All became more irritable, especially with their mothers, and all showed transient setbacks in their beginning independence and self-care. Many of the children had a short-lived return of earlier fears of animals, monsters, and the dark. Mattson and Weisberg (1970, p. 607) noted the "continuously clinging, whiny dependence on the mother" of most of the 2-year-olds, who insisted on as much "physical closeness as possible," such as sitting in their mothers' laps and wanting to be carried. The 3- and 4-year-olds were more likely to withdraw into a "self-contained, undemanding state" such as resting, looking at books, coloring, or watching television. Although less involved with their mothers, these older children made occasional demands and whined briefly if these were not immediately satisfied. These children were the most "independent" in the sample, seemingly detached from others. Yet heightened irritability and short-lived anger were noted in all of the children for 1 to 5 days as their previous vigor returned.

Interestingly, children who were relatively undemanding during the acute phase of their illnesses became irritable, easily frustrated, and anxious over separation during the convalescent period. Such a response may be in recognition of the parents' inability to protect the children from illness. Confrontation with this reality challenges the child's perception of the parent as omnipotent and provokes feelings of helplessness.

Because studies suggest a greater vulnerability for children with chronic illness, it may be hypothesized that a risk factor exists for children whose infections seem chronic or unduly recurrent. The chronicity of illness, more than the incidence of illness, may be of greatest concern (i.e., when the child is struggling with one infection after another with limited intervening periods of good health). Recurrent infections in the child often create stress for the parents and burden the parent-child relationship. In these cases a reevaluation of the child care program, possibly with mental health consultation, is indicated. Research comparing such children in day care with those cared for at home is badly needed.

HELPING CHILDREN THROUGH ILLNESS

Caregiver Support

The central factor in effectively supporting the ongoing development of children with chronic disorders or recurrent health problems is the quality of parental and other caregiver care during illness and afterward. Child development professionals and day care workers list in their own guidelines their knowledge that young children, especially when ill, require familiar caregivers and environments. Separation from parents during illness places an increased burden on the child (Bowlby 1973; Bowlby et al. 1952; Vernon et al. 1965). In the absence of the primary caregiver, an ongoing, well-established relationship with a substitute caregiver is of primary importance in supporting recovery.

Until the child feels renewed confidence in having mastered the anxieties of a vulnerable time, the caring adult enables coping and provides a buffer against severe regression. Psychologically oriented observers recognize that regression and other negative responses are a defense against anxieties. Because regression is most likely to entail the child's loss of his or her most recently acquired skills, the caregiver must recognize the meanings of those skills and their loss to the child. Supportive help to the child includes the adult's conveying that the loss is temporary and that when the child feels better he or she will again participate as before. As the adult's understanding is conveyed to the child, he or she comes to know that the adult can be trusted at times of distress. If the regression is negated or ignored, the child's anxieties in overwhelming circumstances may greatly increase.

In some situations, children's responses to illness or other stress may include unusual developmental progressions. In these cases, comparable understanding is required. Although support for mature behavior is appropriate, the caregiver must also recognize that these behaviors may be a "cover" for anxieties about regression. In these children, regression in other areas may be expected, and this regression will require attention.

Play and Transitional Objects

Children's transitional objects may become particular necessities during a stressful time. The child's use of a special object as a means of comfort at bedtime or at times of loneliness and depression was discussed by Winnicott (1953). In fact, the need for a specific, comforting object or behavior pattern that started at an early age may reappear at a later age during illness or other vulnerable periods.

In addition to the importance of transitional objects, spontaneously developed play during illness—in directions and at a pace set by the child—must be supported and enabled to continue, both in day care and at home. Although the potential curative effects of play were described decades ago by Erikson (1950), adult caregivers still frequently fail to understand subtleties in the latent themes of children's play (Oremland 1986) and thus may miss valuable opportunities to understand what the central issues are for the child. Adult caregivers need to be particularly cognizant of single themes in play that may be clues to important issues the child is pursuing in efforts toward mastery. Certain themes, for example, may indicate that the child needs reassurance that the illness is not his or her fault and does not represent punishment.

During healthy periods, "playing out" the sequence of going to sick-child care, participating there, and being called for by a parent for the return home is a play approach that can help children to prepare for their illness experiences. Other preparation may include the child's visiting the sick bay and reading stories there with the sick care worker, with the parent or regular caregiver present, if possible.

Hospitalized children's play powerfully demonstrates how children attempt to resolve the anxieties associated with illness and various medical procedures (Oremland 1988). Studies of hospitalized children draw attention to the importance of therapeutic play in helping children to prepare for health care experiences such as hospitalization, surgery, or other medical procedures. The basic premise is that the child becomes able to incorporate, a little at a time, that which may be overwhelming if presented all at once, as during the experience itself. An inner preparedness thus can evolve in advance of what is otherwise potentially traumatic (Jessner et al. 1952). In addition, in therapeutic play, the child turns the passive experience of illness into active participation in the process, thus helping himself or herself to cope with anxiety through mastery.

CONCLUSIONS

Although more needs to be learned, much is already known about children's responses to illness, the effects of multiple childhood illnesses at vulnerable developmental periods, and the care of ill children. Theoretical understanding will increase the effectiveness of day care professionals in their care of ill children. Further, mental health consultations to support appropriate parental roles in recurrent episodes of childhood illness may help to alleviate difficulties at those times and afterward.

It is essential to focus on the priorities for the children. When their illnesses are mild, or when they are recuperating and their parents' full-time attention is not possible, day care must meet the particular challenges. Greater understanding of children's responses in these circumstances will allow for more effective approaches that recognize children's emotional as well as physical needs.

REFERENCES

Bowlby J: Attachment and Loss, Vol 2: Separation. New York, Basic Books, 1973

Bowlby J, Robertson J, Rosenbluth D: A two-year-old goes to hospital. Psychoanal Study Child 7:82–94, 1952

Brazelton TB: Working and Caring. Reading, MA, Addison-Wesley, 1987

California Department of Social Services. Unpublished memo on day care centers for ill children. Sacramento, CA, March 1987

Chang A, Harris M, Kelso G, et al: Sick Care Arrangements for Children Enrolled in Day Care. Berkeley, CA, University of California School of Public Health, 1978

Child Day Care Infectious Disease Study Group: Considerations of infectious diseases in day care centers. Pediatr Infect Dis J 4:124–136, 1985

Clinton LH: Guess who stays home with a sick child? Working Mother, Oct 1985, pp 55–64

Erikson E: Childhood and Society. New York, Norton, 1950

Fasciano N: From Wheezles and Sneezles to chicken soup. Working Mother, Oct 1985, pp 62–64

Fredricks B, Hardman R, Morgan G, et al: A Little Bit Under the Weather. Boston, MA, Work/Family Directions, 1985

Freud A: The role of bodily illness in the mental life of children. Psychoanal Study Child 7:69–81, 1952

Hymes JL, Eliot AA: Early Childhood Education: Living History Interviews, Book 2: Care of the Children of Working Mothers. Carmel, CA, Hacienda Press, 1978

Jessner L, Blom GE, Waldfogel S: Emotional implications of tonsillectomy and adenoidectomy. Psychoanal Study Child 7:69–81, 1952

Kahn AJ, Kamerma SB: Child Care: Facing the Hard Choices. Dover, MA, Auburn House, 1987

Mattson A, Weisberg I: Behavioral reactions to minor illness in preschool children. Pediatrics 46:604–610, 1970

Mohlabane N: Infants in day care centers, in sickness and in health. Unpublished master's thesis, Pacific Oaks College, Pasadena, CA, 1983

Oremland E: Helping young children cope with community tragedies. Unpublished manuscript, 1986

Oremland E: Mastering developmental and critical experiences through play and other expressive behaviors in childhood. Children's Health Care 16:150–156, 1988

Oremland E, Oremland J (eds): The Effects of Hospitalization on Children. Springfield, IL, Charles C Thomas, 1973

Pantell RH, Fries JF, Vickery DM: Taking Care of Your Child: A Parent's Guide to Medical Care. Reading, MA, Addison-Wesley, 1982

Schuman S: Day-care associated infection: more than meets the eye (editorial). JAMA 249:76, 1983

Skold K: Working parents and the problem of sick child care. Unpublished report for local grantmakers. Stanford University, Stanford, CA, 1985

Vernon D, Foley J, Sipowicz R, et al: The Psychological Responses of Children to Hospitalization and Illness. Springfield, IL, Charles C Thomas, 1965

Wald ER, Dashefsky B, Byers C, et al: Frequency and severity of infections in day care. J Pediatr 112:540–546, 1988

Winnicott D: Transitional objects and transitional phenomena. Int J Psychoanal 34:89–97, 1953

Work/Family Directions: Guides to Child Care Regulations. Boston, MA, Work/Family Directions, 1985

Part IV

Child Abuse and Day Care

Chapter 12

Sexual Abuse in Day Care

Robert J. Kelly, Ph.D.

In this chapter I will examine some of what we know about the reality of sexual abuse in day care and attempt to answer the following questions: How much and what types of sexual abuse actually occur in day care settings? What is the impact of day care sexual abuse on communities, families, and the victims themselves? How can we best cope with the negative impact of sexual abuse when it does occur?

Public belief in the existence of child sexual abuse in day care settings has followed the path of a steel pendulum. For years it sat inert, in a displaced starting position bounded by public denial and ignorance. It was only in the mid-1980s that media forces, themselves fueled by eye-opening accounts of large-scale child molestation reports, succeeded in pulling an inert public belief to a most uncomfortable and quickly accelerating state of unrest. The forces of fear and paranoia rushed in. During this period, many people believed that child molestation in day care was omnipresent.

Since 1988, most notably in California, it appears that public belief may now be swinging back. With the unsettling potential for false allegations in combination with the seemingly insoluble difficulty of confirmation, public attitudes seem to be retreating toward the more familiar, although unrealistic, position of yesteryear—a position of underbelief.

Of course, public belief comprises many individual belief systems that vacillate at varying speeds and amplitudes. Indeed, the media at times seem to delight in fostering these vacillations, presenting well-timed, contradictory facts and opinion pieces to yank our belief systems back and forth, hindering our attempts to find the truth. Perhaps with increased knowledge, parents and professionals, no matter what their current positions, may begin to overcome the powerful and divisive forces of denial, ignorance, fear, and paranoia by cooperatively moving public belief toward a more accurate and steady position.

INCIDENCE AND TYPES OF DAY CARE ABUSE: THE UNIVERSITY OF NEW HAMPSHIRE STUDY

Undoubtedly our best source of information on the extent of sexual abuse in day care comes from the remarkably thorough national study conducted recently by Finkelhor, Williams, and their colleagues at the University of New Hampshire's (UNH) Family Research Laboratory. Finkelhor et al. (1988) attempted to identify all cases of sexual abuse in day care that were reported in the United States from 1983 to 1985. The study identified 270 centers in which sexual abuse had been substantiated, involving a total of 1,639 victimized children. Since some cases were missed because of problems in the reporting system, the estimated number of substantiated cases was then based on the states with the most complete data. This extrapolation yielded an estimate of 500 to 550 reported and substantiated cases and 2,500 victims for the 3-year period. It became painfully clear that sexual abuse certainly does exist in day care centers.

Finkelhor et al. were quick, however, to encourage us to put this tragic reality into perspective by realizing that there are 229,000 day care facilities nationwide serving seven million children. They estimated that the risk of sexual abuse in day care centers is 5.5 children sexually abused per 10,000 enrolled. This rate is lower than the risk of children being sexually abused in their own households, which the researchers calculated to be 8.9 per 10,000 for children under age 6. They concluded that although a disturbing number of children are sexually abused in day care settings, there is no indication of some special high risk to children in this setting. The researchers attributed the large number of day care molestation cases to the great number of children in day care and to the relatively high risk of sexual abuse to children in all settings.

Overall, the researchers' arguments were realistic and, to some extent, comforting. For a parent considering day care, it can be reassuring to know that the rate of substantiated cases of sexual abuse in day care is less than the rate for "in-home" abuse. And although it is true that this study missed unreported cases, the same is also true for studies estimating abuse in the home.

The UNH study also provides us with much important information about the types of sexual abuse that occur in day care. Some of these data were the result of an in-depth study of a random sample of 43 of the 270 reported cases. The vast majority of the 270 cases (83%) involved only a single perpetrator; more than half (58%) involved someone other than a professional child care worker, such as a janitor, a bus driver, or a child care worker's family member. Finkelhor et al. stated that the multiple perpetrator cases, although less frequent (17%), were clearly the most serious ones, involving the greatest number and the youngest children, the most serious sexual activities, and the highest likelihood of pornography and ritualistic abuse.

The UNH study found that women constituted 40% of the abusers in day care, and they usually perpetrated in conjunction with others. As the researchers noted, this high percentage suggests that knowledge of sexual abuse by women is critical to understanding sexual abuse in day care. But more remarkable is that males, who constituted only an estimated 5% of day care staff, accounted for 60% of the reported perpetrators. Although both men and women were more likely to abuse girls than boys, a slightly larger proportion of the women did abuse at least one boy. Moreover, women in this sample committed more serious offenses than the male perpetrators, including a greater incidence of penetration and more frequent use of force and threats. Finkelhor et al. cautioned that this latter finding may be partly because of a tendency for only the most serious cases of abuse by women to be reported and substantiated.

Unfortunately, perpetrators did not fit any prevailing stereotypes, and only 8% had been previously arrested for a sexual offense. Furthermore, the study was unable to identify categories for day care facilities that might be vulnerable or immune to the threat of abuse. Even traditional indicators such as years in operation, excellence of reputation, and director qualifications did not predict safety from abuse. The few factors that did seem to be associated with less severity included being in a high-crime, inner-city neighborhood and having a large staff. The researchers attributed this unexpected finding to the protective features of increased supervision and a general wariness about suspicious activities in these areas. The risk of abuse also seemed to be reduced in facilities in which parents had ready access to their children, although this feature was by no means fail-safe. Whereas the researchers did find that children seemed to be at somewhat higher risk if they were physically attractive, they concluded that child characteristics were not a major factor in determining who would be abused. In fact, children were no more likely to be abused if they were rich or poor; black, white, Asian, or Hispanic; mature or immature; popular or unpopular.

The abuse episodes detailed in the UNH study often occurred around toileting behavior, with two-thirds of the cases taking place in the bathroom. Although touching and fondling of genitals was the most frequent type of abuse, in 93% of the cases at least one child experienced some form of penetration (including oral, digital, and object). This unsettling statistic is particularly distressing when one considers the young age of these vulnerable victims. Other extreme forms of abuse included children being forced to abuse other children (21% of the cases) and allegations of pornography production (14%) and drug use (13%). Allegations of ritualistic abuse, which the researchers defined as "the invocation of religious, magical, or supernatural symbols or activities," occurred in 13% of the cases.

IMPACT OF DAY CARE SEXUAL ABUSE: THE COMMUNITY, FAMILY, AND CHILD

Scientific research on the phenomenon of child sexual abuse has followed the pace of public belief: motionless for centuries but quickly accelerating within the 1980s. The University of California, Los Angeles (UCLA) Manhattan Beach Project illustrates the varying impact that day care sexual abuse cases can have on communities, families, and victims. In this federally funded study we are comparing the cases of alleged abuse in Manhattan Beach, California (including the McMartin Preschool) with the confirmed Papoose Palace case in Reno, Nevada. We have also included a control group of children from other preschools who have never reported being abused.

In the Papoose Palace case, a single perpetrator, Stephen Boatwright, confessed to having molested more than 60 children. In fact, Boatwright confessed to more sexual activity than was alleged by the child victims during their evaluations (Basta 1986). He is now serving four consecutive life sentences. News of this case shocked and outraged the Reno community. Families whose children had attended Papoose Palace were initially both furious and scared that their children might have been among Boatwright's victims. The victimized children exhibited various emotional and behavioral problems, including depression, anxiety, hyperactivity, and somatic concerns (Basta 1986). The longer term effects, several of which are being investigated in the UCLA study, will always remain something of a mystery. Will any future problems these victimized children encounter be in some way influenced by their childhood trauma?

The Manhattan Beach cases under consideration in the study also included shock and outrage in the community, anger and fear in families, and multiple symptoms among children. More than 80% of the first 62 children in the UCLA study met DSM-III criteria for posttraumatic stress disorder (American Psychiatric Association 1980) during their period of greatest distress. These children were much more fearful than were control children, and those who disclosed to their therapists more involved and more terrorizing types of sexual acts tended to have a greater degree of fearfulness and behavior problems (Waterman et al. 1988). A more recent dissertation (Lusk 1988) on a subset of this sample found that although these children did not differ from controls in terms of IQ, achievement, or locus of control scores, they did exhibit more negative school-related behaviors and attitudes, and the younger children scored lower than their nonabused peers on a measure of self-concept.

The Manhattan Beach cases, however, also involved other elements that did not exist in the Papoose Palace case. Perhaps most important in terms of differential impact is the fact that no one from the Manhattan Beach preschools has confessed to any act of molestation. Without such a confession, suspect as it may be, community and family members have a much more difficult time discerning exactly what did or did not occur. Furthermore, without a confession, the possibility of a long and arduous trial must be considered, in which young, vulnerable victims carry the burden of proof. No such legal case was filed for most of the Manhattan Beach preschools, although all of them have closed. On the other hand, the McMartin Preschool case was the most expensive trial in United States history. Unlike Stephen Boatwright, almost all the alleged perpetrators in the Manhattan Beach cases are free to live in the same community as the alleged victims and families. Indeed, some parents have noted that the experience of suddenly seeing these alleged perpetrators during daily routines such as shopping has been one of the most continuously unsettling aspects of the ordeal.

The absence of a confession, the possibility of a trial, and periodic community sightings of alleged abusers are aspects that the Manhattan Beach cases share with many cases of day care sexual abuse around the country. But the Manhattan Beach cases are also among a minority of cases that include several other aspects that have an overwhelming impact on the community, the families, and the children. First, some of the Manhattan Beach cases were among the 13% of cases identified in the UNH study in which there were allegations of ritualistic abuse. More specifically, the allegations in many of these cases depicted a network of satanic cult members inflicting bizarre, terrorizing acts on child victims. Children reported horrendous sexual acts involving urine, blood, feces, and singing and chanting, as well as the killing of animals and babies. In the UCLA study, two of the most frequently cited excessive fears among Manhattan Beach children were fear of the devil (36%) and fear of hell (26%), compared with roughly 5% or less in the control groups (Kelly et al. 1988). The bizarreness of these alleged activities contributed in part to another atypical aspect: extensive nationwide media coverage, with the nation peering in to see each new development.

The political features of high-visibility cases such as the McMartin Preschool case and the Country Walk case in Florida have been discussed in noteworthy books by Crewdson (1988), Hechler (1988), and Hollingsworth (1986). The McMartin case seems to illustrate best the "pendulum pulling" done by media forces. With the CBS television show "60 Minutes" leading the way, the tone of the media has alternately convicted and acquitted the defendants, a strategy that seems to maximize public interest while emotionally devastating those more personally involved.

REVIEWS OF THE LITERATURE

As for the victims, we are only beginning to understand the impact of sexual abuse on them. Three thorough literature reviews and critiques (Browne and Finkelhor 1986; Conte 1987; Lusk and Waterman 1986) have discussed what has recently been learned about initial and long-term effects, especially on female victims, although none of these reviews were able to find many studies involving day care abuse. Moreover, some excellent recent empirical studies have documented behavioral and emotional effects on young victims, although these too have not focused on abuse that occurred in a day care setting (e.g., Conte and Schuerman 1987; Friedrich et al. 1986, 1987; Tong et al. 1987; White et al. 1988). A notable exception is a recent study by Faller (1988), who found multiple symptoms in many of the 48 children she examined who had been sexually abused in day care.

One important question that we cannot yet answer is whether early age at time of abuse will lead to a more negative impact because of the vulnerability of the child, as suggested by Courtois (1979), Meiselman (1978), and Zivney et al. (1988), or whether a young child's naivete may serve to lessen this impact, as suggested by data presented in the Tufts study (see Gomes-Schwartz et al. 1985). In addition, we know little about the course of effects throughout various developmental periods (Waterman 1986) or the mediating effects of variables such as family response and type of therapy (Briere 1988; Friedrich and Reams 1987; Fromuth 1986; MacFarlane and Waterman 1986; Wyatt and Mickey 1987).

Studies of Specific Day Care Settings and Cross-Sectional Data

In addition to the UCLA study, a number of projects are currently under way to look at the impact of sexual abuse in specific day care settings, such as the Small World Preschool in Niles, Michigan (Mowbray et al. 1988), and the Presidio Day Care Center in San Francisco (Weinberg 1990). Two studies have reported cross-sectional data on day care sexual abuse cases across the country. The UNH national study by Finkelhor et al. (1988) found the following extent of initial psychological symptomatology as measured in 98 subjects: fears (69%), nightmares/sleep disturbances (68%), clinging behavior (53%), sexual acting out/knowledge/interest (46%), bed wetting (36%), crying (35%), aggressive behavior (32%), distrust of adults (29%), school adjustment problems (27%), effect on play behavior (26%), tantrums (25%), toilet training problems (19%), blaming parents (7%), and learning disabilities (5%). Moreover, 45% of all the victims suffered physical injuries related to the sexual acts. These included genital irritation (54%), rectal and/or vaginal trauma (42%), and venereal disease (12%).

The second cross-sectional study compared 67 children abused in 16 day care centers, divided into ritualistic and nonritualistic cohorts, with a comparison group of 67 nonabused children (Kelley 1988). Children in the abuse groups exhibited significantly more behavior problems and lower social competence than did their nonabused peers, with 40% of the abused subjects scoring in the clinical range on behavior problems and 11% in the clinical range on social competence. Moreover, children who had experienced satanic rituals demonstrated significantly more behavior problems than children who were sexually abused without satanic rituals.

As in all studies of sexual abuse, these two studies found that some abused children did not exhibit symptomatology. Although it may be true that some of these children will exhibit symptoms at a later developmental stage, we should avoid the automatic labeling of sexual abuse victims as fearful, problematic children. Moreover, as suggested by the Brief Psychiatric Rating Scale for Children in the UCLA study, children who receive psychotherapy after reporting sexual victimization do show a dramatic decrease in symptomatology over time.

Responding to Sexual Abuse in Day Care

Finkelhor et al. (1988) provided several recommendations concerning the prevention, detection, investigation, and intervention of day care and sexual abuse (see also Glasser, Chapter 13, this volume).

Prevention. The researchers suggested the following:

1. Preventive education for preschool-age children should focus on anti-intimidation training.
2. Day care facilities should institute policy and architectural changes aimed at preventing abuse in and around bathrooms.

3. Parents and licensing officials should pay increased attention to the family members of day care staff and operators.
4. The public should realize that most day care abusers do not fit the stereotypical profile of a pedophile.
5. Parents should be encouraged to seek free access to day care facilities.

Detection. To improve detection of day care abuse, Finkelhor et al. suggested these steps:

1. Increase awareness about the number of female abusers.
2. Teach warning signs to parents, such as genital irritation, unusual sexual knowledge, fearfulness related to day care, and a facility's attempt to deny parental access.
3. Encourage staff members to report their own suspicions of abuse without fear of reprisal.
4. Discourage informal solutions.

Investigation and intervention. The researchers suggested the following:

1. Involve multidisciplinary teams.
2. Increase training for investigators.
3. Attend to the needs of suspected victims and their parents.
4. Include parents in mental health treatment.
5. Foster prosecutorial optimism and skill by educating prosecutors about the strategies used in the many successfully prosecuted cases.
6. Increase awareness about ritualistic abuse.

These recommendations include sound advice that will be helpful for licensing operators, day care directors, staff, and parents seeking or currently employing day care facilities. In an effort to gain additional advice from parents who have already experienced a case of alleged day care sexual abuse, parents in the UCLA study were asked to rate the helpfulness of five categories of coping resources (McCord et al. 1988). For each resource, parents were asked to state whether they utilized the resource, and if so, whether it made the situation "worse," "the same," or "better." In the first category, "Seeking Help from Professionals," more than 90% of the respondents took their child for an initial diagnostic interview. Seventy percent of these rated the interview as helpful, whereas fewer than 7% viewed it as detrimental. Ninety-eight percent of responding parents sought therapy for their child, and 95% of them rated the therapist as helpful, with no one rating the therapist as making the situation worse. In fact, of all the resources inquired about, both mothers and fathers rated the child's therapist as the most helpful resource. Sixty-eight percent of mothers also sought therapy for themselves; of these, 91% rated the therapist as making the situation better, with no therapist being rated as making the situation worse. Although fewer fathers sought therapy for themselves (38%), 92% of them also rated their therapist as helpful, with none rating their therapist as detrimental. Physicians were also rated quite favorably, with most seen as helping and none seen as hurting. However, lawyers, police, and clergy all received mixed reviews from those who utilized these resources, with 11% to 25% rated as making the situation worse.

The second category of coping resources was labeled "seeking help from others." One interesting finding in this category involved a gender difference between parents. Mothers were more likely to seek support from their friends (91%) than from their spouses or partners (82%), whereas fathers were more likely to seek support from their spouses/partners (94%) than from their friends (77%). This finding may be due in part to the fact that there were more single-parent females in the study than single-parent males. Nonetheless, mothers who did seek support from their spouse or partner were much more likely than fathers to view that partner as making things worse (21% versus 3%) and much less likely to view that partner as making things better (69% versus 94%). In general, fathers rated the support they received from other relatives, friends, and support groups more favorably than mothers did. This finding may reflect a tendency for fathers to minimize the problems surrounding the abuse experience.

Respondents varied in their use of resources in the third category, "seeking help from inner sources." "Attempting to forget" and "withdrawing from others" were met with mixed ratings, although "thinking about other things" was viewed as much more helpful than harmful. "Prayer," "meditation," and "yoga" were rated favorably by those choosing to utilize these resources.

The fourth category asked parents to rate the effectiveness of various types of "social action." "Taking an active role in investigating the abuse" and "involvement with the media," which were utilized by approximately one-half of the respondents, were given mixed reviews. On the other hand, favorable ratings were given to "involvement with advocacy programs and organizations," "involvement with legislative change," and "involvement with public education"; no parent who utilized these resources rated them as detrimental. It should be noted that several action groups were formed specifically because of the Manhattan Beach cases, including ACT (Affirming Children's Truths), Believe the Children, Children's Civil Rights Fund, CLOUT (Children's Legislative Organization United by Trauma), and Parents Against Child Abuse.

The final category of coping styles was listed as "miscellaneous resources." As expected, "using alcohol," "using drugs," "using aggression on spouse," and "using aggression on others" were generally seen as negative. Although parents may have tended to rate these coping styles in the socially acceptable direction, approximately one-quarter of mothers and fathers did admit to utilizing alcohol, aggression on spouse, and aggression on others, and close to 10% admitted using drugs. Approximately 85% of the sample tried to educate themselves about sexual abuse, with most of them finding this strategy helpful. Somewhat surprising is the fact that mothers (64%) were much more likely than fathers (44%) to use humor as a coping mechanism. Mothers were also more likely to rate the use of humor as helpful (68%) compared to fathers (27%). No one rated the use of humor as making the situation worse.

Knowledge of Child Development and Judicial Practices

In addition to the recommendations from the UNH national study and the insights of parents in the UCLA study, I also offer one final, and perhaps especially sensitive, suggestion for those who become involved in cases of day care sexual abuse. Defense attorneys seem to be showing us that the best strategy for defending accused abusers is to confuse child witnesses to make them seem unreliable, and then claim that allegations of day care sexual abuse are witch-hunts. In fact, friends of the defense in the McMartin case bought a full-page ad in a local newspaper that read: "Salem, Massachusetts 1692; Manhattan Beach, California 1985." All professionals who deal with cases of day care sexual abuse need to have some knowledge of child development. Children generally tell the truth, although when they are very young we cannot always interpret every word they say in a literal manner.

An example comes from a recent therapy case in which a young sexually abused child told her therapist that her daddy saved her from her abuser. When asked how her daddy was able to enter the locked room, the young girl replied, "He walked through the wall." The therapist followed this response by asking, "Your daddy can't really walk through the wall, can he?" The child responded, "That time he did."

The point of this case report is that sexually abused children can maintain their self-protective escape fantasies without our needing to believe them in a literal fashion. Moreover, the fact that a child reports some literally inaccurate details about the abuse does not mean that he or she was not abused, no matter how a defense attorney may argue this point. In fact, in this one area the judicial court process needs to make major changes, since it is based so strictly on the literal interpretation of witness testimony without adequately considering the developmental factors influencing child language (see Saywitz 1988; Waterman 1986).

Another complicating factor is that some abusers trick their young victims into believing untruths. For example, children from Manhattan Beach preschools reported believing that an observant Satan was present in common objects such as rocks and spiders or that Satan had been placed inside their bodies. We usually are able to identify the more bizarre statements from young children as being the product of mind control rather than literal truth. Unfortunately, there are other, more plausible statements for which we need to consider all possibilities. Thus, if a child reports being taken away in an airplane or a bus, for example, we must consider whether this detail actually occurred, whether the child was tricked into believing it occurred, or whether the child is confused about this detail for some other reason.

CONCLUSIONS

Sexual abuse of young children does exist, and the pendulum of public opinion should no longer be allowed to waiver on this issue. Communities and parents should take steps to prevent, detect, investigate, and intervene on behalf of children, both in the day care setting and in general, to reduce the possibility of such abuse. In addition, when abuse does occur, parents should seek professional counseling for the child victim, as well as for themselves, as appropriate. Finally, the judicial system must be modified to accommodate the testimony of young children. No matter how a defense attorney may try to convince the court otherwise, children usually tell the truth. Professionals must realize, however, that young children's words cannot always be taken literally; their words may require some interpretation because of their stage of development.

REFERENCES

American Psychiatric Association: Diagnostic and Statistical Manual of Mental Disorders, Third Edition. Washington, DC, American Psychiatric Association, 1980

Basta SM: Personality characteristics of molested children. Unpublished doctoral dissertation, University of Reno, Reno, NV, 1986

Briere J: Controlling for family variables in abuse efforts research: a critique of the "partialling" approach. Journal of Interpersonal Violence 3:80–89, 1988

Browne A, Finkelhor D: Impact of child sexual abuse: a review of the research. Psychol Bull 99:66–77, 1986

Conte JR: The effects of sexual abuse on children: a critique and suggestions for future research. Victimology 10:110–130, 1987

Conte JR, Schuerman JR: Factors associated with an increased impact of child sexual abuse. Child Abuse Negl 11:201–211, 1987

Courtois C: The incest experience and its aftermath. Victimology 4:337–347, 1979

Crewdson J: By Silence Betrayed: Sexual Abuse of Children in America. Boston, MA, Little, Brown, 1988

Faller KC: The spectrum of sexual abuse in daycare: an exploratory study. Journal of Family Violence 3:283–298, 1988

Finkelhor D, Williams LM, Burns N: Nursery Crimes: Sexual Abuse in Day Care. Newbury Park, CA, Sage, 1988

Friedrich WN, Reams RA: Course of psychological symptoms in sexually abused young children. Psychotherapy 24:160–170, 1987

Friedrich WN, Urquiza AJ, Beilke R: Behavioral problems in sexually abused young children. J Pediatr Psychol 11:47–57, 1986

Friedrich WN, Beilke R, Urquiza AJ: Children from sexually abusive families: a behavioral comparison. Journal of Interpersonal Violence 2:391–402, 1987

Fromuth ME: The relationship of child sexual abuse with later psychological and sexual adjustment in a sample of college women. Child Abuse Negl 10:5–16, 1986

Gomes-Schwartz B, Horowitz J, Sauzier M: Severity of emotional distress among sexually abused preschool, school-age, and adolescent children. Hosp Community Psychiatry 36:503–508, 1985

Hechler D: The Battle and the Backlash: The Child Sexual Abuse War. Lexington, MA, Lexington Books, 1988

Hollingsworth J: Unspeakable Acts. Chicago, IL, Congdon and Weed, 1986

Kelley SJ: Responses of children to sexual abuse and satanic ritualistic abuse in day care centers. Paper presented at the National Symposium on Child Victimization, Anaheim, CA, April 1988

Kelly RJ, Waterman J, Oliveri M, et al: Powerlessness and subsequent fears in victims of alleged ritualistic child sexual abuse. Paper presented at the International Conference on Child Abuse and Neglect, Rio de Janeiro, September 1988

Lusk R: Cognitive and school-related differences in allegedly sexually abused and non-abused children. Unpublished doctoral dissertation, University of California, Los Angeles, 1988

Lusk R, Waterman J: Effects of sexual abuse on children, in Sexual Abuse of Young Children. Edited by MacFarlane K, Waterman J. New York, Guilford, 1986, pp 3–12

McCord J, Oliveri M, Waterman J, et al: Coping patterns of parents whose children reported being molested in preschool. Paper presented at the International Conference on Child Abuse and Neglect, Rio de Janeiro, September 1988

MacFarlane K, Waterman J: Sexual Abuse of Young Children. New York, Guilford, 1986

Meiselman K: Incest: A Psychological Study of the Causes and Effects With Treatment Recommendations. San Francisco, CA, Jossey-Bass, 1978

Mowbray C, Bybee D, Valliere P: Community and agency responses to a large scale incident of day care sexual abuse. Paper presented at the National Symposium on Child Victimization, Anaheim, CA, April 1988

Saywitz KJ: Children's conceptions of the legal system: "court is a place to play basketball," in Perspectives on Children's Testimony. Edited by Ceci SJ, Ross DF, Toglia MP. New York, Springer-Verlag, 1988, pp 131–157

Tong L, Oates K, McDowell M: Personality development following sexual abuse. Child Abuse Negl 11:371–383, 1987

Waterman J: Developmental considerations, in Sexual Abuse of Young Children. Edited by MacFarlane K, Waterman J. New York, Guilford, 1986, pp 15–29

Waterman J, Kelly RJ, McCord J, et al: Therapists' descriptions of alleged molestations in Manhattan Beach preschools. Paper presented at the National Symposium on Child Victimization, Anaheim, CA, April 1988

Weinberg G: Stress, coping, and adaptation following a day care abuse crisis: the preschooler and his family. Unpublished doctoral dissertation, University of California, Berkeley, CA, 1990

White S, Halpin BM, Strom GA, et al: Behavioral comparisons of young sexually abused, neglected, and nonreferred children. J Clinical Child Psychology 17:53–61, 1988

Wyatt GE, Mickey MR: Ameliorating the effects of child sexual abuse: an exploratory study of support by parents and others. Journal of Interpersonal Violence 2:403–415, 1987

Zivney OA, Nash MR, Hulsey TL: Sexual abuse in early versus late childhood: different patterns of pathology as revealed on the Rorschach. Psychotherapy 25:99–106, 1988

Chapter 13

Toward the Prevention of Child Abuse in Day Care

Martin Glasser, M.D., F.A.P.A.

According to the University of New Hampshire national study of child abuse and neglect in the United States, approximately 7% of all child maltreatment known to professionals involves sexual abuse (U.S. Department of Health and Human Services 1980). Put differently, the incidence of such sexually abused children is estimated to be 100,000 to 500,000 children each year (Allen 1986). Twenty-five percent of reported cases concern preschool-age children. The number of children reported to have been abused in child care settings is not clear, but it appears to be a significant minority (less than 2% of all reported cases) (Contralto 1986).

In the past decade, several day care centers were discovered to have children who had been both physically and sexually abused. Media coverage (see Kelly, Chapter 12, this volume) and the subsequent impact on insurance for all day care centers have highlighted this topic and brought it to the attention of child care providers, social welfare agencies, civil and criminal courts, and parents.

In this chapter I will discuss guidelines to help parents evaluate a prospective center. I will also offer suggestions for prevention of child exploitation in a day care setting and discuss the behavioral changes associated with child abuse in the preschool-age child, as well as assessment, intervention, and rehabilitation of the child.

The consequences of sexual abuse depend on the age and developmental stage of the child; the nature of the abusive situation; circumstances surrounding the disclosure, investigation, and disposition of the case; and how people and institutions in the child's life respond to the child. The impact on children who have been sexually exploited has been extensively studied since the late 1960s. Research included descriptions of children's coping defenses and later adaptation (Finkelhor 1984; Mrazek and Mrazek 1980; U.S. Department of Health and Human Services 1980).

In the 1980s laws were introduced to reduce the probability of child abuse by caregivers. Educational programs for child care providers, parents, and preschool- and school-age children have been targeted to prevent, or in some cases expose, child sexual abuse as early as 3 years of age.

PREVENTION

Programs to prevent child abuse in the day care setting focus on three areas: 1) early identification and diagnosis, 2) treatment, and 3) education (U.S. Department of Health, Education, and Welfare 1976). Parents are the focal point for all these intervention strategies—their participation and monitoring are essential to the success of the program.

Early Identification and Diagnosis

This approach requires that each community establish guidelines for care. It relies on the reporting of any suspected abuse, on prompt response to any concern initiated by a parent or provider, and having available a sensitive and expert team of evaluators. It also depends on the cooperation of legislators to establish guidelines for the operation of day care centers and mandates 24-hour staffing of the protective services section of the local department of social welfare.

The health care system must make the assessment of possible child abuse a health priority by offering training to the examining physicians, developing a child-oriented facility for examination of child victims, and coordinating the evaluation of the child with the required agencies (district attorney, police, public welfare, public health, mental health, forensic health, and specialized treatment staff). When such an approach is established in the community, the number of possible child abuse cases that are identified should increase.

Treatment

The treatment phase provides the child and his or her family with the necessary medical, psychological, and emotional care. Other assistance to the family should include long-term psychiatric services, emergency loans, visits by a parent aide, and other services appropriate to rehabilitate the child within the family constellation. Funding for these special services has been made more available through programs initiated by community groups. In addition, many states collect funds from convicted felons as part of victim witness assistance programs.

Education

The education component of prevention includes general public awareness, the training of professionals, and working with parents and children to assist them in identifying abuse. Some examples of historical findings suggestive of abuse are listed in Table 13-1. Early childhood education programs have in common four objectives (Borkin and Frank 1986; Conte 1985):

1. The establishment of the concept of private areas of the body that children have a right to control. Included is the difference between touching that is "okay" and touching that is "not okay."
2. The right to say no to an adult who is doing something to the child that seems strange, intrusive, or harmful.
3. The importance of trusting one's own feelings if an adult's activities seem "bad."
4. The need to tell a trusted adult if someone has touched the child inappropriately and to keep telling until someone believes the report.

Although these programs are now often found in the school-age setting, research shows only slight potential benefit to preschoolers (children aged 3 years or younger). In the 4- to 5-year-old age group, the program described by Conte (1985) found some changes in awareness after participation in the program, but Conte also stated the following:

> To date there is no evidence describing the long-term effects of prevention training in terms of either positive effects, such as increased assertiveness,

Table 13-1. Historical findings suggestive of abuse

Frequent injury to child explained by peer interaction, play, or self-inducement

Medical injury not compatible with explanation offered by day care provider

Delay in reporting or attempt to receive medical care for child after injury

Change in explanation of how an injury occurred

prevention of sexual abuse, or greater person safety, nor of negative effects such as increased fearfulness, anxiety or a generalized distrust of adults." (p. 320)

The most helpful component in prevention is parents' involvement in the program: communicating with other parents about possible questions or concerns, drop-in visits to monitor the program, and the interaction of the child with staff and peers. In fact, after the selection of a day care facility, monitoring the facility is perhaps the most powerful deterrent to abuse.

STATE AND SOCIETAL GUIDELINES

Most states mandate that all group day care programs allow parents free access for unannounced visits. Table 13-2 shows an example statement of consent that each center must give to parents. When observing center activities, parents should pay special attention to the children's affect, interactions with the staff, and the ability of the staff to relate to the children in an empathetic manner.

Guidelines for the physical site, staffing requirements (maximal staff-child ratio), and criminal screening for day care program operators are set forth by each state through its licensing procedures (Department of Social Services, State of California 1987). Most states require inspection of group day care facilities before a state license may be obtained.

Therefore, licensed facilities have met the minimal state requirements, and there appears to be a lower incidence of abuse in such licensed centers. However, licensing guidelines vary from state to state (see Miller, Chapter 15, this volume). Also, training requirements do not follow a uniform standard from state to state; yet the training of staff is intimately linked to the quality of care (see Howes, Chapter 2, this volume). A study of abuse in North Carolina day care centers found that centers that had lower standards of training and were subject to less frequent monitoring were five times more likely to have serious complaints brought against them than programs with higher standards and more frequent monitoring (Russell and Clifford 1987). Furthermore, complaints against unregistered

Table 13-2. Example statement of parents' right to visit and inspect day care program

1. Parents or guardians have the right, upon presentation of identification, to enter and inspect preschool facilities, without advance notice to provider.

2. The law prohibits discrimination or retaliation against a parent electing to inspect the center.

3. All parents must be notified of this right in writing.

family day care homes were likely to be three times as severe as those filed against registered homes (Russell and Clifford 1987).

If family group day care center is in a neighbor's home, or if a parent brings a caregiver into the child's own home, many states now offer a fingerprinting clearance to inform the parent of any past criminal offenses. This service is especially important because previous felony convictions for child abuse significantly increase the chances of further victimization of children.

BEHAVIORAL CHANGES IN ABUSE

The preschool-age child lacks abstract understanding of the reason why he or she was emotionally or physically abused. A common reaction is the displacement of his or her feelings of vulnerability and helplessness with the magical belief that he or she is "bad" and therefore deserves the punishment.

Although the signs of neglect differ somewhat in cases of physical or sexual abuse, from the child's perspective, any harm that has been experienced under the care of an adult produces feelings of distrust and fear toward other adults and even siblings. The result is a generalized distancing from caregivers and parents, mood lability, isolation and constriction of affect, and behavioral symptomatology (Green 1985). The general behaviors of distress observed in abused children include fears, sleep disturbances, clinging, enuresis, and encopresis.

The behavior of the child in day care can often alert parents to either neglect or abuse. The child in diapers with a persistent diaper rash or fear and distress upon being changed beyond what is developmentally expected, the persistently thirsty or hungry child, the child who intensely protests drop-off beyond the initial adjustment period or who appears apathetic upon pickup are all possible signs for concern.

The child who has been exposed to sexually explicit material or who has been sexually abused can behave in what may resemble adult erotic behavior. Such behavior includes approaching parents or caregivers and attempting to hold or fondle their genitals or becoming preoccupied with their own genitals in open, frequent masturbation.

Sexual abuse is frequently identified through the presence of venereal disease, which can be sexually transmitted to children. Vaginal discharge is often the only physical symptom, and its presence should alert parents to the need for a prompt medical examination. Any unusual findings in diapers or underwear should be saved for medical examination. Canavan (1981) recommended a thorough physical examination regardless of the amount of time lapsed since the last sexual contact. Signs and symptoms of trauma and infection should be carefully assessed by medical personnel on physical examination. Tables 13-3 and 13-4 list findings suggestive of physical and sexual abuse.

INTERVENTION

When it is discovered that a child has been abused in the day care setting, several factors should be considered to understand the degree of emotional damage that the child may experience in the discovery period and during the treatment and rehabilitation phases. The rehabilitation of the child actually begins with the discovery, and each subsequent contact with a significant adult has a potential effect that is either beneficial or detrimental.

Six factors influence the abused child's emotional reaction and recovery: 1) the child's experience of the abuse, 2) the repetition of the abusive act,

Table 13-3. Behaviors of preschool children suggestive of abuse

Behaviors suggestive of increased anxiety

Clinging
Sleep disturbances
Change in toileting skills
Mood lability
Biting at fingers and nails
Loss of developmental skills
Change in eating habits
Increase in fears or phobias

Behaviors suggestive of neglect

Persistent thirst or hunger
Hesitation to enter program at drop-off and apathetic response at pickup
Change in pattern of interaction with parents, siblings, and peers
Defiant behavior to parents with inappropriate expressions of anger
Aggression to adults, siblings, and peers
Lack of discrimination between adults and strangers
Change in play activities, with new major themes of aggression and violence

Specific behaviors found in sexual abuse

Approaching parents or other adults in erotic manner
Attempting to touch or manipulate genitals or mimic adult erotic activities
Preoccupation with own genitalia or open masturbation of frequent or "driven" quality
Excessive preoccupation with self, parents, or peers concerning sexual issues
Avoidance of using toilets or complaints of pain or discomfort upon urination
Complaints of itching or discomfort around perineal area
Fecal soiling or encopresis, daytime urinary incontinence, or onset of nighttime wetting (enuresis)
Protest at time of changing diaper, or assuming unusual position of legs at changing time
Persistent cyclic vomiting of a nonorganic origin
Play behavior revealing erotic, sexualized play with dolls

Table 13-4. Physical findings suggestive of abuse

Findings suggestive of physical abuse

Recurrent injuries to head and neck; small hemorrhages or marks
Bruises on arms or legs suggestive of hand or pressure inducement
Injuries discovered by X-ray, or "coincidental" injuries such as spiral fractures not
  previously reported
Failure to thrive, or a developmental delay

Findings suggestive of sexual abuse

Swollen or bruised genitalia
Blood on underwear
Discharge from vagina found to be sexually transmitted disease, or infection unusual in
  child
Anal irritation or trauma that is persistent and unexplained
Pain on urination or defecation
Difficulty in ambulation due to pain in genitals
General health complaints such as stomachaches, generalized malaise, or somatic
  concerns

3) the circumstances of the discovery, 4) the physical repercussions of the discovery, 5) the reaction of "significant others," and 6) psychotherapeutic intervention. These factors are presented with clinical examples in the following sections to promote an understanding of them.

Common behaviors at the time of disclosure that can persist through the treatment and rehabilitation phases include regressive symptoms such as fear of darkness or isolation; clinging to parents, peers, or siblings; desire to sleep with parents; enuresis and encopresis; and preoccupation with the person who may punish them now that the abusive events are disclosed. Some children also may have transient feelings that parents or siblings will consider them "bad" for what they have revealed.

The Child's Experience of the Abuse

The history of the abusive event must be reconstructed to learn how the child experienced it. This task should be attempted by allowing the child, in his or her own words and without adult assistance or prompting, to describe the events. Clarification or additional explanation of sexual abuse or physical abuse in adult abstract terms can often confuse the child and only add to the burden of his or her guilt or discomfort during the disclosure phase.

The child's perception of the event may occur with minimal physical or emotional trauma despite law enforcement agencies and the parents' own reactions to the event. The child's experience of stress is highly variable and individualized. Therefore, great care must be taken not to increase stress, create behavioral problems, and prolong rehabilitation during the legal investigation.

Clinical Example 1

A 3-year-old girl was in a family group day care program that was supervised by the owner of the program, a woman whose husband came home each day to have lunch and was left in charge of the children while she went shopping. The husband would take the child into his bedroom, remove her diaper, and fondle her genitalia. The child did not understand why the man touched her in this manner and was able to tell her mother later that she did not like this man to change her diapers.

Repetition of the Abusive Act

The experience of an isolated event can have a strikingly different impact on the child than an act that is repeated multiple times.

Clinical Example 2

The day care provider told all her preschool children that she would not tolerate their need to use the bathroom more than once in the morning. For this reason, she withheld fluids and punished a child each time he or she had an "accident." Over time, the children who remained in this center became increasingly more traumatized, and many who left the center had persistent problems with sphincter control.

Circumstances of the Discovery

The time of the discovery and the circumstances surrounding the exposure of abuse can influence the emotional outcome of the preschool child. Previous threats to coerce the child not to reveal the abusive act, the acceptance of the child's story as fact, and the ability to assure the child that the bad person who was the perpetrator is "locked up" and not able to come back and hurt the child are all factors that may influence the emotional state of the child. Ideally, the initial interview should be conducted in a location that is either familiar to the child or at least is nonthreatening, with all agencies cooperating to gather the child's story at the same time.

Clinical Example 3

A preschool girl was brought to the emergency room because of a physical injury she incurred in the day care facility. The explanation from the day care center did not appear compatible with the severity and nature of the injury. The parents were called, and a law enforcement official was also summoned. The child, although severely bruised, was not in serious medical jeopardy, yet she was kept in the examining room and was asked by many people, including the day care provider, to validate the presented explanation while the doctor and the police officer openly debated the "real explanation." The turmoil of the medical and forensic system appeared emotionally traumatic and unnecessary for this child.

The following case illustrates a contrast in the management of the child and her family.

Clinical Example 4

A 5-year-old girl was brought to the receiving facility after the parent noticed, upon returning home from day care, a blood stain on the child's underwear and swollen genitalia. The child was in no immediate medical distress and was taken into a playroom where she played with toys and was introduced to the interview staff. The parents of the child were interviewed in another room. After the parents felt that they could rejoin their child and support her through the exam, they came into the playroom. The exam was performed with the mother holding the child on her lap. The child and her mother spent the remainder of the night in a hospital room, and the swabs of the perineal area were collected the next morning while the child remained in her bed. The rest of the forensic exam and the history were easily obtained in the child's hospital room when both the child and the parents were less anxious and fearful.

Physical Repercussions of the Discovery

Some exploitative acts to a preschool child can result in hospitalization to assess injury and on rare occasions require surgical intervention. Although this type of medical intervention may be necessary and life-saving, the child often perceives it as punishment and is hence further traumatized. A frequent fantasy of the child is that the perpetrator has arranged this punishment for "telling." If the injury results in a long-term disability, the child and family can have a significantly more difficult time in the resolution of the emotional trauma and in the rehabilitation of the child.

Clinical Example 5

A 2½-year-old boy was in a day care setting with his 5-year-old sister. Because of his irritability and age, he was often verbally reprimanded by the day care provider and on several occasions was physically shaken with her hands around his neck, resulting in multiple small hemorrhages (petechial) around his face and neck. On one occasion the trauma was so great that it caused a retinal hemorrhage resulting in blindness to one eye. Because of his age, his memory of the trauma was not clear. Yet his increasing awareness of his disability and the filtered memory that was available to him through his parents and his sister made his recovery slow, and his emotional rehabilitation was prolonged over several years.

Reaction of Other Persons

The events that occur after discovery of abuse can lead to the introduction to the child of numerous adult strangers, including police officers, medical providers, investigators, social workers, lawyers, and mental health counselors. The intensity of passion the adults feel toward the injury to the child and the anger toward the adult who perpetrated the injury is often rapidly perceived by the child.

Initially, the ability to assist the child and also offer a separate site for the parents to express their rage and distress is helpful to both the child and the parents. When the preschool child sees his or her mother and father crying and angry, the child often misinterprets the emotional state of the parents as anger toward the child for being "bad."

Clinical Example 6

A 1½-year-old boy was present in a day care setting where several children were abused. The child had been enrolled in the program for only 1 day when the center was closed because of the discovery of abuse of other children. The mother of this child was angry and felt guilty because the center she had chosen was dangerous, even though her child had experienced no apparent injury. The mother became a community organizer to help gather information for the police and the subsequent criminal trial. Meetings were held in her home, with the mother participating in several media presentations as a "victim's mother." When this child was examined at age 4, he appeared as emotionally damaged as other children who indeed had been victimized. At 5 years of age, the child exhibited behavioral problems that appeared to be related to the filtered memory recreated by his parents.

The preceding example is in contrast to a child who had been in the same abusive setting for more than 2 years and had experienced multiple injuries. In this case, though, the parents quickly reestablished a trusting relationship between themselves and their child, offered a strong and cohesive family setting, and placed the child in supportive psychotherapy with their participation. This child's behavioral problems were rapidly resolved, and he appeared asymptomatic 2 years later.

Psychotherapeutic Intervention

The emotional adaptation to trauma has entered the psychiatric nosology as a separate clinical syndrome: the posttraumatic stress disorder (DSM-III; American Psychiatric Association 1980). In children who are victims of abuse, this syndrome has immediate effects as well as potential long-term effects. Green (1978a, 1978b, 1985) has described the psychological defenses that children use when confronted with physical abuse. These defenses include denial, isolation of the emotion, and projection resulting in symptom formation of fears and avoidance.

The ability to reconstitute emotionally depends on the availability of adults who will allow the child to express his or her feelings, utilize adaptive mechanisms, and reexperience unresolved feelings through reenactment (Terr 1981). The supportive role of the parents in this process is essential, yet the child often struggles with ambivalent feelings toward the parents, desiring their support while experiencing anger toward the parents for having placed him or her in a situation that resulted in abuse. The therapist is in an excellent position to assist both the child and the parents during the disclosure period. The utilization of play therapy can allow the child to "express in play" (Terr 1981) a repetitive theme related to the experience of the trauma. As Terr (1981, p. 745) documented in a follow-up of the traumatic kidnapping of a school bus in Chowchilla, California: "The connection between post-traumatic play and the trauma remains unconscious until it is interpreted by the therapist." In other words, offering only the opportunity to reenact the trauma or a related theme cannot provide the emotional resolution necessary until the child's residual conflicts are identified and interpreted in the therapeutic play session.

The parents' role in the therapeutic situation is to reinforce the attachment they have already established with their child. The tendency of a parent to become fixated on a specific component of the trauma or the need to encourage the child to reexperience the events verbally can interfere with the child's capacity to adapt and defend against the intrusive memories of the trauma. The collaboration between the therapist and parents is therefore essential to allow the preschool child to continue development and to resolve the conflicts that have resulted from the trauma.

When the preschool child enters elementary school, during times of family stress, and at the time of entering puberty, conflicts concerning the trauma may again surface in the form of symptomatology (Goodwin 1985). Entering psychotherapy at these times is often helpful to the child who must deal with a higher level of abstraction and hence resolution.

THE EFFECT OF LEGAL PROCEEDINGS ON THE CHILD

The need for the child to participate in criminal or civil court proceedings can interfere with the child's healing process. Since the criminal proceedings follow the trauma by many months, the child must temporarily reexperience the trauma in an adversarial setting. Although some states now allow for either a videotape of the child's testimony or allow the child to be interviewed in the judge's chambers, other courts insist that the child face the accused perpetrator and testify in an open courtroom. The cross-examination and questioning often raise latent issues of guilt and anger toward the parents for not protecting the child (see also Kelly, Chapter 12, this volume). Civil proceedings, if initiated, can follow several years after the trauma. The need to recall the traumatic events for the court in this setting can also cause a temporary regression in the child who has developed appropriate coping skills to deal with the traumatic event.

In some cases, the child victim can resolve the conflict during the disclosure phase and rapidly return to continuing development with a minimal amount of intervention. These resilient children can enter the courtroom, offer testimony about the perpetrator, and address the issues surrounding the event and prosecution with only transient distress. The child who continues to have intrusive recall of the event, sleep disturbances, emotional constriction, fears, phobias, and mood volatility resembles adult victims of similar trauma and fits the criteria of the posttraumatic stress disorder. Such a child requires referral to a child mental health professional.

Because of the necessary involvement of the legal system, the traditional role of the therapist as evaluator is expanded in such instances to include the family and the mandated agencies (social service, juvenile and criminal court, police, district attorney, and public health). The prelitigation phase also places pressure on the therapist to uncover and report, in order to identify or add evidence toward prosecution of the perpetrator.

The therapist is thus placed in a situation of forming a therapeutic alliance with the child and family while appropriately participating in the forensic issues that arise. Countertransference issues often must be explored to minimize projection of the therapist's feelings onto the child during a time when many adult evaluators are influencing the child's emotional state.

CONCLUSIONS

Abuse of the preschool-age child in the day care setting brings emotional turmoil to the family and child and can often create emotional sequelae over a period of time, depending on the nature of the trauma and the reaction of others. Appropriate support from the child's family, therapy, and agencies that work with victimized children can all help speed the abused child's recovery and rehabilitation.

Furthermore, it must be emphasized that the preschool-age child is heavily influenced by his or her parents' emotional state upon discovery of abuse. Yet the parents must deal with their own intense emotions of rage, guilt, disgust, shame, and dismay while attempting to assist and support their child, the identified victim. Intervention programs must focus on offering the parents immediate opportunities to express their feelings at the time of disclosure, often away from the child. Continuing support through parents' support groups, individual and couples therapy, and if necessary, family therapy to assist the parents in their emotional conflict present valuable resources for parents, enabling them to be able to continue to support and assist their child.

REFERENCES

Allen J: Child sexual abuse and day care. Presentation at the National Association of Young Children, 1986

American Psychiatric Association: Diagnostic and Statistical Manual of Mental Disorders, 3rd Edition. Washington, DC, American Psychiatric Association, 1980

Borkin J, Frank L: Sexual abuse prevention for preschoolers: a pilot program. Child Welfare 65:75–82, 1986

Canavan JW: Social child abuse, in Child Abuse and Neglect: A Medical Reference. Edited by Ellerstein NS. New York, John Wiley, 1981, pp 233–252

Conte JR: An evaluation of a program to prevent the sexual victimization of young children. Child Abuse Negl 9:319–328, 1985

Contralto S: Child abuse and the politics of care. Journal of Education 168:70–79, 1986

Department of Social Services, State of California: Licensing Manual for Day Care. Sacramento, CA, Department of Social Services, 1987

Finkelhor D: Child Sexual Abuse: New Theory and Research. New York, Free Press, 1984

Goodwin J: Post-traumatic symptoms in incest victims, in Post-Traumatic Stress Disorders in Children. Edited by Eth S, Pynoos RS. Washington, DC, American Psychiatric Press, 1985, pp 155–168

Green A: Psychiatric treatment of abused children. J Am Acad Child Psychiatry 17:356–371, 1978a

Green A: Self destructive behavior in battered children. Am J Psychiatry 135:579–582, 1978b

Green A: Children traumatized by physical abuse, in Post-Traumatic Stress Disorder in Children. Edited by Eth S, Pynoos RS. Washington, DC, American Psychiatric Press, 1985, pp 133–154

Mrazek PR, Mrazek DA: The effects of child sexual abuse: methodological considerations, in Sexually Abused Children and Their Families. Edited by Beezley P, Mrazek PR, Kempe C. Oxford, Pergamon Press, 1980

Russell SD, Clifford RN: Child abuse and neglect in North Carolina day care programs. Child Welfare 66(2):149–163, 1987

Terr L: Forbidden games. J Am Acad Child Psychiatry 20:741–760, 1981

U.S. Department of Health, Education, and Welfare: Child abuse and neglect: the community team approach to case management and prevention (DHEW Publ No OHD-75-30075). Washington, DC, DHEW, 1976

U.S. Department of Health and Human Services. National Center on Child Abuse and Neglect: Sexual Abuse of Children: Selected Readings. Washington, DC, DHHS, 1980

Chapter 14

Working With Maltreated Children and Families in Day Care Settings

Catherine Ayoub, M.N., Ed.M., Penelope Grace, D.S.W., and Carolyn M. Newberger, Ed.D.

Identification of child maltreatment and intervention with the maltreated child and his or her family are complex and difficult tasks. Day care workers are in a unique position to provide support and education not only to the child but also to the parents and the community. Such support requires knowledge of and sensitivity to both the special needs of children and the needs and realities of families. In this chapter we will first present information about child maltreatment, including definitions, indicators, and parental and societal variables. Then we will present guidelines for identifying and working with maltreated children in day care settings.

Maltreatment falls into a number of categories, including neglect, physical abuse, sexual abuse, and emotional abuse. These categories are not mutually exclusive, however, and patterns of maltreatment may change in form and severity as the child develops or circumstances change. Even with categories there is a great deal of variation. Child maltreatment is perhaps best thought of as "a symptom of family dysfunction resulting from a complex causal process" (Newberger et al. 1980). Great care must be taken in each individual evaluation to avoid stereotyping or laying blame.

233

Child abuse occurs for a variety of complex, interacting reasons. Among these are parent and child temperaments, cognitive capacities, parental knowledge and awareness, social and economic conditions, family structure and interaction patterns, community resources, and operating societal norms.

FORMS OF CHILD MALTREATMENT AND THEIR MANIFESTATIONS

In this section we will discuss the major forms of child maltreatment: emotional abuse, neglect, physical abuse, and sexual abuse.

Emotional Abuse

Of the various forms of child maltreatment, emotional abuse is both the most prevalent and the most difficult to identify with certainty. Emotional abuse frequently accompanies physical and sexual abuse; it can also exist in isolation. It may be continuous or episodic, and it includes verbal and emotional assault, close confinement, and threatened harm. Emotional neglect is best described as inadequate nurturance or affection, permitting socially maladaptive behavior, and not providing other forms of necessary care (U.S. Department of Health and Human Services 1981).

The reactions of infants and young children to emotional abuse often include a slowing down of development and/or pervasive sadness, anger, or apathy. The developmental impact of maltreatment is most often seen in language delays in the young child. Gross and fine motor development may also be delayed.

Autoerotic activities may become significant. Thumb sucking may be preferred over sucking for nourishment. Self-stimulation through repetitive behaviors such as twirling may be present. Maltreated babies may appear attached to no one, and they may lack curiosity and interest in their surroundings.

Because behaviors indicative of emotional neglect vary, they are difficult to pinpoint. The toddler who is emotionally abused may be clingy or withdrawn. He or she frequently has separation problems of one extreme or the other. Egeland and Sroufe (1981) found that emotionally neglected children aged 12 to 18 months were more anxious in their attachment to their mothers than were the children in a control group. At 2 years, these children were described as angry, frustrated, and noncompliant.

At 42 months, the emotionally abused children demonstrated low self-esteem and poor ego control. They were more apathetic and withdrawn, yet they could also be hyperactive and distractible. In general, these children lacked enthusiasm and had difficulty pulling themselves together to complete a task (Egeland et al. 1983).

Emotional abuse derails the child's sense of mastery and competence. The push to conquer the environment is fueled by curiosity, autonomy, and a positive sense of self, all of which are often damaged in these children.

Specific areas of interaction may trigger parental anger and disapproval. Particular developmental issues such as toilet training or infant feeding are common areas of difficulty and may become the locus of the parent-child interaction. In other cases, the emotionally abusive relationship is widespread, crossing all areas of the parent-child interaction.

One of the primary characteristics of emotional abuse is that it involves interactions that deprive the child of his or her respect as a human being. The child's speech, dress, or actions may be ridiculed. Verbal expressions of emotional abuse may include harsh criticism, harassment, ridicule, or inappropriate demands. Many children are told repeatedly that they are worthless, bad, or irresponsible. Overt rejection of this kind, reinforced daily, is terribly damaging to the developing human psyche.

The abused child is often the target of displaced anger that breeds in the family. The child may indeed become a scapegoat for many family problems; he or she thus allows parents to avoid marital difficulties or other family conflicts. In families in which the child is keeping individual or family anxiety from intensifying, change is difficult. If the scapegoated child is removed from the family system, there is an increased likelihood that another scapegoat, possibly another child, will be found.

Negative messages may be relayed to the child directly or indirectly. Indirect messages can leave the child with no way to respond. For example, a parent repeatedly says, "Good children never wet their beds," to a child who is a bed wetter. When the child wets his bed, the parent says nothing but sighs deeply. The message is clearly conveyed, but the child is not allowed the opportunity for direct response to the parental message.

Children may be deprived of peer interaction, educational opportunities, or social experiences because their parents see them as threatening or inappropriate. Children who are never allowed to play outside or to see peers suffer from a form of emotional abuse.

Another significant area of emotional maltreatment involves children who are not direct victims of either overt or passive abuse but who are witnesses to violence against intimate family members, most typically their mother. Domestic violence, specifically the battering of women by their partners, occurs in a substantial number of American households. The psychological consequences for these children vary from very aggressive behavior to complete submission and hopelessness. The level of impairment can approach and even exceed that of children who are directly physically victimized (Jaffe et al. 1986).

In situations of indirect violence, the child can be further victimized by the human service and judicial systems. When the nonviolent parent leaves the relationship, the children can be placed in positions of heightened vulnerability through judicial rulings of unsupervised visitation with the violent parent. In extreme cases, children have been placed in the custody of a murdering parent. How does any child, much less a preschool child, understand being put under the control of someone who is willing to injure or even kill a family member? We believe that a child cannot logically reconcile these acts with feelings of self-worth or safety.

Neglect

The definition of child neglect is fraught with ambiguity. It is typically defined by the economically advantaged and is most frequently applied to the economically disadvantaged. Although some components of neglect can be operationally defined, most legal definitions are intentionally vague to allow for a broad range of case-by-case judgments. This definitional latitude entrusts a great deal of authority to child-protection service agencies, with attendant risks for overzealousness or underconcern.

Standards of neglect are culturally derived. Some situations have little ambiguity. Many others leave families vulnerable to standards that may speak more to an ideal than to essential components of child care.

Understanding the socioeconomic stressors and the familial factors that interact to create a given outcome is vital. Children who come to day care with poor hygiene may reflect extremely diverse situations. A parent may be blatantly neglectful and make no effort to wash the child. But multiple contributing factors often erode parental caregiving, such as poverty, inadequate housing, and severe familial stresses.

Neglect involves an omission of care. It can be divided into several categories: physical neglect, medical neglect, and safety and supervision neglect. Although it is convenient to describe neglect in these separate groupings, they are by no means mutually exclusive. A child can and often does suffer from more than one form of neglect or may be alternately abused and neglected.

Neglect may be acute or chronic. Acute neglect is more likely to occur when the family or parent is under additional stress, such as loss of employment, a significant death, or a geographic move. In these cases, the parental care usually improves when the crisis is past.

Chronic neglect, however, likely reflects limitations in the caregiver's awareness of the child's needs or in the caregiver's ability to respond to those needs. For example, serious emotional or physical illness or substance abuse can reduce the parent's capacity to provide basic care. In these situations, the parent may have an awareness of the child's needs and be able to meet them adequately when he or she is not ill or inebriated.

Environmental stress in neglectful families also tends to be higher than it is in other families. Environmental conditions such as poverty, poor housing, and unemployment can have the same effects on the child as failures in parental care. The effects of these social conditions have been shown to produce symptoms of developmental risk that are similar to those of abuse victims (Elmer 1977).

Parental factors that can contribute to neglect include lack of judgment, lack of motivation, and lack of knowledge of the basics of children's needs. Lack of parental awareness of the child's perspective appears to be implicated in child neglect. Newberger and Cook (1981) found significant differences between neglectful mothers and controls in their ability to see their children as having needs separate from their own. In some cases the lack of awareness of the child's needs is focused on one area. A child can be well cared for physically and neglected emotionally. Others may be warmly and lovingly nurtured most of the time, but occasionally they may be left in dangerous and unsupervised situations.

The younger the child, the more vulnerable he or she is to chronic neglect and the more severe are the consequences. Once the child can get to the refrigerator for himself or herself, use the bathroom, or work in other ways to meet basic needs, he or she may do better.

The physical and developmental manifestations of neglect in a child require careful identification and treatment. These signs may be subtle and are often overlooked; because they are cumulative, they can be easily missed in a single observation.

Physical neglect. Physical neglect includes conditions in which children are lacking in basic food, shelter, or clothing. It involves problems with physical hygiene, inappropriate dress, unsanitary surroundings, substandard housing, and lack of nutrition. It is important to look to societal as well as familial problems in assessing neglect. Many of these signs of neglect are also signs of poverty. Increasing numbers of families are being forced to live in substandard conditions in this country. Homeless families crowd the nation's shelters, forced to live side by side with the mentally ill. Parents may fully understand their children's needs and the negative impact of living in these environments, but they may have neither the financial resources nor the political influence to change their situation. A guaranteed standard of living is not among the nation's priorities. Therefore, the following signs and symptoms must always be considered in the context of the family's social and economic realities.

A child's personal hygiene and physical care may show the following signs of neglect. The hair may be uncombed, greasy, and matted. The child may have dirt encrusted on the skin or embedded in skin folds. He or she may have foul-smelling body odor and feces or discharge material in the genital area. The ears may be packed with wax and dirt, and the fingernails may be uncut and dirty. Lack of dental care may be evident by green or brown matter on the teeth and foul breath from decay. Soiled clothing may be worn for several days or weeks. Clothing that is always oversized or undersized to the point where it impedes the child's activity is a concern. It may be torn and held together with pins; clothes may be missing (socks and underwear are most common). Clothing inappropriate to the weather may also be a sign of neglect.

Children in these situations are often further victimized through ridicule by peers for their appearance or smell. They may be ostracized by classmates and teachers alike for continuous hygiene or dress problems.

Children may also suffer from nutritional neglect. They may be left to obtain their own food or to feed themselves. Meals may be provided sporadically with little routine. The content of the meal may be improper for the child's age and development.

Children's safety is at risk when they are exposed to unusual environmental hazards or are inadequately supervised in environments that pose only ordinary hazards. Of concern are children who are left alone, shuffled from caregiver to caregiver, or repeatedly left in the care of others who are not properly instructed or do not provide adequate supervision.

Often children have accidents that could have been prevented only by unusual prediction and timing on the part of the parent. Some accidents, however, are preventable through adequate supervision. Inadequate supervision can mean allowing a child to explore in dangerous areas without a parent present, exposing the child to harmful products or poisons, or leaving the young child to care for himself or herself. Injuries that occur as a result of inadequate supervision are most common in children under 3 years of age. Infants and toddlers are the most vulnerable to injury and require the most supervision.

Medical care neglect. Medical care neglect involves the omission of medical evaluation or treatment, resulting in physical or emotional damage to the child. As with physical neglect, there are levels of medical care neglect.

Pediatricians suggest that no child should go through the first 5 years of life without medical care. Many states require that children be immunized before they enter school. Such a requirement provides an automatic endpoint to the time children can go without basic immunizations and physical assessment. In doing so, this requirement legislates a minimum health care standard.

Some parents refuse well-child care, specifically immunizations, on religious or cultural grounds. These families are given special consideration, but only after information about the risks to the nonimmunized child are nonjudgmentally presented.

Many cases of medical neglect are not clear-cut. The child may not be in immediate danger or the effects of withholding treatment may not be known. In many cases, parents have limited access to the medical care system. Without health insurance, medical costs can be prohibitive. Health care is received on an emergency basis, with little exposure to preventive services. Among the chronically impoverished, medical care is synonymous with the hospital, and the hospital is often perceived as the place to give birth or to die.

Families need patience and understanding around these issues. Although basic care needs must be met, it is important not to infantilize the parents in an effort to get them to obtain medical care for their children.

Physical Abuse

Physical abuse is frequently defined as "any physical injury inflicted on a child by other than accidental means by a person responsible for his health or welfare" (U.S. Department of Health and Human Services 1977). Because the injuries are physical, they frequently require medical evaluation. The physical manifestations of child abuse are one indicator used by legal and social systems to assess severity and danger to the child.

Important considerations in the identification of physical abuse include the age of the child and the location, extent, severity, and age of the injuries. The younger the child, the more dependent he or she is on the parent for basic needs. The younger child is also most vulnerable to injury if a caregiver physically lashes out. Approximately two-thirds of all children with reportable abuse are under 3 years of age.

Physical violence against a child may occur just once, or it may be a repetitive pattern of parental behavior. Multiple injuries in different stages of healing may suggest ongoing physical maltreatment of the child. Children who are subjected to chronic but less physically endangering violence may suffer as many (or more) problems in their development as children who survive a single, serious inflicted injury. Using physical findings as the central diagnostic yardstick in child abuse, however, can be dangerous. Parent and child can be better served if physical findings are understood as only one feature of the complex situation that includes developmental, emotional, historical, and environmental factors.

Injuries characteristic of physical abuse. The injuries of reportable abuse are many. Major categories of injury are discussed here to provide a working knowledge of these physical manifestations. Injuries can involve trauma to the skin and subcutaneous tissue, including bruises, abrasions, hematomas (swellings containing blood), bites, and burns; injuries to the head and central nervous system; internal injuries, including chest and abdominal injuries; and injuries to the skeletal system.

Injuries may be caused by blunt force such as a blow with the hand, foot, or a blunt instrument (belt, hairbrush, lamp cord). Injuries may result from shaking or throwing a child. Foreign substances may come in contact with the child's skin and cause thermal injuries (scalds or chemical burns), or objects may be placed over or around the child causing asphyxia (choking, suffocating).

Soft tissue injury is the most common physical manifestation of abuse in the young child. Injuries to the genitals, buttocks, cheeks, thighs, neck, and back are more likely to have been inflicted, whereas injuries to the shins, knees, elbows, and hands are more likely to be a result of childhood accidents (Ellerstein 1981). The location of such injuries must be placed within a developmental context. A bruised hand in a 1-month-old infant is viewed with more concern than a bruised hand in a 3-year-old.

Between 40% and 70% of children identified as physically abused show some external evidence of trauma to the face and head (Klein 1982). Children with bilateral black eyes should be evaluated carefully, for accidental injury usually occurs to only one side of the face. Marks on the side of the face, particularly those that are linear in shape (a clear area surrounded by a series of four or five finger marks), suggest that a child was slapped. In the case of a fall, the prominent portions of the face—the forehead and the chin—are likely to be scraped and bruised. If the child is struck, the pattern of injury follows the points of contact, with more vivid bruising over the bony prominences.

Injuries to the mouth are not uncommon. Most frequently seen is a torn frenulum (under the tongue), which results from either a direct blow or forced feeding. If the split frenulum is accompanied by broken teeth, cut lips, or fractures of the facial bone, a direct blow is likely. The absence of other surrounding injuries suggests forced feeding. A frenulum tear in a child who is not walking is pathognomonic in the absence of a clear explanation of an accident (Bernat 1981). Bruises at either side of the mouth may be the result of repeated gagging.

Injury to the genitalia or the buttocks and inner thighs is often indicative of abuse. Children are sometimes punished for bed-wetting or masturbating by tying or pinching their penises or by biting their genitals or inner thighs. Severe bruising to the buttocks and legs in the characteristic shape of a weapon (switch, flyswatter, lamp cord, wooden spoon, hairbrush, paddle) is evidence of excessive discipline. (Because corporal punishment commonly includes spanking, this type of injury is frequently dismissed by professionals.)

The human hand can leave its mark anywhere on the body if enough force is used. Grab marks can be seen on the cheeks as the adult attempts to get the child to eat or take medicine, or on the upper arms or chest (encirclement bruises) as a child is caught and shaken. Pinch marks from poking, which appear as crescent-shaped bruises, can be found on numerous parts of the body. Patterns of fingertip bruising on the upper arms, face, or buttocks are of concern. Linear or fingertip marks on the neck may indicate choking. Linear circular bruises or scars around the neck or the extremities may be due to ropes or cord used to restrain the child.

The other major category of inflicted trauma to the soft tissue is burns. Scaldings are the most frequent type of inflicted burn. These are typically immersion burns, usually a result of children being held in hot water in a bathtub, sink, or other container. Characteristics of these burns are uniformity and the evidence of a demarcation line indicating which area of skin was exposed to the hot liquid. Burns to the trunk, buttocks, genital area, and upper thighs are indicative of dunking. Flexion areas of the body, such as the hip and back of the knees, are characteristically spared. Immersion burns involving the extremities typically demonstrate a "stocking" or "glove" distribution. With immersion burns, noncontiguous burn spots are minimal or absent, as the child is held down in the water, making it hard for him or her to splash.

Contact burns result when an object is placed on the skin: grid burns from floor or wall heaters, circular burns from stove burners or hot plates, and linear burns from radiators are typical. Isolated burns on the buttocks, palms of the hands, or soles of the feet are particularly suspicious. Another kind of contact burn is from cigarettes. Inflicted cigarette burns are frequently confused with impetiginous lesions, and careful evaluation is recommended.

Injuries to the head and central nervous system make up the second major group of physical abuse indicators. These injuries include cerebral contusion, retinal hemorrhages, subdural hematomas (when children are violently shaken), spinal injury, and asphyxia.

Abdominal injuries are the most common cause of death in abused children. Blunt trauma to the abdomen can bruise or rupture any number of vital abdominal organs or the tissue surrounding them, creating profound shock or death. Internal organs, including the kidney, spleen, pancreas, stomach, and intestine, may be compressed or crushed. A child who is punched or kicked in the abdomen is highly vulnerable to rupture of the stomach or colon. Crushing force such as is created when a child is thrown or struck can lacerate the pancreas, liver, or spleen. Symptoms of abdominal injuries are recurrent vomiting, abdominal swelling, and tenderness.

Skeletal injuries result from direct blows, bursting, shaking, or squeezing. The infant skull—thin and pliable with open fontanelle and patent suture lines—is particularly vulnerable to blunt trauma. A direct blow can result in diastatic, bursting fracture. Pointed objects can cause localized areas of bony depression or perforation. A spiral fracture of a lower extremity in which a twisting force is used is highly indicative of inflicted trauma.

Close confinement includes torturous restrictions of the child's movement. Such confinement involves many forms of physical restraint, including tying a child's arms or legs together, binding a child to a chair or bed, or confining a child to a closet or similar enclosure for prolonged periods of time.

The family context.   Physical injuries do not exist in isolation. Other past or present injuries, the history of this injury, the condition and developmental status of the child, and family stresses must all be considered when there is concern about possible child abuse. It is important for day care providers to talk with parents in a caring way that lets them know that the provider notices the injuries and is concerned.

Some general characteristics of families with an abused child are worth mentioning. A delay in treatment can be indicative of abuse or neglect. Also of concern are parents who state that they have no idea how the accident occurred, who minimize the injury or the child's response to it, or who provide an explanation that is not compatible with the nature of the injury or with the age or activity level of the child. Parents may insist on explanations that are clearly implausible, or they may deny any responsibility for the child's injuries. *It is not the role of the day care provider to challenge a parent on the truthfulness of his or her story or to demand details about the exact nature of the instrument used or the time, place, or circumstances of the incident.* Rather, this time is a time to express concern about the child and family in a caring, supportive way and, if child abuse is suspected, to inform the parent of the obligation to report. Further investigation is then in the hands of the agency charged with that task. To the extent possible, the day care provider needs to remain a supportive presence in the child and parents' life.

Sexual Abuse

According to the national incidence study of child abuse and neglect, approximately 7% of all child maltreatment known to professionals involves sexual abuse (U.S. Department of Health and Human Services 1981).

These cases may be only a fraction of the actual number, for sexual abuse is often a closely guarded family secret that is not divulged until there is a major disruption or crisis in the family system.

In the past, the degree of force used was the central determinant of the severity of a sexual abuse incident. But in most cases of sexual child abuse, force is not necessary because the child knows and has some trust in the assailant. Of all sexually abused children, the number molested by a parent or guardian, or other family member, usually male, may be as high as 80% (Sigroi 1975). In these cases, the abuse is likely to go on for months or years and to be marked by secrecy enforced through various means, including threats or blaming the child. Physical force is not typically present. A parent may or may not know, or may or may not believe the child or take action to stop the abuse. Sexual assault by a stranger tends to be a single isolated event, frequently involving physical force, to which the child responds by telling a supportive family member (for further discussion, see Glasser, Chapter 13, and Kelly, Chapter 12, this volume).

Behavior characteristic of sexually abused young children is nonspecific except for hypersexualized behavior, which is considered a specific indicator of exposure to sexual material or involvement in sexual activity. Young children in particular do not engage in specific sexualized behavior unless they have been exposed to it. Other frequently identified, nonspecific behavioral sequelae of sexual abuse in young children include anxiety, fear, shame, guilt, depression, and feelings of loss and grief. A number of the emotional responses described in the "Emotional Abuse" section of this chapter also are common.

The consequences of sexual abuse depend on the age and developmental stage of the child, the nature of the abusive situation, circumstances surrounding the disclosure, investigation and disposition of the case, and how persons and institutions in the child's life respond to the child. If the abusive interaction is part of a larger picture of family dysfunction, then consequences are thought to be more serious than those usually present following an isolated incident outside the family.

Many children involved in incestuous relationships are removed from their homes, increasing their trauma. They may feel responsible for the destruction of their families and fear that they have been alienated from them permanently.

In general, positive physical findings are present in only about one-third of sexually abused children. Young children who are penetrated may have enlarged anal or vaginal openings, infections of the mouth, venereal disease, or other scars.

When children disclose sexual abuse in a day care setting, great care should be taken to listen to them, to avoid leading questions, and to obtain help. Young children who have limited understanding of time and place may tell the story a bit at a time. They may act it out with toys or engage in sexually suggestive activities with classmates. In all cases, this activity and distress should be taken very seriously.

Most experts suggest careful examination of clothing and fingernails, particularly if the incident is recent. Any unusual findings in diapers or underwear should be saved for medical authorities. The child should not be wiped or bathed until after an exam.

Suspicions of sexual abuse raise staff anxiety more than any other form of maltreatment. The lack of hard evidence in the majority of cases tends to create additional distress. Accurate and prompt notification of mandated authorities and care in handling both the disclosures and the belongings of the child are paramount.

WORKING WITH PARENTS AND FAMILIES

Histories of parents are as varied as the children they bring to day care settings. Recognizing and understanding the needs and capabilities of every parent are crucial to providing care to their children.

Each parent brings unique capabilities, vulnerabilities, past experiences, and expectations to the family. Some parents have had very traumatic childhoods. Some parents have been physically abused (Steele and Pollock 1968), others emotionally injured, and still others victims of extreme hardship. Other parents have physical limitations that make parenting more difficult and complicated. Still others face obstacles such as abject poverty, violent marital relationships, multiple crises, cognitive limitations, and misinformation about children and child care that impede the development of their best capabilities as parents.

Many parents who maltreat their children also love their children and would like to be good parents. For a variety of reasons, some within their control and influence and others beyond it, they fall short of this goal. Identifying significant impeding issues and joining the parent in addressing them is one of the most direct and effective ways to help the child.

It is important to assist the parent in maintaining appropriate autonomy and control in the parent-child relationship as well as in other relationships and circumstances in the parent's life. To the extent possible, empower the parent, and identify and solve problems together. Communicate respect for the parent and the parent's own ways of coping and adapting to his or her unique realities. When supported and respected as a person, a parent is more likely to use the day care setting as a resource to develop the confidence and skills needed to interact successfully with other persons and institutions in his or her life.

Although it is important for day care personnel to be able to identify possible maltreatment, *child protective agencies*—not day care centers—

are responsible for investigating reports of suspected abuse and initiating any legal action on behalf of the child. It is inappropriate and possibly even harmful for day care staff to take a judgmental position in regard to the family. Such a posture invades the relationship between staff and child. It is a terrible emotional burden for a child to be caught between loyalty to the family and loyalty to teachers and staff who disapprove of the family. However the child chooses to resolve such a conflict, it involves a loss. Day care staff must be especially careful to treat parents with respect, understanding, and recognition of their authority in regard to their children.

A particularly vulnerable group of parents is women who are themselves victims of violence. Parental victimization harms children in two ways: the child is a witness to violence, which carries its own serious developmental consequences (Jaffe et al. 1986); and the victimized parent's role of caregiver may be affected.

Battered women are confronted with a multitude of issues that require particular care and planning to overcome. Household practices may need to be adapted to placate the batterer and to prevent violence toward the children. Otherwise, the battered woman may be forced to leave home. She may still be vulnerable to violence if the batterer finds her. She will typically be court ordered to make the children available for visitation and may even lose custody if she cannot establish herself in an approved setting.

It is important to keep the possibility of interspousal violence in mind while working with the family. Insisting that the family or couple meet may heighten the risk for a parent who has let a child care worker know that she has been victimized. The bringing of problems to the parents' attention collectively may be used by the batterer as an excuse for further violence.

If there is evidence of child maltreatment, it is important to inform the victimized woman of any intentions to file a protective service report so that she may take necessary protective action. It is also good practice to inform any parent when a protective report is made. Strengthening the victimized parent maximizes the potential for a positive family resolution.

Knowledge of family violence is also important in understanding the child's behavior and in helping the parent, as is shown in the following example:

In a Boston day care center, the teachers noticed a marked behavior change in 2½-year-old Jeremy. Jeremy had been an engaging child, sensitive to the needs of peers and cooperative with staff. But he became increasingly aggressive, oppositional, and excessively active. Jeremy's mother informed the teacher that she was having the child assessed for hyperactivity and was hopeful that he would be placed on medication. In a meeting with Jeremy's mother and the center's consultants, the relatively sudden changes in the child's behavior were noted. Questions were asked about possible changes in the home environment. Jeremy's mother explained that her live-in partner had lost his job in construction and was home full-time. He had become an emotional tinderbox, falling into violent and unpredictable rages. Jeremy appeared to be acting out the chaos he experienced at home. His high level of activity was, in turn, being used as a focal point by the batterer. In a desperate attempt to protect Jeremy, his mother hoped that tranquilizing him would remove him as a target of her partner's violence.

Once the center staff understood the issues that Jeremy's mother was struggling with, they were able to help her start solving her problems in a constructive way. She was referred to a service program for battered women. Center staff helped her discuss her situation with her protective service worker and were able to help her address her son's anxiety, reframing it as a normal response to a frightening and very confusing home environment.

Sometimes parents are not amenable to intervention by day care staff. They may want to restrict their involvement with staff. They may even respond to expressed concerns about the child's well-being by removing the child from the program. Especially with situations such as these, it is helpful for staff to receive mental health consultation and support.

REPORTING CHILD MALTREATMENT

Day care teachers are often the first to notice problems associated with child maltreatment. All 50 states include in their reporting statutes, either by direct reference or in more general language, a requirement for day care professionals to report suspected child abuse and neglect to the mandated state agency. Consequently, each center or family provider should have a process and an organizational structure to handle identification, reporting, and follow-up of suspected cases of child abuse or neglect. Decisions about who reports, when they do so, and with what supports should be worked out in advance. Written policies should be reviewed with all staff.

It is the obligation of each staff member to know about the nature and signs of child maltreatment. Child maltreatment is a symptom of dysfunction that results from complex processes, making each situation unique. It requires acknowledgment of the complicated issues that surround any episode. Providers should know enough to question unusual injuries, behavioral distress, and developmental difficulties that appear related to parental care or to mistreatment of the child. This perception requires training and the availability of consultants (in medicine, law, mental health) who may be called on for guidance and support.

Access to a competent multidisciplinary team can expedite help for the child and the family as well as serve as important support to day care personnel. This team can be an ad hoc group of local professionals who could come together as needed or an already established unit in another institution, such as the local hospital or mental health center. Contact with these professionals ideally should take place before an incident and can occur through a liaison person as well as through educational experiences where these other professionals are present. Individual, face-to-face contact is always helpful. In centers in which children are being seen by protective services, regular conferences should be held not only with parents, but also with protective services and other providers as well.

Institutional responsibility includes the development of a specific written policy that details staff action and responsibilities when maltreatment is suspected. A uniform format for reporting is helpful; thus all information is recorded and processed in a similar fashion. Documentation in maltreatment situations is of utmost importance, and external injuries and behavioral observations should be described carefully and objectively. Any actions or statements of the child should be recorded, as should those of parents. Who talked to whom, when, and where must be recorded precisely. Any physical evidence of maltreatment—diapers that contain possible evidence of sexual abuse, dangerous objects that a child presents such as drugs, sharp objects, and so forth—should be kept and given to medical or protective service authorities.

Those individuals who know the child best should be encouraged to participate in the process of identification, assessment, and reporting. They should never have to undertake this task alone. In our opinion, all reports should be brought to the attention of a senior administrative person. This individual, usually the program director, should be available to discuss the teacher's concerns and to help implement the reporting process.

Several critical steps aid decision making within the reporting process. The first is information gathering. This step should begin as soon as an injury or indicator is identified, and it includes observation of the child and communication with the parent(s). If there is physical injury, medical assessment is imperative. This process may involve informal consultation with the medical person on staff and/or a request to the parent to have the child seen medically, with permission from the parent for the day care center to receive information from the physician about his or her findings.

Waiting to make a report can be detrimental not only in terms of documentation, but also because the child may remain at risk. Staff and administrative personnel must have a set procedure for action that includes careful but immediate intervention.

Parental involvement in the reporting process is recommended whenever possible. There should be one staff member who assumes primary responsibility for working with the parent. It is frequently a difficult and uncomfortable step for this person to speak with the parent about the day care center's concerns. Much of the apprehension surrounding this process, however, can be alleviated by explaining to the family what the reporting process is and is not. First, reporting is required by law when it is suspected that a child may be at risk. It does not usually mean that a child will be removed from home. It is a referral for help for a family in which there is a child in distress.

The reporting process can often serve as an important stimulus for a family to begin to acknowledge that there is a problem that needs to be addressed. On a number of occasions, after initial anger, family members turn to the reporting providers for support. Some families react with relief. In all situations there is the risk that the family will be angry at the day care center and that they will remove the child. Although this concern is usually a consideration in reporting, it should not be used as a reason for failing to make a report.

Day care staff can be extremely helpful in assisting a family through the official investigation process that follows a report. The staff person working with the parent should have knowledge of the investigative process in the community in order to help the parent understand what is going to happen and, if the parent wishes, be with the parent during the process.

It is hoped that after a report is filed, the child will continue in day care. Special contact with parents is often helpful to map out the course for future care. This activity should be supportive and assure the parent of the center's continuing care for both the parent and the child and that the parent will continue to be informed and included if any new concerns arise. If a child is placed in foster care, the day care center may be the only point of continuity. Especially in these circumstances, the center staff is of critical importance to the child as he or she struggles to cope with the changes.

Reporting child maltreatment is never a comfortable process. It can be made more effective and helpful through policy, procedure, and personal contacts that support the goal of protecting the child as well as getting services for the family. Reporting can benefit both child and family if knowledgeable, sensitive professionals are involved and have support from colleagues in other parts of the child protective, medical, and legal system. Glasser (see Chapter 13, this volume) explores the role of the child psychiatrist in this process, which has significant therapeutic and preventive implications.

MALTREATED CHILDREN IN GROUP SETTINGS

Each child is a unique individual whose understanding of and interaction with the environment is a product of many factors, including the child's personality, developmental level, cognitive capacity and experiential history, and the nature of the immediate environment. Numerous attempts have been made to identify within these elements particular signs and symptoms of maltreatment and to determine how they influence ensuing development (Wolfe and Mosh 1983). Some insights can be gained from this research.

For example, Kinard (1982) found that maltreated children under the age of 3 are likely to exhibit more emotional problems than those maltreated at a later age: these younger children had fewer coping mechanisms for defending against stresses in their lives. Main and George (1985) found that maltreated toddlers responded to distress in peers with aggression, fear, anger, or attempts at a mechanical comforting movement. In contrast with their peers, maltreated children were less likely to display empathic or genuinely comforting behavior toward the distressed peer.

Child behaviors are to be viewed collectively, as patterns providing clues about a child's approach to the world. No single behavior has definitive meaning or a predictable cause. When a child is observed over time, the meaning and stability of particular behavioral sequences can become more evident.

If the symbolic meaning of an act is understood, intervention to alter or extinguish it can be more effective. Rituals, for example, are often important coping mechanisms in unsafe or unstable environments. Seemingly insignificant items (a coin, a piece of paper) can become precious objects of transition between home and day care. It is important not to diminish their value or to insist that they be removed. Similarly, a child who tries to hide items in his or her pockets may need a concrete reminder of the day care setting to carry home.

Maltreated children often approach normal environmental tasks with limited emotional resources. Trust in relationships may be impaired. For some children this lack of trust produces high anxiety when they are exposed to anything new, or even in making routine transitions between activities. For others, it creates an absence of "normal" anxiety about new situations.

Children with histories of maltreatment may also tend toward extremes in relationships with adults. For example, a child may cling indiscriminately to one adult after another or immediately climb into a stranger's lap. In contrast, other maltreated children may have difficulty seeking or accepting comfort from caregivers. All of these patterns can be understood as ways of coping with deficits in children's primary intimacy relationships.

It is important to offer children struggling with these issues opportunities to explore close relationships both through play and with day care staff. That there be one primary caregiver in the center who is available to the child with reasonable reliability is vital. It is particularly important that there be a consistent response to a child when anxiety or other signs of distress are displayed. Routines are comforting for most children. They can be particularly comforting for most unpredictable environments. Routines and verbal preparation, which allow children to move through transitions with knowledge of what to expect, can be a vital element in building trust.

Maltreated children also often feel unsafe. This feeling has many different manifestations, including withdrawal, expressions of fear, and aggression. Children need to be told clearly with words and actions that they will not be allowed to hurt themselves or their peers, and that no one else in the day care setting will be allowed to hurt them. It is sometimes difficult for staff to feel comfortable disciplining children who they know are victims of deprivation or violence. For the child, this discipline may be experienced as another form of abandonment and of confirmation that violence cannot be controlled—that the world is a dangerous place. Kind, clear, firm, and reasonable limits are an important part of a therapeutic environment.

A natural developmental task of children in day care is learning appropriate ways to get their needs met, including learning to delay gratification. All young children find it difficult to wait for food once they are aware of their hunger. For children whose experiences include irregular feeding, feeling hungry can create a panic reaction. They may become frantic, grabbing for food and trying to swallow too rapidly, risking choking. They may hoard food in the mouth or clothing.

If possible, the time between the arrival of food and its service should be minimized. Children who have experienced deprivation may need gentle restraint, with an ample supply of food maintained within their vision. They may need a special activity to help them wait or a role in the service such as putting napkins on the table. The mealtime should be as relaxed as possible, with plenty of time for eating and social interaction; then it becomes a pleasurable experience rather than a desperate struggle for gratification.

For some children, day care provides a singular opportunity to learn age-appropriate behavior. At one end of the spectrum are children who are infantilized or whose emotional development has been delayed in some other way. At the other end are parentified children, who have had to assume responsibility and sensitivities beyond their years.

As this discussion has indicated, working with maltreated children in day care settings does not require major changes in approach or curriculum but rather a reframing of activities to help children with their individual issues. In theory this task is not a departure from practice with other day care participants. What is different is the continual need to think about what patterns of behavior mean to the child and how they are used by the child to cope with fears, anxieties, and expectations generated by his or her life experiences. This activity can best be accomplished when a center has the opportunity for regular mental health consultation.

> Two-year-old Monique was described by her teachers as overactive, unable to sit through a meal or to join her peers in "circle activities." She became easily frustrated, but she pushed away anyone who tried to assist her. Instead, she would fall down and cry. Her teachers tried rewarding her for even small successes and minimized efforts to correct her, but there was no improvement.
>
> When observed by consultants, Monique was noted to be hypervigilant, monitoring anxiously the activities around her. She would position herself in the corner of the room, and when anyone approached, she would defend herself by surrendering, crying, and falling to the ground. It was discovered that this child lived in a very violent home. Her father battered her mother, and several siblings had been placed in foster care because they had been maltreated by the parents. Monique also had an older sibling who behaved aggressively toward her. Her behavior in day care could be understood as survival efforts that she had developed to cope with her difficult home environment.
>
> In working with Monique, it was important to help her maintain the behaviors she needed to protect herself at home while providing an experience of safety at the center. Monique's place at the table was changed to a corner position. "Circle activities" were done in an ellipse with her place against the wall. When staff persons approached Monique they announced their intentions and moved very slowly. They encouraged her efforts and minimized their control over the situation. Within several months, Monique was less fearful and more trusting, although she still reverted to her old patterns when new situations arose. (It is worth noting that this child's home situation was being monitored by the local protective service agency, and foster care was not then considered appropriate.)

As this case illustrates, a child's behavior can have many different meanings. What seemed like a short attention span was really a survival tool. This understanding enabled Monique's teachers to address the issues underlying her hypervigilance and emotional fragility. In the day care environment, they were able to provide Monique with alternative interpretations of others' actions toward her, thereby expanding the repertoire of responses she could make.

CONCLUSIONS

As a primary focus for increasing numbers of young children, the day care center has considerable impact on the socialization of children entrusted to its care. This function is especially important for children who have been maltreated. Day care can provide the opportunity for a child to experience a different approach to trust, mastery, and interaction with peers and adults, all critical activities of early childhood. By doing so, it has the potential to provide the additional support the child needs to survive and overcome the difficulties that are part of his or her experience. A day care program that is sensitive to a maltreated child's special needs as well as to the needs of the family can make a considerable difference in all their lives.

REFERENCES

Bernat JE: Bite marks and oral manifestations of child abuse and neglect, in Child Abuse and Neglect: A Medical Reference. Edited by Ellerstein NS. New York, John Wiley, 1981, pp 141–164

Canavan JW: Social child abuse, in Child Abuse and Neglect: A Medical Reference. Edited by Ellerstein NS. New York, John Wiley, 1981, pp 233–252

Egeland B, Sroufe A: Developmental sequelae of maltreatment in infancy, in New Directions for Child Development: Developmental Perspectives of Child Maltreatment. Edited by Rizley R, Cicchetti D. San Francisco, CA, Jossey-Bass, 1981, pp 77–92

Egeland B, Sroufe LA, Erickson M: The developmental consequences of different patterns of maltreatment. Child Abuse Negl 7:459–467, 1983

Ellerstein NS (ed): Child Abuse and Neglect: A Medical Reference. New York, John Wiley, 1981

Elmer E: Fragile Families, Troubled Families: The Aftermath of Infant Trauma. Pittsburgh, PA, University of Pittsburgh Press, 1977

Jaffe P, Wolfe D, Wilson S, et al: Similarities in behavioral and social maladjustment among child victims and witnesses to family violence. Am J Orthopsychiatry 56:142–146, 1986

Kinard M: Experiencing child abuse: effects on emotional adjustment. Am J Orthopsychiatry 52:82–91, 1982

Klein DM: Central nervous system injuries, in Child Abuse and Neglect: A Medical Reference. Edited by Ellerstein NS. New York, John Wiley, 1982

Main M, George C: Responses of abused and disadvantaged toddlers to distress in agemates: a study in the day care setting. Developmental Psychology 21:407–412, 1985

Newberger CM, Cook S: Parental awareness and child abuse neglect: studies of urban and rural parents. Paper presented at the National Conference for Family Violence Researchers, University of New Hampshire, Durham, NH, 1981

Newberger E, Hyde J, Holter H, et al: Child abuse and neglect, in Behavioral Pediatrics: Psychosocial Aspects of Child Health Care. Edited by Friedman S, Haekelman R. New York, McGraw-Hill, 1980, pp 329–338

Sigroi SM: Sexual molestation in children. Children Today 4(3):18–21, 1975

Steele B, Pollock C: A psychiatric study of parents who abuse infants and small children, in The Battered Child, 2nd Edition. Edited by Helfer R, Kempe H. Chicago, IL, University of Chicago Press, 1968, pp 89–134

U.S. Department of Health and Human Services. National Center for Child Abuse and Neglect: Child abuse and neglect state reporting laws (DHHS Publ No OHDS-80-30265). Washington, DC, DHHS, 1977

U.S. Department of Health and Human Services. National Center on Child Abuse and Neglect: Study finding on National Study of Incidence and Severity of Child Abuse and Neglect (DHHS Publ No OHDS-81-30325). Washington, DC, DHHS, 1981

Wolfe D, Mosh M: Behavioral comparisons of children from abusive and distressed homes. Journal of Counseling and Clinical Psychology 51:702–708, 1983

Part V

National Policy and Day Care

Chapter 15

The Expanding Federal Role in Child Care

Congressman George Miller (D-California)

In the late 1980s the public policy discussion on child care moved beyond questioning the need for governmental involvement to the highly charged debate about the extent and nature of that involvement. Once considered a second-class issue on Capitol Hill, child care has traveled the long road to legitimacy as a political issue and policy issue, finally rewarding the attention paid to it for decades by the child development community. In the early 1990s, the framework for a broad national child care policy will almost certainly be put in place.

The attention currently lavished on child care marks a sharp departure in policymakers' thinking. For most of the 1980s, the public policy debate was dominated by a stance articulated most forcefully by President Ronald Reagan and his supporters. This philosophy holds that reinvigorating the U.S. economy necessitates dismantling the infrastructure of domestic social programs; that responsibility for childrearing resides with church and family, not with the federal government; and that women, despite their economic commitments, should assume full-time care for their children. While policymakers debated these issues, the need for, and consensus around, a national child care policy grew because of changes in family structure, the increased presence of women in the paid labor force, and the dramatic impoverishment of children, factors that show no signs of abating in the foreseeable future.

At the same time, social scientists strengthened their evidence of the importance of early childhood care and education in assuring social and economic success in adulthood. Federal early childhood development programs such as Head Start and the Supplemental Feeding Program for Women, Infants, and Children (WIC) have been demonstrated to improve the academic and health status of participants, thereby obviating the need for more expensive assistance programs later in a child's life. Similarly, researchers have found that high-quality child care enhances both cognitive and social development.

In this chapter I will review the advances and retreats in federal child care policy over the past 60 years, with special attention to the decade of the 1980s. I begin with an historical summary of previous child care initiatives, ending with the era of "benign neglect" under President Reagan. I will explore the demographic and economic changes that have increased the demand for child care, issues of child care demand and supply, the short supply of high-quality care, and evidence of the value of such care. Then I will return to the growing constituency for child care policy that has developed in recent years, and, finally, to the most recent federal initiatives that have emerged.

LESSONS FROM PREVIOUS FEDERAL CHILD CARE PROGRAMS

The earliest federal initiatives on child care involved the establishment of day care programs under the Federal Emergency Relief Administration and Works Progress Administration (WPA), pillars of the New Deal. Rather than cut back social programs to fuel economic growth, as was done in the 1980s, these New Deal efforts, guided by Keynesian economic theory, saw social spending as a way to provide employment and expand the economy. The WPA nurseries, for example, were justified as a source of jobs for unemployed teachers as well as a bulwark against the worst deprivations that young children suffered during the Great Depression (Kerr 1973). In fact, the reasons offered for instituting nurseries under WPA were much like those that would be offered 30 years later for founding the Head Start program: they would enhance opportunity and improve educational outcomes for a specially targeted group of educationally disadvantaged children.

Federal support for child care expanded dramatically during World War II but did not form a stable basis for postwar child care policy. Whereas in the WPA era, child care was seen as a service for only the poorest families and children, by the middle of the war it was seen as a necessity for the war effort. With the rise in access to "good jobs at good wages" in manufacturing and defense-related employment, women flooded into the paid labor force during the war (Milkman 1987). However, federal policy lagged behind this transformation in the demography of the workplace, and wartime production suffered as a result. Seventy-five percent of women war workers were married and 3 million of them were full-time housewives; absenteeism and job turnover were rampant and directly affected wartime production (Chafe 1972).

Until Congress acted to provide funding for child care centers in 1942, the child care market during World War II presented a more extreme version of what we see today: tales abounded of inadequate care, latchkey children, and injuries to unsupervised young people. According to the contemporary literature, "[t]he locked car became a surrogate babysitter; and in many places bands of children roamed the streets while their mothers worked" (Kerr 1973, p. 163). One social worker in the San Fernando Valley found 45 infants locked in cars in a war plant parking lot; the number of child neglect cases in Norfolk, Virginia, tripled (Chafe 1972).

Despite the need for child care during World War II, the initial resistance to federal involvement was strong. When that involvement finally arrived, it was both limited and couched in rhetoric that downplayed any endorsement of women's work outside the home. For example, even as it was directing employers to establish child care services and flexible work arrangements for their women employees, the U.S. War Manpower Commission declared that "the first responsibility of women, in war as in peace, is to give suitable care in their own homes to their children" (Kerr 1973, p. 163). Later in the same year, the Congress and the President approved the Community Facilities Act, or Lanham Act, of 1942, which provided matching funding for localities that could demonstrate that they needed child care centers to support production for the war. By February 1944, centers funded under the Lanham Act served only 65,717 children; by the spring of 1945, these centers still served only 100,000 children, meeting less than 10% of the estimated need (Chafe 1972).

Although the quantity of child care provided under the Lanham Act represented a significant improvement over that offered before the war, the federal government insisted that its only interest in providing child care funds lay in maintaining wartime production. As a result, the justification for federally subsidized child care evaporated with the end of the war (Chafe 1972; Hartmann 1982).

At the end of the war, many women withdrew from the paid labor force, either voluntarily or involuntarily (Milkman 1987). Federal policy both reacted to, and exacerbated, this trend by dismantling its funding for the Lanham centers. Fears of an economic depression and of hostility from male workers motivated the national government to encourage women to leave the outside-the-home labor force (Michel 1987).

Funding for child day care reemerged under a variety of auspices in the 1960s and 1970s. An emphasis on equality of opportunity and carefully targeting federal resources made child care of various kinds part of the move for a "Great Society." Unlike Lanham Act programs, however, and like WPA nurseries, these programs targeted specific groups of children, with distinctions in programs for the poor and nonpoor.

Funding for child care, primarily for economically disadvantaged children, was expanded through a variety of legislative initiatives including the Social Security Amendments of 1962 and 1967, the Head Start program inaugurated in 1964 under the Economic Opportunity Act, Title VII of the 1965 Housing and Urban Development Act, and the 1965 Model Cities Act (Kerr 1973). Federal assistance for the day care needs of middle-class families was created through tax credits and deductions for child care as a business expense. The Revenue Act of 1971, the Tax Reduction Act of 1975, and the Tax Reform Act of 1976 liberalized federal income tax provisions for nonpoor working families (Robins and Weiner 1978).

Beyond funding and tax credits for child care, Congress in the 1960s and 1970s introduced a number of important child welfare programs that resulted in a significant drop in child poverty: WIC, created as a pilot program in 1972 and expanded nationally in 1975; Title XX of the Social Security Act, which funds day care, protective services, and home care, in 1974; the Child Care Food Program in 1968; the Elementary and Secondary Education Act in 1965; and the Education for All Handicapped Children Act in 1975. All these social programs addressed the special needs of different groups of children—the disabled, the educationally disadvantaged, and the poor—but did not comprise an organized strategy of child and family support. Services were fragmented, resources were limited, and political support was unsteady.

The only comprehensive child care legislation ever seriously considered by Congress was the Comprehensive Child Development Act of 1971, introduced by Sen. Walter Mondale (D-Minnesota), to establish a federally funded system of child care. The bill passed both houses of Congress but was vetoed by President Richard Nixon as "the most radical piece of legislation to emerge from the 92nd Congress." He claimed it would commit "the vast moral authority of the national government to the side of communal approaches to child rearing over and against the family centered approach" (Zigler and Goodman 1982, p. 345).

THE REAGAN YEARS

Ronald Reagan, like Franklin Roosevelt 50 years earlier, came to power pledging to promote full employment, economic opportunity, and a strong economy. Yet Reagan pursued a very different political path in seeking these goals. In the Roosevelt era, full employment and eliminating poverty through government involvement were considered central to regaining economic strength. In the 1980s, the same welfare state credited earlier with strengthening the American economy by providing consumers with money to spend was blamed for draining the federal bank, bleeding the taxpayer, and boosting the federal deficit.

As a result, rather than continuing the development of social initiatives for children, the Reagan administration reversed course, arguing that deep cuts in children's and other social welfare programs were necessary to improve economic growth. Keynesian-style spending under Reagan occurred largely under the auspices of the defense program. Because children's programs lacked powerful political and popular support, programs like Title XX and WIC could not be protected as easily from budget cuts as more comprehensive, widely used programs with more powerful constituencies, like Social Security. Estimates indicate that federal expenditures for child care for low-income families declined 36.4% in real terms between 1980 and 1988. After adjusting for inflation, the 1988 funds for Title XX were less than half of those for pre-Block Grant programs in 1977 (Children's Defense Fund 1988). Since there is no single source of federal funding for child care, cuts came from a variety of federal programs including Title XX, Aid to Families with Dependent Children (AFDC), and Head Start.

Cuts in child care services were comparable to those in other children's programs under Reagan. Several programs were eliminated altogether or merged into underfunded block grants. As the House Select Committee on Children, Youth, and Families found in its ground-breaking report, "U.S. Children and Their Families: Current Conditions and Recent Trends, 1989," on a host of measures, the Reagan years took a drastic toll on millions of American children and families (U.S. Congress 1989). Not only were the "truly needy" among American children not spared the effects of program cuts, but they were often the special targets of these cuts. Hundreds of thousands of economically disadvantaged children lost access to health care because of program changes and funding reductions proposed by Reagan and enacted in 1981 (Children's Defense Fund 1988). Chapter I, the federal program funding compensatory education, served one-third fewer poor children at the end of the 1980s than at the beginning (Children's Defense Fund 1988). Since 1982, participation in the Food Stamp program—in which three out of five recipient families contain children—has declined 14% (U.S. Congress 1989, pp. 272–273).

Even as children declined as a proportion of the American population, they remained the poorest age group in the United States. More were poor and living at even lower income levels in 1988 than in 1979; nearly as many were poor after 6 years of "recovery" as in the depths of the recession of 1982 (U.S. Bureau of the Census 1989). The record shows that throughout the 1980s, the educational, medical, and developmental well-being of children, especially poor children and their families, was sacrificed in the name of stimulating economic growth and reducing the size of federal involvement in domestic policy.

Under the Reagan administration, the belief that private sector initiatives are the most effective vehicle for meeting people's needs gained new validity, and this notion was applied to child care to some extent. Credits to encourage corporations to set up child care services for employees were incorporated into the tax code through the Economic Recovery Tax Act of 1981. As of 1987, however, fewer than 1% of medium- and large-sized firms provided any sort of child care services to their employees (Conference Board 1989).

DEMOGRAPHIC AND ECONOMIC CHANGES INCREASE CHILD CARE DEMAND

At the same time Reagan administration policies withdrew child care assistance from low-income families, people at all income levels found themselves needing child care outside the family. Because of a combination of demographic, social, and economic changes, the majority of parents are now unable to provide full-time care for their children. Between 1947 and 1973, median family income rose in real terms, setting a record in each consecutive year. During this period, many primary wage earners earned enough to support their spouse and children. Since 1973, the so-called family wage has eroded substantially. According to the congressional Joint Economic Committee, mean real family income declined by 8% between 1973 and 1984. If mothers had not gone to work during this period, then the loss in family income would have been more than three times greater (Levy and Michel 1985; U.S. Congress 1986).

Data from the Bureau of Labor Statistics suggest that the decline in real family income is not a temporary phenomenon. Between 1986 and the year 2000, service industries will account for virtually all of the projected growth in new jobs (U.S. Bureau of Labor Statistics 1987; U.S. Department of Labor 1989). Nearly half of these jobs today are located in the retail trade and other personal services industries, and they pay an average annual income of $11,754. These jobs also offer limited, if any, benefits such as health insurance and retirement plans, further reducing purchasing power. They also offer very limited opportunities for advancement (Schoen 1987; Service Employees International Union 1987). If current job and wage trends continue, young families starting out in the late 1980s can expect to earn 25% less in real wages throughout their lifetimes than did their parents (Schoen 1987).

Increasingly, in two-parent families, both adults must work to provide their children with basic economic security. In 1986, 14% of married working women with children were married to men who earned less than $10,000; 43% were married to men who earned less than $20,000; and 54% were married to men who earned less than $25,000. The 1988 poverty threshold for a family of four was $12,091 and the 1986 median income for families with children was $29,303 (U.S. Bureau of the Census 1989; U.S. Bureau of Labor Statistics 1987).

By 1987, more than 51 million women were in the work force, with an unprecedented 53% of all married women with infants under 1 year of age on the job or looking for work. In 1988, women with children under 6 years of age formed the largest group entering the work force (U.S. Congress 1989). This dramatic shift in women's participation in the labor force is primarily attributable to structural changes in the nation's job market, the decline in the value of real earnings, and the changing composition of American families (see, e.g., U.S. Congress 1987). With the majority of women economically unable to provide in-home care for their children, even if they might choose that option, most families find themselves seeking child care just as they seek housing, health care coverage, or any other basic necessity.

DEMAND FOR CHILD CARE FAR OUTSTRIPS SUPPLY

In the early 1980s members of Congress were increasingly compelled to recognize the difficulties besetting American families. In 1983, an impressive majority in the U.S. House of Representatives created the Select Committee on Children, Youth, and Families and charged it to investigate the status and needs of American children and families. Subsequently, the Senate established a children's caucus for members interested in these issues. After the 1986 election, when control of the Senate returned to the Democrats, the Committee on Labor and Human Resources reorganized two subcommittees into the Subcommittee on Children, Family, Drugs, and Alcoholism.

In the Select Committee's first year, in hearings across the country, it quickly became apparent that the lack of safe, quality child care was a pressing concern among parents in every part of the country, at every income level, and in every ethnic group: young professionals as well as low-income parents faced often overwhelming problems in finding child care. No group of parents had many acceptable options in carrying out their responsibilities as primary caregivers. Many parents were being forced to choose repeatedly between going to work and caring for their children and were in many cases able to do neither task to their satisfaction (U.S. Congress 1984).

For the vast majority of families, child care has become a financial burden that devours a considerable portion of their income. In 1986, U.S. families spent an average of nearly 10% of total family income on child care, which was comparable to average family expenditures for food. As one indication in the change in family expenditures, the poverty line was designed around food needs (the so-called Orshansky Index equals the Department of Agriculture's "Thrifty Food Plan" times 3), but it in no way accounts for child care costs. Poor families in the United States spend roughly 20% to 26% of their total income on child care (Hofferth 1987).

In 1987, approximately 28.3 million American children under the age of 15 were in need of some type of child care while their parents worked. Existing spaces in licensed child care centers and regulated family day care homes, however, could accommodate only 2.9 million children—scarcely more than 10% of the estimated need (Children's Foundation 1987; U.S. Bureau of the Census 1987; calculations by the Select Committee on Children, Youth, and Families). The other 25.4 million were cared for by relatives, in unlicensed centers, or by no one at all. The status of the majority of these children is uncertain because no comprehensive research exists on child care facilities. What is certain is that for the millions of parents who need child care services, assuring the quality of that care has become paramount.

THE FRUSTRATING SEARCH FOR QUALITY CARE

Since the overwhelming majority of parents must work to support their children, parents need to be able to ensure that their children are receiving care that provides for their health, safety, and educational development. Experts agree on the key ingredients of quality care: skilled child care workers, parental involvement, and enforcement of standards of health, safety, and staff-child ratios (U.S. Congress 1984).

At present, states are responsible for setting child care standards and for monitoring and enforcing those standards. As a result, standards for child care—including staff-child ratios, minimum health and safety requirements, registration or licensure requirements for family day care homes, and even the rights of parents to visit their children—vary dramatically from state to state. Regulations are spotty, unequal, and incomplete.

The staff-child ratio is a key indicator of the quality of child care, especially for infants. As of 1986, only three states met the recognized standard of one staff person to care for three infants (Young and Zigler 1986). Eleven states permit five or more infants in family day care without an assistant (Morgan 1987).

Only 18 states guarantee parents the right to conduct an unannounced visit to their children's child care center, and even fewer states (11) guarantee that same right to parents whose children are in family day care homes (Morgan 1987). Only 22 states formally license family day care homes (Children's Foundation 1987). Five states have either no method of regulating family day care or only a voluntary registration process. A handful of other states regulate only state-funded centers (Morgan 1987).

The problems of availability and quality in child care are exacerbated by the pitifully low wages paid to child care workers. More than 70% of the nation's child care workers have annual earnings below the poverty level; the resultant high job turnover diminishes the quality and continuity of care. New findings from the National Child Care Staffing Study (Whitebook et al. 1990)—the first comprehensive profile in a decade of child care training, salaries, and quality—reveal shockingly low salary levels and high turnover rates for the women who work in child care. Child care workers earn just $5.35 an hour on average; for full-time, year-round work this comes to a total of $9,363—less than the poverty line for a family of three. Wages in child care have declined in recent years, even as demand has expanded dramatically. As a result, turnover among workers has tripled in the last decade, from 15% to 41% (Whitebook et al. 1990). These findings are particularly startling when combined with the evidence that high turnover levels in child care lead to limited cognitive and social development for children (Whitebook et al. 1990).

Because of the haphazard state of child care regulation, we have no comprehensive data on the type and quality of care that children are receiving. For instance, it is estimated that 75% to 95% of all home-based child care providers are unlicensed or unregulated by the state. Some of the data that are available are unsettling: a recent report from a county social services department in North Carolina found that five out of the six reports of child abuse in day care homes occurred in unlicensed homes. A follow-up statewide study found that complaints against unregistered homes were three times as likely to be severe as those against registered homes (Russell and Clifford 1987).

The presence of a state license is no guarantee that a child care facility is safe. Because of limited resources, many states have inadequate monitoring and investigation programs. According to a recent state survey, the number of complaints to state licensing officers has increased in most states, leaving less staff time for routine visits. Some states even decreased the number of licensing staff; as a result, 18 states inspect child care programs only once a year and four states less often than once a year (Morgan 1987). Even some of the most dramatic abuse cases in recent years have occurred in licensed facilities. In Fairfax, Virginia, a woman registered with the county to provide child care was recently convicted of neglect in the poisoning death of an infant in her care. Such a tragedy highlighted Virginia's weak regulatory and enforcement scheme for family day care providers. Between 1978 and 1984, 42 children were allegedly abused at the McMartin Preschool, a licensed child care program in a Los Angeles suburb. At the time, the California Department of Social Services inspected licensed child care centers only once every 3 years. It took national media attention and the advent of such a crisis for California to mandate yearly inspections.

Child care standards and regulation are a long-term bone of contention among those who formulate policy. Still, research indicates that in most states, the present regulatory systems are not giving parents the help they need in assuring that their children will receive safe, healthy, and developmentally appropriate care.

QUALITY CHILD CARE CONFERS A VARIETY OF BENEFITS

Many policymakers think of child care as providing custodial care for children while their parents work. Researchers have found, however, that good-quality care provides a wide variety of benefits for children—even very young children—besides custodial care. For instance, latchkey children who attend after-school programs show marked academic improvements and increased self-esteem (U.S. Congress 1984).

Child care has also proved crucial to the success of programs to encourage single mothers to leave the public assistance rolls. The Massachusetts Employment and Training Choices (ET-Choices) program spends half of its $57-million budget to pay for child care expenses for participants. "People are participating in ET-Choices because the training and education opportunities are good, and because child care is provided. Without child care assistance it just wouldn't be possible" (Sanders 1987, p. 29). As of 1987, 86% of ET-Choices participants who had left welfare were still off welfare 1 year later. In all the major work and welfare demonstration programs conducted in recent years, child care has proven crucial to success (Gueron 1987).

Although child care is not widely available for handicapped or disabled children, researchers conclude that even temporary, "respite" child care plays a positive role in reducing the financial and emotional stresses experienced by families with a disabled child (U.S. Congress 1984). Child care also serves as a useful tool in efforts to reduce abuse or neglect by parents and in reducing the need for expensive, disruptive, and often tragic foster care placements. Some social service agencies reserve child care slots for children in protective custody, and others provide "crisis nurseries" and drop-in centers where parents who fear they are about to abuse their children may leave them temporarily. Families with regular access to child care have the lowest rates of substantiated child abuse reports, at 6% for those who have full-time child care compared with 38% for those who have no regular child care (Kotch and Parke 1986).

DEVELOPING A CHILD CARE CONSTITUENCY

Although parents have always counted the care and education of their children among their highest priorities, policymakers have been slow to recognize that child care has become an essential service for the majority of American families. For most, child care is as important as education, housing, and health care, which have long received substantial federal support. As early as 1970, the White House Conference on Children found that quality day care was the number one need of American children and families. But both the 1971 effort by Senator Mondale and a 1978 effort by Sen. Alan Cranston (D-California) to promote a federal child care initiative found the community of interest still fragmented and polarized.

Finally, in 1984, the House Select Committee on Children, Youth, and Families began a national and comprehensive initiative on child care. The committee found, and helped create, a far warmer climate for discussion of child care than that found by legislators in 1970 or 1978 (U.S. Congress 1984).

The most remarkable result of the committee's efforts has been the emergence for the first time of a broad-based bipartisan constituency in favor of a national child care initiative. In 1984 more than 65 national organizations, as well as both liberal and conservative members of the Select Committee, endorsed the development of a broad range of child care options. Since then, unions and other private sector agencies have joined the drive for child care legislation. By the late 1980s, public opinion polls had begun to reflect the depth of grass roots support for child care that emerged in the committee's findings. A 1987 Harris poll found that 73% of the respondents would be willing to increase their taxes to support child care. In a 1987 Yankelovich poll, 53% of the individuals surveyed answered that government should do more to provide for child day care (Wallis 1987). Evidence mounted that the pressing need of families for child care broke down ideological and, to some degree, budgetary opposition to passing new legislation.

Countermanding the trend toward consensus were the pressures of the deficit. Mounting federal debt and subsequent attempts by Congress and the Reagan-Bush administrations to reverse its growth made legislators reluctant to initiate new social programs. An ideological commitment to "no new taxes," made during the 1988 campaign by then-candidate Bush, further served to constrain the debate over social spending. Congress was reluctant to propose new taxes, while existing dedicated taxes such as those for Social Security were well protected by their politically formidable constituencies.

This, essentially, is the situation in which we find ourselves today. On the one hand, policymakers have received a strong mandate from the public and national organizations to expand their commitment to child care. Many legislators have answered this mandate, warming gradually to the idea of a federal child care initiative. However, budgetary concerns have held others back; both budgetary and lingering ideological questions have made it difficult to reach a consensus on policy that matches the consensus on need.

But policymakers with a serious commitment to child care can find a way out of this quandary. No one denies that comprehensive child care is an expensive proposition. However, in the federal budget ($1.05 trillion for fiscal year 1988) there is ample opportunity to allocate even several billion dollars a year for programs that help local governments and the private sector increase the availability of child care and create a long-term funding mechanism that makes high-quality child care available to every family. The budget question is not so much fiscal as it is philosophical: Are we ready to make access to child care a national priority?

Long-term thinking also offers a way out of the fiscal quagmire. Without exception, evaluations of early childhood education and health programs have demonstrated that public investments in early childhood development can lead to significant budget savings later on (U.S. Congress 1985, 1988). For example, every dollar spent on early prevention and intervention in a preschool education program like Head Start can save six dollars against the later costs of remedial education, welfare, and crime (Berrueta-Clement et al. 1984; U.S. Congress 1985). The same logic, by which policy investments early in the life course produce savings later on, applies even more powerfully to comprehensive, quality child care than it does to Head Start.

SEARCHING FOR A LEGISLATIVE RESPONSE

Reflecting both the undoubted consensus around child care need and the more reluctant consensus on the budgetary good sense of federal child care support, there was a rush of legislative activity around child care in the middle and late 1980s. In 1984 I introduced the first new, comprehensive child care bill in the decade, the Child Care Opportunities for Families Act, into the 99th Congress. Since then, both Democrat and Republican policymakers have submitted legislation utilizing an array of different schemes to expand or redirect federal funding, and give states incentives to improve the quality and supply of child care.

The legislative proposals of the middle 1980s included vouchers for poor working families, funding mechanisms that would allow states to expand child care systems across the board and give the federal government responsibility for setting quality standards, child care block grants to fund new services and resolve liability insurance issues, and demonstration programs using school facilities as the bases for universally available child care (see Zigler and Freedman, Chapter 1, this volume). All these proposals acknowledged that the federal government had to invest leadership responsibility and funding in a national child care policy commensurate with the need for services. This funding would have to answer the demand with a wide variety of programs and facilities but also insist on maintaining high standards of availability and quality.

Congress also addressed the issue of child care in the course of reforming AFDC, the nation's major "welfare" program. The Family Support Act (FSA) of 1988 is the first national welfare plan to mandate child care provision for women making the transition from welfare to work. The act, which requires that people who receive income grants participate in employment and training programs, also guarantees child care assistance to those who participate. In addition, FSA eases the transition from welfare to work by extending child care assistance to participants for up to 9 months after they have entered the mainstream labor force and ceased receiving welfare payments. Although the fate of this provision depends on state-level implementation, on this point welfare reform has recognized the needs of working women.

At this writing, House and Senate conferees are negotiating an agreement based on the child care bills that have survived the legislative process to this point. Although the initiatives differ on the amounts awarded for general child care, the expansion of Head Start from a part-day to a full-day program, the presence and stringency of quality standards, the use of teachers and school sites, the appropriate role of sectarian and religious child care providers, and other issues, all the initiatives under consideration agree on core points. They all provide for at least the beginnings of comprehensive service provision, limited to no single income group or category of vulnerable children; all agree on the need for state and local level flexibility in a framework of federal financing and debated degrees of regulation; and none mandates a single type of child care site, provider, or financing. The inclusion of tax credits in all of the bills under consideration—a particular concern of conservatives—implicitly recognizes the fact that many parents choose to raise their children full-time, in their own homes; however, in the subsidies available for both family day care homes and center-based care and schools is the recognition that many parents choose to do, or must do, otherwise.

A HEALTHY FUTURE FOR CHILDREN AND FOR THE UNITED STATES ECONOMY

Assuring the maximum development of our children is directly tied to national and international concerns. One of the most significant economic shifts of the past decade has been the transformation of the United States from the world's biggest creditor nation to its largest debtor. Since the United States has had difficulty competing in traditional manufacturing with developing countries where cheap labor is abundant, the nation's future economic expansion depends on developing and marketing more sophisticated products and services and training a highly skilled work force to perform these jobs.

Regaining global economic strength requires substantial investments in human, as well as manufacturing, capital. This imperative is especially challenging for two reasons. First, tomorrow's economy will depend on workers who are more highly trained and educated than in the past but who, in greater numbers, will be starting school with greater income and educational deficits. One out of every four of today's preschoolers lives in poverty, one in five is at risk of becoming a teen parent, and one in seven is at risk of dropping out of school (Children's Defense Fund 1988). In 1987, nearly 1 million young people left public schools without graduating. Fewer than half of high school seniors read at levels considered adequate to carry out even moderately complex tasks; 80% have inadequate writing skills (Committee for Economic Development 1987). Lacking basic skills, these "at-risk" youth will be ill-equipped to handle the kinds of jobs necessary to assure the health of the United States economy.

Second, the future labor pool is shrinking. In 1983, for the first time, the number of Americans over the age of 65 outnumbered the number of teenagers. Although only 10 years ago young adults accounted for one-quarter of the United States population, by 1995 they will account for 16%, reducing by 25% the size of the entry-level labor force. Assuming the economy continues to expand at a moderate pace, business will be forced to delve deeper into the labor market of at-risk youth (Education Commission of the States 1985). A report by the Committee for Economic Development, a research organization of corporate America, argues that "if the United States is to be a world class economy in the next century, then we had best begin preparing them now to have a world class work force" (Committee for Economic Development 1985, p. 2).

Child care that is affordable and safe, and enhances the social and cognitive development of young children improves the ability of families to provide for the economic security of their children. At the same time, it prepares young children for adulthood, allowing them to perform effectively in the labor market and to establish stable families of their own.

CONCLUSIONS

Whether the houses of Congress negotiate their differences on child care legislation and the President signs the act they approve are the immediate concerns at this writing. But these concerns beg the larger question—whether the combined weight of desperate need, indubitable research findings, and broad policy consensus can work to provide a level of federal support for child care unparalleled since at least the Lanham Act during World War II. We must also ask whether, unlike our treatment of programs supported by the WPA or Lanham Act, we are now prepared to sustain federal support for child care over the long term, in good economic times as well as bad, and in periods of obvious crisis as well as those in which the need is more subdued.

We came far enough in the 1980s to set a policy framework in place, but we have still to ensure that the promise of that framework is fulfilled: that legislation is backed with fiscal resources, that child care personnel are trained and compensated so that they can provide adequate services, and that a flexible but firm regulatory structure ensures safe and nurturing child care environments in every state of the union. As we have seen, child care is no longer a second-class political issue. Our challenge is to make it a first-class service for American families.

REFERENCES

Berrueta-Clement JR, Schweinhart L, Barnett S: Changed Lives: The Effects of the Perry Preschool Program on Youth Through Age 19. Ypsilanti, MI, High/Scope Press, 1984

Chafe WH: The American Woman: Her Changing Social, Economic, and Political Roles, 1920–1970. New York, Oxford University Press, 1972

Children's Defense Fund: A Children's Defense Budget FY 1989: An Analysis of Our Nation's Investment in Children. Washington, DC, Children's Defense Fund, 1988

Children's Foundation, Family Day Care Advocacy Project: 1987 Family Day Care Licensing Study. Washington, DC, Children's Foundation, 1987

Committee For Economic Development: Children in Need: Investment Strategies for the Educationally Disadvantaged. Davis, CA, International Dialogue Press, 1987

Conference Board, Work and Family Information Center: Prevalence of employer-sponsored child care. Unpublished manuscript, June 1989

Education Commission of the States, Business Advisory Commission: Reconnecting Youth. Denver, CO, ECS-BAC, 1985

Gueron J: Reforming Welfare With Work. New York, Manpower Demonstration Research Corporation/Ford Foundation, 1987

Hartmann S: The Home Front and Beyond: American Women in the 1940s. Boston, MA, Twayne Publishers, 1982

Hofferth SL (Health Scientist Administrator, Demographic and Behavioral Sciences Branch, Center for Population Research): Testimony before U.S. Congress, House, Select Committee on Children, Youth, and Families hearing, American Families in Tomorrow's Economy, Washington, DC, July 1, 1987

Kerr V: Child care's long American history, in Child Care, Who Cares? Foreign and Domestic Infant and Early Childhood Development Policies. Edited by Roby PA. New York, Basic Books, 1973, pp 157–171

Kotch JB, Parke TL: Family and social factors associated with a substantiation of child abuse and neglect reports. Journal of Family Violence 1(2):167–176, 1986

Levy FS, Michel RC: The economic future of the baby boom. U.S. Congress, Joint Economic Committee. Washington, DC, U.S. Government Printing Office, 1985

Michel S: American women and the discourse of the democratic family, in Behind the Lines. Edited by Higonnet M. New Haven, Yale University Press, 1987, pp 154–167

Milkman R: Gender at Work: The Dynamics of Job Segregation by Sex During World War II. Urbana, IL, University of Illinois Press, 1987

Morgan G: National State of Child Care Regulation, 1986. Watertown, MA, Work/Family Directions, 1987

Robins P, Weiner S: Child Care and Public Policy. Lexington, MA, Lexington Books, 1978

Russell SD, Clifford RM: Child abuse and neglect in North Carolina day care programs. Child Welfare 66:149–163, 1987

Sanders R (Director of Voucher Day Care, Department of Social Services, Commonwealth of Massachusetts): Testimony before U.S. Congress, House, Select Committee on Children, Youth, and Families hearing, Child Care: Key to Employment in a Changing Economy. Washington, DC, March 10, 1987

Schoen C (Research Economist, Services Employees International Union): Testimony before U.S. Congress, House, Select Committee on Children, Youth, and Families hearing, American Families in Tomorrow's Economy. Washington, DC, July 1, 1987

Service Employees International Union: Solutions for the New Workforce. Prepared for Solutions for the New Workforce: A National Conference on Policy Options, Washington, DC, 1987

U.S. Bureau of the Census: Who's Minding the Kids? Current Population Reports, Household Economic Studies, Series P-70, No 9. Washington, DC, U.S. Bureau of the Census, 1987

U.S. Bureau of the Census: Money Income and Poverty Status in the United States: 1988. Washington, DC, U.S. Government Printing Office, 1989

U.S. Bureau of Labor Statistics: Current Population Survey. Washington, DC, 1987

U.S. Congress. Joint Economic Committee: Working mothers are preserving family living standards. Washington, DC, U.S. Government Printing Office, 1986

U.S. Congress. House. Select Committee on Children, Youth, and Families: Families and Child Care: Improving the Options. Washington, DC, U.S. Government Printing Office, 1984

U.S. Congress. House. Select Committee on Children, Youth, and Families: Opportunities for Success: Cost-Effective Programs for Children. Washington, DC, U.S. Government Printing Office, 1985

U.S. Congress. House. Select Committee on Children, Youth, and Families: American Families in Tomorrow's Economy. Washington, DC, U.S. Government Printing Office, 1987

U.S. Congress. House. Select Committee on Children, Youth, and Families: Opportunities for Success: Cost-Effective Programs Update, 1988. Washington, DC, U.S. Government Printing Office, 1988

U.S. Congress. House. Select Committee on Children, Youth, and Families: U.S. Children and Their Families: Current Conditions and Recent Trends, 1989. Washington, DC, U.S. Government Printing Office, 1989

U.S. Department of Labor: Outlook 2000. Monthly Labor Review, Nov 1989, pp 3–74

Wallis C: The child-care dilemma. Time, June 22, 1987, pp 54–60

Whitebook M, Howes C, Phillips D: Who Cares? Child Care Teachers and the Quality of Care in America. Final Report of The National Child Care Staffing Study. Oakland, CA, Child Care Employee Project, 1990

Young KT, Zigler F: Infant and Toddler Day Care: Regulations and Policy Implications. New York, American Orthopsychiatric Association, 1986

Zigler E, Goodman J: The battle for day care in America: a view from the trenches, in Day Care: Scientific and Social Policy Issues. Edited by Zigler EF, Gordon EW. Dover, MA, Auburn House, 1982, pp 338–350

Chapter 16

Child Care Law and Child Care Advocacy

Carol S. Stevenson

The lack of a national day care policy and a corresponding sound legal framework for the development of day care services in the United States originates in part from a national ambivalence about accepting the changing role of women and the changing makeup of the American family. Often the legal difficulties encountered by day care programs are an indirect manifestation of a societal belief that a woman's proper place is in the home, caring for children without pay, and that only parents can properly care for their children. This country's lack of acceptance of out-of-home child care is revealed both by its failure to consider day care as a social institution and by the imposition of inappropriate constraints on the development of day care services (Grubb 1985).

In the 1980s there was a resurgence of public interest in the issue of child day care. Because the number of families who need day care services has grown so dramatically, and because the "baby boom" generation is in its prime childbearing years, the child care issue has received widespread attention in the popular media and in political forums at the national, state, and local levels.

To date there is no comprehensive national policy about child day care or support of working parents, and the attention has mainly resulted in piecemeal policy initiatives at the state and local levels (Blank and Wilkin

1986). Often as the result of interest at the gubernatorial level, a number of states have developed comprehensive day care initiatives and have been successful in passing new laws and appropriating additional funds to serve the growing need (Governor's Office of Human Resources 1987). In addition, private groups have done much to enhance the face of day care. Whereas many such efforts have resulted in successful approaches to the delivery of child care services, a true solution to the underlying systemic problems with the provision of child care in the United States will require a greater devotion of resources and a broad-based consensus about how those resources are to be utilized (U.S. Congress 1984).

NEW FEDERAL LEGISLATION

In 1987 the first comprehensive federal child care bill since the 1970s was introduced in Congress. Calling for a $2.5-billion appropriation, the Act for Better Child Care (known as the ABC bill) primarily will provide subsidies, to be administered by the states, for child care costs for low-income families. The ABC bill also addresses quality, licensing standards and procedures, worker salaries and training, and the establishment of child care resource and referral agencies.

The long overdue introduction of the ABC bill is a beginning. Even its proposed appropriation will meet only a tiny fraction of the need for financial assistance for families who use child care services. For example, it is estimated that California's share of the appropriation will be approximately $221 million—almost doubling what that state currently spends from its general fund for subsidized child care services. Yet the more than $330 million that California currently spends annually on direct child care services meets only 10% of that state's need (California Assembly Office of Research 1986).

The ABC bill begins to address one of the major questions facing child care advocates: Who will pay for the services? To build a comprehensive system of available care, two other questions must be answered: Where will the service be located and how will it be regulated? Miller (Chapter 15, this volume) reviews other federal legislation and addresses the central question of who will pay for child care.

WHO WILL PAY FOR CHILD CARE

Parent Fees

Currently, most of the cost of nonparental child care is paid directly by parents. With fees ranging from $20 to $200 per week, the cost of child care is a substantial portion or beyond the means of the family budget (California Child Care Resource and Referral Network 1986; U.S. Bureau of the Census 1985). A family living on a subsistence income must rely on unpaid child care arrangements, sacrifice other necessities in order to pay for child care, or hope to find help through some form of subsidized care.

Because public resources devoted to child care services are inadequate, the ability of parents to pay for care and the needs of children are often pitted against the needs of child care workers to earn a living wage. The low pay of child care workers is a hidden subsidy of child care services (see also Phillips and Whitebook, Chapter 7, this volume).

Government Support

The federal and state governments currently spend money on child care in a variety of ways. The public policy purposes of the expenditures can generally be justified in either of two ways: because they enable parents to work, or because they enhance the education and development for certain at-risk populations of children. The inability of policymakers to see the interrelatedness of these two purposes has at times resulted in programs that do not reach the population they are intended to serve and in inadequate allocation of resources to deliver services.

Enabling Parents to Work

Dependent care tax credit. The single largest source of public assistance for child care is an indirect one: the federal dependent care tax credit. Internal Revenue Service data show that in 1984 more than 7.5 million taxpayers claimed the credit and received more than $2.6 billion in tax benefits (U.S. Department of the Treasury 1986). The federal credit offsets dependent care expenses necessary to enable parents to work. The amount of the credit is based on the family's adjusted gross income. Unfortunately, few families receive the maximum credit allowable because those with annual incomes under $10,000 usually cannot afford to incur the maximum allowable expenditures of $2,400 for one child or $4,800 for two or more children. The average credit received by families in 1983 was approximately $322.19. Because the credit is an after-the-fact reimbursement, it does little to help low-income families meet the month-to-month expenses of day care or enable them to purchase more expensive care. Moreover, financial support of child care through the credit has little impact on the wages of child care providers or the operating budgets of child care programs.

Program subsidies. The Title XX Social Services Block Grant is the major source of federal funds available to states to meet the child care needs of low-income children and families. Forty-four states and the District of Columbia use Title XX funds matched with state revenues to provide child care assistance. Because of severe funding cuts in the early 1980s, the federal Title XX appropriation for 1987 was, after adjusting for inflation, only 75% of the 1981 level (Blank and Wilkin 1986).

Since Title XX funds are administered as a block grant to the states, the amount spent on child care is within each state's discretion. In 1986, approximately $790 million in Title XX funds was spent on child care services by the states. The requirements for Title XX expenditures are quite flexible, allowing states to serve families eligible for Aid to Families with Dependent Children (AFDC), as well as teen parents, parents in job training programs, and children in need of protective services. Children from infancy through school age can be served with these funds.

States vary greatly in the amount of state general revenues spent on child care. A number of states have increased their funding for child care programs over the past several years, either by adding funds to supplement the Title XX funding or through new initiatives with separate funding mechanisms. The extent of state involvement depends, in large part, on the health of the state's economy.

AFDC child care payments. The cost of child care is an allowable expense under the AFDC program. The costs of care, up to $160 per month, can be "disregarded" from the earned income of the recipient in the computation of a monthly grant amount. There are no readily accessible data on the amount expended on the child care disregard. In practice, the AFDC disregard is a flawed approach for helping low-income families pay for child care. The $160-per-month maximum is inadequate to purchase decent full-time care in most parts of the country. The after-the-fact reimbursement is impractical because it requires recipients to prepurchase care with an income that barely covers the more basic needs for heat, food, shelter, and clothing.

In states where welfare reform legislation has passed, child care has been identified as a key component to successful employment and training of welfare recipients. The Massachusetts Employment and Training Choices (ET-Choices) program pays for child care throughout the training period and up to 1 year after a recipient is employed, an expenditure of $21.4 million in 1987. The provision of transitional child care is essential for successful movement from welfare to work.

Tax treatment of employer-supported child care. Child care assistance provided by an employer to an employee through a dependent care assistance plan is a tax-free benefit to the employee and tax deductible to the employer. This favorable treatment of dependent care as an employee benefit has been in effect since 1981. Currently, approximately 2,000 employers (of the 6 million employers in the United States) offer some form of child care assistance to their employees.

The most popular forms of child care assistance offered by employers are resource and referral services and the creation of salary reduction programs, which allow employees to pay for their child care expenses with pretax dollars. Neither of these forms of assistance requires a large financial outlay or continuous funding of a new, costly benefit. But the institution of any form of child care assistance by an employer heralds a workplace recognition of conflicts between work and family that are a major stress on American families. If dependent care assistance is offered as a salary reduction plan, it must meet certain statutory requirements.

Policies That Support Healthy Child Development

The following child care programs are motivated not by the need to assist in the payment for child care while parents are at work but by the special needs of certain populations of at-risk children. Whether those children are at risk of academic failure, abuse, or neglect or because of a physical handicap, the programs that have been designed to serve them do not always take into account that the parents of these children need to work. In the vast majority of these programs, program quality and standards are among the highest available to any population of children, yet the failure of policy to view the child's need for appropriate care and parents' need for gainful employment as integrally related has at times created programs that inadequately serve the families most in need.

Head Start. Head Start delivers comprehensive educational, health, nutritional, social, and other services to economically disadvantaged children pursuant to federal program standards. With an appropriation of close to $1 billion, it is the largest federal program expenditure for preschool care. Begun during the 1960s' War on Poverty, Head Start programs are designed to give underprivileged children an opportunity to develop skills that will enhance their readiness for kindergarten. Although the program exclusively serves income-eligible families, only 15% of Head Start programs operate for a full workday. For working parents, taking advantage of Head Start often means making double child care arrangements.

Early childhood initiatives in the public schools. Since the early 1980s, research on the positive effects of early childhood education and efforts at education reform have served to justify state expenditures for early educational intervention. Currently, 26 states have begun such an initiative; prior to 1980, only 8 states had provided state revenues for state prekindergarten programs. State investment in early childhood education is made by expanding Head Start programs, providing parent education programs, or (most commonly) providing funds for pilot or statewide prekindergarten programs. Two-thirds of the state programs are targeted for at-risk children or children with other conditions such as limited English proficiency or school readiness. Only four states permit children to be served for the full working day. Comprehensive coordination between these school-based educational programs and day care funding and services does not take place in the majority of the states (Marx and Seligson 1987).

Increased services to handicapped preschoolers. A recently enacted federal bill appropriates money to states that implement statewide early education programs for all handicapped preschoolers. The law mandates services to moderately handicapped children, expanding greatly the number of handicapped children who can be served. Individual education programs must be developed to meet the unique needs of each preschool child and his or her family. The provisions of this law are a good example of a policy that addresses a child's needs in the context of his or her family. For example, parents who do not choose to enroll their child in a preschool program or in special education can receive in-home services.

In brief, the devotion of adequate financial resources to the provision of decent quality child care services must be the primary concern of every child care advocate in coming years. For families who cannot afford care and for children who are caring for themselves and each other, change cannot come soon enough. The provision of free labor for child care will not come by finding senior citizens to volunteer or immigrants to work below the minimum wage. Raising our children has a different economic cost today, and this cost must be addressed at every level of social policy planning.

HOW WILL CHILD CARE BE REGULATED?

Child care programs are currently regulated independently by each of the 50 states. For a comprehensive comparison of the licensing standards of various states see Morgan (1987); for an overview of the legal issues in regulating child care see Grubb (1985). There are no federal child care standards. Child care centers, which usually include preschools and nursery schools, have different regulations than family day care homes do. Standards, which vary considerably, include staff-child ratios, staff qualifications, and requirements for the physical facility. In determining the effect of regulation on the quality of care, the level of regulatory enforcement is as important as the standards. In a number of states, a higher standard is required of programs that are funded by the state. Other sources of child care funding, such as Head Start, have independent performance standards that exceed licensing requirements.

Licensing requirements serve as minimum standards—a level of operation below which no program can operate legally. It is critical that both consumers and advocates understand that licensing standards should not be used as the sole measure of quality in programs.

Typically, policymakers show an interest in licensing only in response to crisis. For example, following the media sensationalism surrounding child abuse cases in child care centers, lawmakers wanted to be able to "fix" child care with more stringent regulation. Numerous bills were introduced that increased the screening of child care workers and enhanced the penalties for licensing violations. Little or no concern was given to the cost or the effect of these requirements on the actual safety of child care facilities. Child care services are rarely regulated with regard for the complexities of providing the service or with a recognition of all the players involved.

Parents' Role in Regulation

The legal aspects of the parents' role in the development, delivery, and regulation of child care services have been given scant attention. The trilateral legal relationship among parent, child, and state becomes quadrilateral with the addition of a paid caregiver. Parental guilt, coupled with a shortage of services, has in the past effectively stifled much voicing of parental discontent with the status quo. Perhaps the most positive outcomes of the concerns about child abuse in day care have been the increased scrutiny of programs by parents, an increased willingness to voice complaints about substandard programs, and the establishment of statutory rights in some states to enter and inspect facilities where one's children are in care. Particularly in family day care homes, where the sheer number of homes—each caring for small numbers of children—precludes frequent monitoring by the state, the role of parents as monitors is critical.

Child care resource and referral agencies educate parents about what to look for in programs and about the need to continue to be observant of the program and their child's response to it. The tremendous growth of child care resource and referral agencies since 1982 is one of the most positive signs for the development of accessible child care services. In good-quality day care, parents and providers form a mutually beneficial partnership to care for the children. Likewise, parents and the licensing agency must work together to adequately regulate child care.

Cost Versus Quality

High standards mean more expensive care. Advocates for lower standards cite the current high cost of services to parents to support their position. Private child care programs that want to keep the current ratios argue that if staff-child ratios are increased, the additional costs will be borne by parent fees, effectively pricing lower middle-class families out of the paid child care market. Likewise, say conservative lawmakers, if we want to serve more children in subsidized child care, we should just lower the staff-child ratio so that more services could be provided with the same expenditure of dollars.

These arguments are insidious because they pit the families who need child care against both the child care workers and the best interests of the children. Public consensus is required if standards are to be upgraded. Such consensus can be reached only if policymakers are willing to tackle the need for sufficient resources to make child care affordable while simultaneously working to improve standards.

Licensing and Religious Exemptions

Another troubling aspect of the regulation of child care is the continuing effort of certain church-sponsored child care to become exempt from any regulation. The vast majority of church-housed and church-sponsored child care programs accept the need to be regulated and have no problem meeting licensing standards in their programs. Some Christian groups, however, vehemently assert that the regulation of child care programs in their churches violates their First Amendment rights to practice religion freely. The licensing standard most commonly objected to is the prohibition against corporal punishment. Twelve states specifically exempt church-sponsored child care programs from their licensing requirements. In states in which no exemption exists, some church-based programs have challenged the licensing requirements in court. For the most part, the licensing laws have been upheld as necessary to a compelling state interest in protecting the health and safety of children and not an infringement on the church members' First Amendment rights (Sanger 1985).

In sum, the regulation of child care is in a constant state of flux. It is at the whim of public perception about the safety of child care programs, the need for the state's protection, and the availability of public resources. Forty-one states have updated their requirements for child care centers in the past 5 years, 19 since 1985. As more and more children spend their time in child care, the importance of child care regulation should become more widely accepted. In theory, everyone agrees about the importance of adequately regulating child care. In practice, few policymakers are willing to allocate public resources to make certain that standards are routinely enforced. Involving the state in the delicate and intimate relationship between a family and their paid caregiver requires sensitivity and common sense. Although the consumers of child care need protection from unscrupulous operators, the providers of care need fair and equitable treatment by the state.

WHERE WILL CHILD CARE BE LOCATED?

In addition to state licensing schemes, child care is regulated at the local level through municipal and county zoning ordinances and through local building and fire code requirements. These requirements, often both overlapping and contradictory, effectively operate to ban licensed child care in some localities. The need for acceptance of child care programs in our neighborhoods and communities, indeed in our own backyards, is as critical as it is obvious.

Zoning and Family Day Care

The prohibition of family day care due to restrictive and often expensive local zoning requirements has impeded the development of regulated day care in many parts of the country (Pegg 1985). Neighborhood fears of the encroachment of nonresidential uses into residential neighborhoods, coupled with often expensive and intimidating permit procedures, have hampered the growth and legitimization of family day care in many communities. Twelve states currently have laws that prohibit localities from restricting family day care in residential zones. Almost all of these laws have been passed since 1986. Once a state preempts local law in this area, advocates and providers still face the challenge of implementing the law at the local level. Finding acceptance for the home-based care of children in family day care in every community in the United States is necessary if the need for child care is ever to be met.

Child Care in New Developments

As part of its Downtown Plan, San Francisco passed a landmark ordinance in 1985 requiring developers of new office and hotel space either to set aside square footage for child care facilities or to contribute money to an affordable child care fund. The ordinance was justified on the basis of the increased need for child care generated by the increased employment of parents in new commercial and hotel developments. The San Francisco ordinance has not yet generated any new child care spaces because of overall stringent limits on growth and the fact that many of the office buildings currently under construction were approved prior to the passage of the ordinance. (See Cohen 1987 for an overview of methods for including child care in the land use and development process.) Seattle offers developers a density bonus for including space for a number of public benefits, including child care, in new commercial developments. In Seattle, several developers have taken advantage of the bonus for day care and three new projects in the downtown area now include space for child care centers.

In addition, in a number of locations developers are beginning to view the provision of space for child care services as an amenity that will give them a competitive edge in attracting new tenants. Ideally, the dedication of space for child care will work hand in hand with a commitment on the part of employer-tenants to assist in underwriting the cost of the service. The community need for a particular type of service should be carefully assessed prior to devotion of resources. The ability of the employees within a particular development to pay for the care must also be taken into consideration.

CONCLUSIONS

Child care services in the United States are housed and operated in diverse settings. Family day care homes in residential neighborhoods, proprietary chains on convenient commuter routes, nonprofit programs in church basements, and afterschool programs on public school sites are some of the most familiar locations for child care in the United States.

To achieve a comprehensive system do we need more uniformity, or can these diverse types of care coexist? The strength of the current diversity is in the choice it gives parents seeking care for their young children. Providing optimum out-of-home care to preschoolers requires a great deal of attention to individual, family, and cultural differences.

Can we develop payment mechanisms flexible enough, yet accountable enough, to allow resources to go to a variety of programs? Can the regulation of child care be comprehensive and yet fair handed so that the majority of care operates within the system in which it is accessible to more families? Can child care resource and referral agencies serve as the community-based center of this complex delivery system? How should they be funded?

These are the issues to which advocates must find answers if we are to have adequate child care in place before this generation of children are grown. The need has been acknowledged and accepted. The hard work of finding ways to meet that need and providing for both the children and the caregivers continues.

REFERENCES

Blank H, Wilkin A: State Child Care Fact Book 1986. Washington, DC, Children's Defense Fund, 1986

California, Legislature, Assembly, Office of Research: California 2000: A People in Transition—Major Issues Affecting Human Resources. Sacramento, CA, Joint Publications, June 1986

California Child Care Resource and Referral Network: Preliminary Child Care Cost Results from the California Child Care Resource and Referral Network Inventory of Child Care Facilities, San Francisco, CA, August 1986

Cohen AJ (ed): Planning for Child Care: A Compendium for Child Care Advocates Seeking the Inclusion of Child Care in the Land Use/Development Process, San Francisco, CA, Child Care Law Center, 1987

Governor's Office of Human Resources, Commonwealth of Massachusetts: Partnerships for Day Care: Final Report of the Governor's Day Care Partnership Initiative, Boston, MA, June 1987

Grubb E: Day care regulation: legal and policy issues. Santa Clara Law Review 25 (2–3):303, 1985

Marx F, Seligson M: Current Early Childhood Initiatives in the States: Preliminary Findings from the Public School Early Childhood Study. Wellesley, MA, Wellesley College Center for Research on Women, 1987

Morgan G: The National State of Child Care Regulations 1986. Boston, MA, Work/Family Directions, 1987

Pegg L: Family day care homes: local barriers demonstrate needed change. Santa Clara Law Review 25(2–3):481, 1985

Sanger C: Day Care Center Licensing and Religious Exemptions: An Overview for Providers. San Francisco, CA, Child Care Law Center, 1985

U.S. Bureau of the Census: Comparative weekly costs for child care in seven major cities as of January 1985, in Making Child Care Work: Managing for Quality. Household After-Tax Income Reports for 1980–1985. Washington, DC, U.S. Government Printing Office, 1985

U.S. Congress. House. Select Committee on Children, Youth, and Families: Child Care: Beginning A National Initiative. April 4, 1984, Hearings. Washington, DC, U.S. Government Printing Office, 1984

U.S. Department of the Treasury. Internal Revenue Service. Statistics of Income Division: Individual Income Tax Returns 1984. Publ No 1304. Washington, DC, 1986

Index

Abuse. *See* Child abuse
Access to programs, 119, 207, 212, 222, 265, 281
Act for Better Child Care (ABC bill), 276
Adult-child ratio, 27–28, 96–97, 116, 169, 265
Advocacy
  developing a child care constituency, 267–268
  issues, 275–284
  parents' role, 281
  and sexual abuse, 213
Affirming Children's Truths (ACT), 213
Age at entry into day care, 24, 31, 55–56, 60, 61, 106, 117
  See also Infant day care
Aggression
  and attachment, 85, 86
  and child care providers, 91, 150, 154
  comparison study of toddlers, 150, 153, 154, 156
  and infant day care, 29, 30, 39–41, 51–62
Aid to Families with Dependent Children (AFDC), 261, 269, 278
Ainsworth Strange Situation, 22–23, 45, 46, 50–51, 87, 111, 147
American Academy of Pediatrics, 180, 182, 185
Anxiety-based model of child development, 71–73
Association of Child Care Providers, 123
At-risk children, 9, 76, 259, 268, 270–271, 277, 279–280
  See also Head Start
Attachment
  effects of day care, 14, 22–24, 46–51, 93–95, 96
  nonconcordant, 24

primacy of parental, 94, 105, 108, 154
research review, 42–51
and social behavior of day care infants at older ages, 51–62
and stability of care, 8, 25–26, 117
theory, 72–73, 86–89
See also Separation

Battered women, 235–236, 245–246
Before- and after-school programs. *See* School-based child care
Believe the Children, 213
Boatwright, Stephen, 208
Brief Psychiatric Rating Scale for Children, 211
Budget deficit, 268
Bush administration, 268

California Sick Child Care Task Force, 195
Caplan, Gerald, 4
Caregivers. *See* Child care providers
Carter administration, 13
Centers for Disease Control (CDC), 181, 182, 187
Child abuse
  and access to programs, 207, 212, 222, 265, 281
  and adult-child ratio, 28
  and attachment, 31
  behavioral changes, 223–224, 225, 249
  child's perception of, 225–226
  education, 211, 220, 221–222
  factors influencing recovery, 224–225
  identification, 220
  intervention, 224–229
  legal proceedings' effects, 229–230
  and licensed day care, 222–223, 265–266
  parental, 105, 246–248